"The best remedy for those who are afraid, lonely, or unhappy is to go outside, somewhere where they can be quite alone with the heavens, nature, and God."

from The Diary of Anne Frank

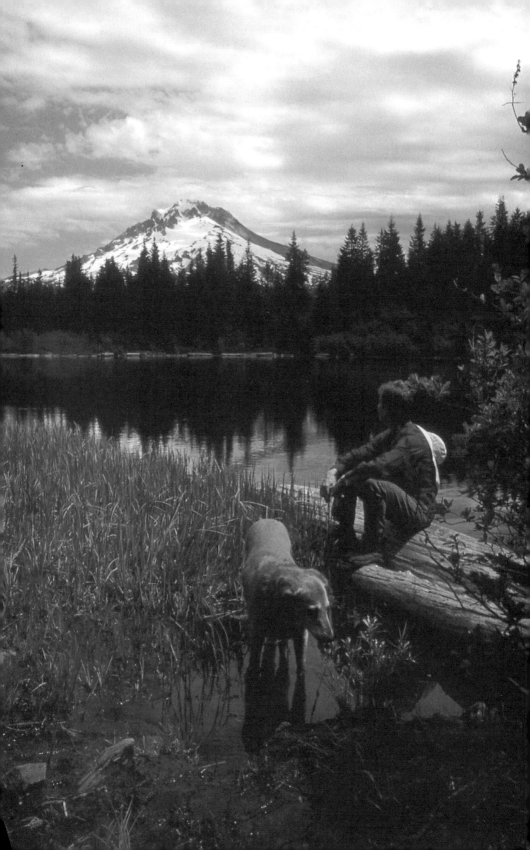

Afoot & Afield

Portland/Vancouver

A comprehensive hiking guide

Douglas Lorain

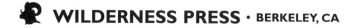 **WILDERNESS PRESS** · BERKELEY, CA

Mirror Lake (Chapter 6: Trip 32)

Afoot & Afield Portland/Vancouver: A Comprehensive Hiking Guide

1st EDITION June 2003
2nd EDITION March 2008

Copyright © 2003, 2008 by Douglas Lorain

Front cover photo copyright © 2008 by Douglas Lorain
Interior photos: Douglas Lorain
Maps: Douglas Lorain
Cover design: Andreas Schueller and Larry B. Van Dyke
Book design and layout: Andreas Schueller and Larry B. Van Dyke
Book editor: Laura Shauger

ISBN 978-0-89997-468-2
UPC 7-19609-97468-0

Manufactured in Canada

Published by: **Wilderness Press**
1200 5th Street
Berkeley, CA 94710
(800) 443-7227; FAX (510) 558-1696
info@wildernesspress.com
www.wildernesspress.com

Visit our website for a complete listing of our books and for ordering information.

Cover photo: Mt. Hood from Hood River Mountain (Chapter 5: Trip 25)

SAFETY NOTICE: Although Wilderness Press and the author have made every attempt to ensure that the information in this book is accurate at press time, they are not responsible for any loss, damage, injury, or inconvenience that may occur to anyone while using this book. You are responsible for your own safety and health while in the wilderness. The fact that a trail is described in this book does not mean that it will be safe for you. Be aware that trail conditions can change from day to day. Always check local conditions and know your own limitations.

Acknowledgments

I have no scapegoat to take the blame for the inevitable mistakes that occur in the preparation of any guidebook. All errors and omissions fall entirely at my own booted feet. Nonetheless, a few people deserve to be mentioned for their help in making this book happen.

For her love, support, and assistance with every aspect of this book (and in my life), top honors go to my wife, Becky Lovejoy.

For her assistance with all things botanical and for putting up with me as a sibling, I thank Christine Ebrahimi.

For introducing a fresh perspective on useful outdoor books, my appreciation goes to Trevor and Kathy Todd.

I also thank Brianna James, without whose friendship and support this book (and many other things) would not be possible.

Finally, thanks to the people at Wilderness Press who, to my amazement, were nice enough to publish my books in the first place. Special mention must go to Tom Winnett, Mike Jones, Jannie Dresser, Jaan Hitt, Roslyn Bullas, Larry B. Van Dyke, and Laura Shauger. They all deserve more recognition than they usually get for turning my preliminary efforts into something that is readable, useful, and attractive for you, the reader.

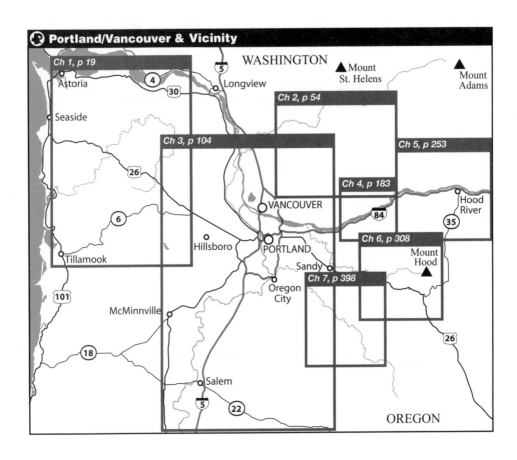

WASHINGTON

▲ Mount
St. Helens

▲ Mount
Adams

5

4

30

Astoria

Longview

Seaside

26

6

VANCOUVER

Hood
River

84

35

Tillamook

Hillsboro

PORTLAND

Mount
Hood
▲

101

Sandy

Oregon
City

McMinnville

26

18

Salem

5

22

OREGON

Contents

Preface

Outdoor lovers in the Portland/Vancouver metropolitan area are among the most fortunate in the country. Within a one-hour drive from their homes, they can hit the trail through dense old-growth forests, walk beside spectacular waterfalls, climb to viewpoints above massive glaciers, explore wetlands that are home to waterfowl and bald eagles, traipse through wildflower-covered meadows, or wander through the quiet forests of a 5000-acre park right in the city of Portland. Few other cities in the country have such a wide assortment of opportunities.

My goal in writing this book was to provide the first comprehensive guide to every worthwhile walk of at least 1 mile, on still-wild public lands, and accessible by a drive of an hour or less from Portland. The one-hour driving time is from somewhere in the major cities and suburbs of the greater Portland/Vancouver area. That does not mean that every drive will be less than one hour for every resident. If you live in Hillsboro, it may take you up to 45 minutes just to get to Gresham, on the other side of the metropolitan area, before you start the one-hour drive to Mt. Hood. Nonetheless, every trip has a short enough drive time to qualify as a good spur-of-the-moment adventure.

The hikes range in difficulty from simple strolls through urban preserves to rugged climbs in the Columbia River Gorge and on glacier-clad Mt. Hood. There are paths here familiar to every Portland hiker as well as dozens of new routes never covered in any guidebook. They have in common a convenient proximity to Portland and a wild character that allows city residents to "get away from it all."

A large percentage of these hikes are open year-round. So this guide also serves as a winter hikes manual. The northwest's notoriously soggy winters often make trails muddy. With waterproof boots and the proper attitude, however, hikers can enjoy many fine trails all year.

Many worthwhile urban and semi-urban walks have been excluded because they don't qualify as "wild." If you are looking for a quick leg-stretcher, and don't mind a landscape that features manicured lawns or picnic tables, then try any of the many easy hikes in city parks and greenways. Often these routes follow paved trails that hikers share with joggers and bicyclists. Among the best of these options are the Fanno Creek Greenway in Beaverton, the Fernhill wetlands in Forest Grove, the network of trails around Washington Park's arboretum, the quiet trails on the campus of Reed College, the riverside paths in Willamette Park and Oaks Bottom, several new trails in the Tualatin River National Wildlife Refuge, the rapidly expanding collection of paths on Gresham Butte, and the Salmon Creek Greenway in Clark County.

Trails that do not qualify as "wild" also include pleasant routes that feature wild scenery but are located near major roads or go through and around golf courses, such as those at Skamania Lodge or at Glendoveer and Rose City golf clubs.

I have hiked every trip in this book at least once and most of them several times. However, roads and trails do constantly change. New routes are built, old trails cease to be maintained or are simply abandoned, and floods and landslides obliterate some routes. Your comments on recent developments or changes are welcome. Please write to me in care of Wilderness Press at mail@wildernesspress.com.

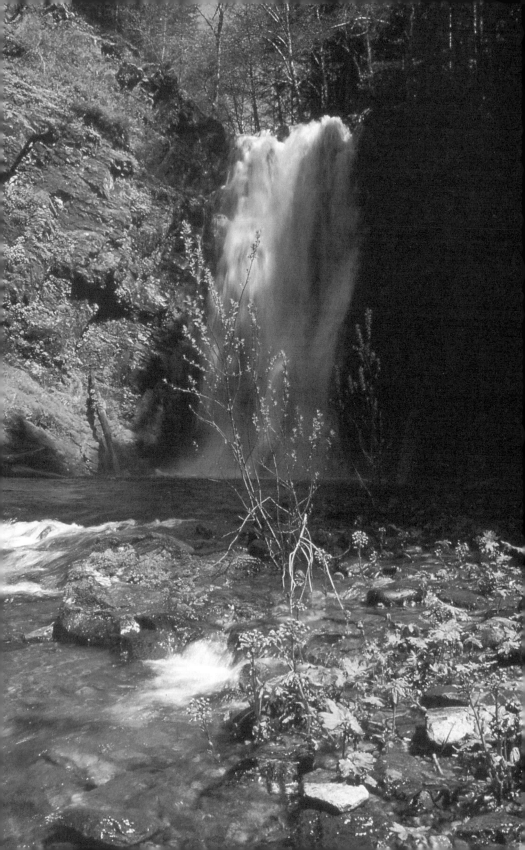

The Second Edition
& Its 60 New Hikes

It is time, all you enthusiastic hikers out there, for the much anticipated second edition of *Afoot & Afield Portland/Vancouver*. Those familiar with the first edition will find several changes and significant improvements. First of all, every map has been redone, updated, and significantly improved to be more user friendly. Most trips now have their own map while others are shown on a map with other nearby trails, and many more landmarks and details are shown to help visitors follow the trail. In addition, the organizational format and numbering system has been streamlined to make it much easier for you to find hikes in the area you are interested in visiting.

Easily the most important feature of the second edition, however, is that it includes 60 brand-new adventures to spectacular destinations in every corner of our region, almost all of which come with the bonus of solitude being a virtual certainty. Every Portland/Vancouver area outdoor lover, no matter how many years they have been hiking local trails, is guaranteed to find numerous great hikes that they have never taken and probably didn't even know existed. Among these new hikes are trips to a truly superb waterfall on remote North Siouxon Creek in Southwest Washington, several trails exploring the sunny and flower-covered slopes of the eastern Columbia River Gorge, a hike to a virtually unknown clifftop viewpoint in the Clackamas River country that will absolutely blow your (hiking) socks off,

details on how to find a new trail up previously closed Fish Creek Mountain, paths leading to remote and beautiful fishing spots in the almost unknown canyons of Roaring River and South fork Clackamas River, descriptions of little-traveled routes in usually crowded areas like Silver Falls and Oxbow parks, several newly constructed trails in the Coast Range's Clatsop State Forest, and literally dozens more. In addition, every hike from the first edition of the book has been updated, and 10 of them have undergone major revisions due to trailheads being relocated and/or the trails themselves being completely rerouted.

With all these additions, the book now describes nearly 200 hikes within an hour's drive of the city, so it is safe to say that nothing has been excluded. The goal was to include absolutely every local "wild" trail, making this book the comprehensive "bible" for all nearby hikes. You no longer have to own several different books or check several different sources to find a suitable trail or a description of a particular route you want to hike. If you can't find it here, it either doesn't exist or isn't legally accessible. So, get out those hiking boots and hit the trails, my fellow pedestrians. You are fortunate enough to live in a city with almost unlimited options for enjoying your favorite activity in beautiful surroundings. And you now own a guide that details every one of those options. The outdoors is yours to explore and savor. See you on the trails!

Chinook Falls, Siouxon Creek area (Chapter 2: Trip 3)

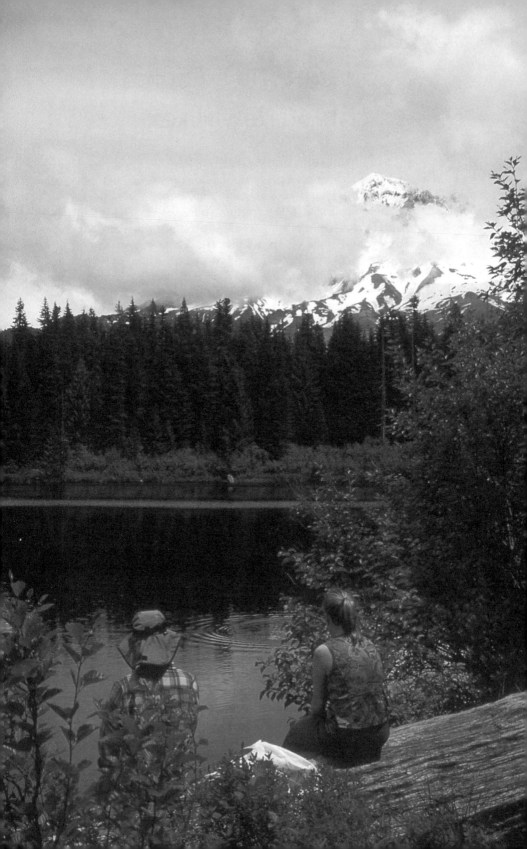

Introducing the Portland/Vancouver Area

In most cities, a book like this would begin with something like "welcome to the wildlands beyond the city's familiar concrete jungle." But no Portland/Vancouver resident would recognize or agree with that characterization because this is a city still firmly tied to Mother Nature. One reason for this, of course, is that often Ma Nature literally hits you in the face with rain as soon as you walk out the door—a humbling and a useful reminder of just who's in charge here. But even when it isn't raining, the natural world is still constantly in evidence. It's just a short drive from anywhere in the greater Portland area to forests so wild that you are more likely to see elk than other people. On the city's skyline sits not only Mt. Hood, the signature landmark of our region, but four other wild volcanic peaks: Mounts Adams, Jefferson, Rainier, and St. Helens. Parts of the Columbia River Gorge, only 30 minutes from the downtown skyscrapers, remain as wild today as when Meriwether Lewis and William Clark passed through the region in 1805.

But Portland is not only surrounded by wild country, it manages to include wilderness right in the city limits. The enormity of Forest Park, the largest forested city park in the world, provides country that is wilder than many designated wilderness areas. In the towering evergreens that stand in virtually every city neighborhood live gray squirrels, raccoons, great horned owls, and other wildlife. Endangered peregrine falcons live amid the downtown buildings and bridges. People even fish for salmon in the Willamette River in downtown Portland. So Portland is truly a city where you can never really escape the natural world—and that's just the way we like it.

Every Imaginable Shade of Green: The Local Flora

I once had a friend who moved from the Pacific Northwest to Phoenix, Arizona. He liked his new environment but would constantly comment about how much he missed the color green. All the rain the Portland area gets ensures that even in the dry months of late summer it always stays green. Washington may officially be the Evergreen State, but it's Portland that takes the honor as the evergreen city.

All that greenery is composed of thousands of plant species inhabiting dozens of different environments. Professional botanists recognize a wide range of plant communities throughout our area. The average hiker, however, won't notice most of these because the same species are predominant throughout the region. Once you learn to recognize these relatively few species, you are well on your way to

Bunchberry blossoms

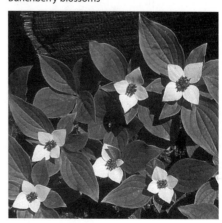

feeling like an expert and getting more enjoyment from your travels.

As all of us umbrella-toting Portlanders already know, we live in a virtual rain forest. That forest is made up of a canopy of big trees with several layers of understory species.

Douglas fir is by far the most abundant species on the forest's top floor. Point at any random conifer on most of the trails in this book and there is roughly a 75 percent chance that the tree is a Douglas fir. At lower elevations the second most common species is the western hemlock, a beautiful evergreen with tiny needles and drooping limbs. At the highest elevations of the Cascade Mountains, the hemlock family banner is taken up by a close relative, the mountain hemlock. A similar thing happens with cedars. At lower elevations look for western red cedar, while in the high country Alaska yellow cedar takes over. With the true firs you should recognize grand fir down low, Pacific silver fir and noble fir at mid-elevations, and subalpine fir up high. Other evergreen species of note include Engelmann spruce, western white pine, and lodgepole pine.

Deciduous trees are less common than conifers, but they mix with the evergreens at all lower elevations, and in some areas leafy trees actually outnumber those with needles. Especially abundant are bigleaf maple and red alder. On the drier hills you will find woodlands of Oregon white oak, while in the wet bottomlands of the river valleys there are black cottonwoods. From mid-October to mid-November both bigleaf maple and black cottonwood grace the area with their bright yellow leaves.

Get off the elevator at the second floor of our forests, and the doors will open up to a whole array of smaller tree species. Most notable of these is the vine maple, another great fall-color species. This short understory tree has many-pointed leaves that turn a striking reddish-orange color in October. Another second-story species is the Pacific yew, a fascinating conifer that lives in shady forests and uses red berrylike fruits, instead of cones, to reproduce. Pacific dogwood, with its showy white blossoms in April and May, also deserves mention. Other common small trees on the second story include Pacific willow, Sitka alder, black hawthorn, and Oregon ash.

Below these small trees is a layer of large and small shrubs. Once again, unless you want to be an expert, you need only to learn a handful of the most common species. Many of the larger shrubs are berries, like salmonberry, thimbleberry, and blackberry, all of which have tasty edible fruit in season. Other common large shrubs include elderberry (both red and blue varieties), serviceberry, snowberry, and devil's club. Probably the most abundant large shrub at mid-elevations in the Cascades is the Pacific rhododendron. From May to early July, the showy pink blossoms of this evergreen plant put on displays that can even make clear-cuts look good—well, almost.

Moving down to the forest's ground floor takes us to the low-growing shrubs. The most important member of this group, especially for your taste buds, is the huckleberry. From mid-August until mid-September the positively delicious berries of this abundant mid- to high-elevation plant will slow the berry-picking hiker's progress to a crawl. Other common low shrubs include kinnnikinnick, salal, and, in the alpine zone, both pink and white heather. No list of low shrubs would be complete without mentioning one of the most abundant members of the group, the yellow-blooming Oregon grape.

The plants most closely associated with the floor of our forests are ferns. Experts recognize numerous species but, once again, the novice only needs to know four or five common varieties. Sword fern, easily the most common type, is a hardy but strikingly beautiful evergreen fern so abundant in this area that it is often taken for granted. Sunnier areas invariably feature bracken fern, while wetter places have lots of maidenhair and lady fern. The final fern species that the average hiker will want to learn to recognize is the licorice fern. This common species is what botanists term *epiphytic*, which means that instead of growing out of the ground like its relatives, the licorice fern grows directly out of tree trunks and rocks.

Everybody loves flowers and many people go hiking specifically to enjoy the sight and smell of blossoms. From March through September, there are always flowers to enjoy somewhere in our region. Wildflowers, however, are difficult to categorize, because so many different kinds of plants, including many listed above, produce flowers. If we restrict this group to just the smaller, ground-level types (as most people do), then you can look like an expert by knowing just a few dozen species. When hiking in dense forests, you won't see great displays of wildflowers, but you will find scattered blooms that help to brighten the shady forest floor. Look for yellow wood violet, the relatively rare pink calypso orchid, and several varieties of white flowers, including trillium, queen's cup, bunchberry, twinflower, and vanilla leaf.

If you want to see great wildflower displays, get out of the forest and head for the meadows. In the lower-elevation valleys, you need to find one of those increasingly rare places that has yet to be paved over or plowed under. The most striking flower in these fields is blue camas, a plant that was once an important food source for Native Americans.

There is greater variety in the mountains. Depending on the elevation, the higher meadows provide spectacular displays any time from mid-June through mid-August. Just as the snow melts, the ground comes alive with the blossoms of glacier lily, avalanche lily, and western pasqueflower. A little later, you enjoy cinquefoil, lupine, paintbrush, spiraea, shooting star, yarrow, and, perhaps most notable of all, beargrass. By the end of summer, the meadows still have some flowers, especially asters, goldenrods, and blue gentians, which bloom well into September.

The banks of creeks feature lush vegetation and a unique array of water-loving flowering plants. Of particular note are yellow monkeyflower and pink Lewis monkeyflower, false Solomon's seal, and bleeding heart. Dry and rocky places have wildflowers better adapted to these environments. Here you may find yellow stonecrop, blue larkspur, lavender cliff penstemon, and the whites of pearly everlasting, prairie star, and cats ear, among others.

If wildflowers lead the brigade of popular plants, then the least popular plant, poison oak, also deserves mention. This species is most common in dry, sunny places, but it can also be found in denser forests. You should be especially wary of this rash-producing menace when you are hiking in the eastern Columbia River Gorge. Poison oak comes in a variety of forms, sometimes growing as a vine and sometimes as a low bush, but it always has lobed, often shiny leaves, that grow in groups of three. Hikers who travel with the family pet need to remember that, no matter how smart you think Rover is, he probably isn't bright enough to recognize

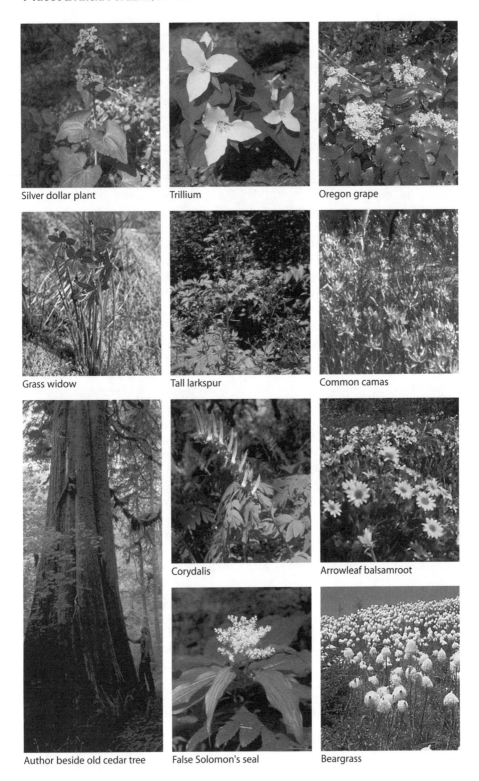

Silver dollar plant

Trillium

Oregon grape

Grass widow

Tall larkspur

Common camas

Author beside old cedar tree

Corydalis

Arrowleaf balsamroot

False Solomon's seal

Beargrass

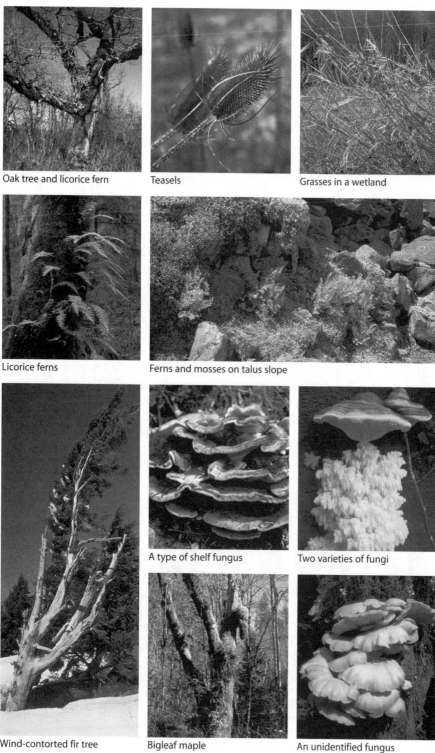

Oak tree and licorice fern

Teasels

Grasses in a wetland

Licorice ferns

Ferns and mosses on talus slope

A type of shelf fungus

Two varieties of fungi

Wind-contorted fir tree

Bigleaf maple

An unidentified fungus

and avoid poison oak. Many unsuspecting pet owners have picked up a nasty rash from merely petting their dog after a hike in poison-oak country.

Various species of moss grow abundantly in our forests. Trying to identify these species is beyond the interest level of most hikers. It's worth pointing out, however, that the old adage about moss growing only on the north side of a tree does not work around here. If you get lost and try to navigate by this old trick, you'll be in big trouble because in this wet environment moss grows on *all* sides of the trees.

Mushrooms and fungi are an area of special interest for many Northwest hikers. Our forests feature several dozen varieties growing out of the ground, out of old stumps, and even out of living trees. Many species are edible, and collecting mushrooms is a fun activity. Do not, however, eat any mushrooms unless you are experienced and completely confident in your ability to identify the various species. There are several poisonous types in our area, and every year people get sick, and some even die, from eating the wrong mushrooms.

Fur, Feathers, Scales, & Slime: The Local Fauna

Hikers aren't the only creatures leaving footprints on our area trails. By far the most common large mammal you will encounter, apart from *Homo sapiens* and their canine companions, is the black-tailed deer. Even on trips within the city limits, you are likely to see deer tracks, and every hiker who spends time in the backcountry will see lots of deer. Next on the list of large mammals is the Roosevelt elk. It's always a thrill to catch a glimpse of these large, impressive animals. The most likely area to observe elk is in the Coast Range. Other large mammals prowling area forests include black bears and mountain lions, but the average hiker would be extraordinarily fortunate to see either.

Smaller mammals are another story. In the right habitat, every hiker will see chipmunks, Douglas squirrels, and pikas. Some representative examples of the other common smaller mammals in our area are porcupines, beavers, raccoons, skunks, coyotes, red and gray foxes, marmots, and snowshoe hares. Hikers who

A type of shelf fungus on a log along the Clackamas River

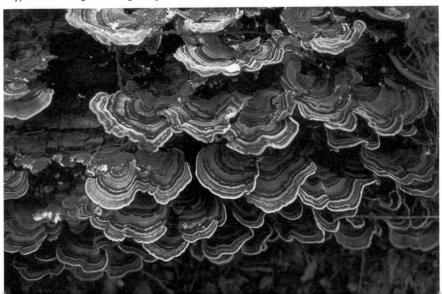

are quiet stand a better chance of seeing these, and all other, wildlife.

As is true throughout the world, insects are, by far, the most common form of wildlife in our area. Apart from admiring butterflies, however, most hikers think of insects only when they are forced to swat bothersome mosquitoes. Higher on the food chain are spiders. The thick vegetation and the abundance of insects for prey ensure that spiders are quite common. The most important result of this fact is that the first person to hike a trail in the morning must negotiate an obstacle course of webs. You will spend considerable time (and a lifetime's vocabulary of swear words) wiping the webs off your face, hair, and clothing. My advice is to wave a walking stick in front of you or, better yet, convince your hiking partner to take the lead. Another good option is to hike in the winter, when spiders are less active and build fewer webs.

After insects, our most common and conspicuous form of wildlife is birds. The feathered menagerie includes a wide range of colors, sizes, and forms. Tiny rufous hummingbirds zip past looking for flowers to visit, while various species of chickadees, wrens, warblers, and sparrows, among others, fill the forests with song. Easily the most common bird in the mountains is the dark-eyed junco, formerly called the Oregon junco and still termed that by the average proud Oregonian. During the winter months, these happy, clicking birds with black heads come down to the valleys and are among the most common residents at backyard feeding stations.

Great blue herons are probably the most conspicuous large birds in the Portland area. Every Portlander is familiar with this, the city's official bird. These tall and delicately beautiful avians are often seen flying overhead, prowling for food along streams or beside ponds, or just standing around in dry fields hunting for mice. Other large birds of note include Canada geese and various species of ducks, which spend their winters in the mild climate of the Willamette Valley; ospreys and bald eagles, which can often be seen on larger lakes and rivers; and red-tailed hawks, easily our most abundant flying predators.

The Pacific Northwest is home to eight salamander species, one of the highest such concentrations in the world. Our wet forests host some fascinating and beautiful species, including the long-toed salamander, the tiny Oregon ensatina, and the aptly named Pacific giant salamander, which actually barks. Due to their secretive nature, however, you will rarely see any salamanders. The sole exception to this rule is the roughskin newt, an interesting and abundant representative of the group that can be found in almost any pond, lake, or slow-moving stream. A fact unknown to even most experienced outdoor lovers is that the roughskin newt is poisonous. Their skin emits a toxin that, if ingested, can be deadly. Fortunately, the poison cannot penetrate your skin. But be sure to wash your hands after handling a newt.

Other amphibians also take well to this damp environment. You will encounter several species of frogs, the most common of which are the Pacific treefrog, the western toad, and the red-legged frog. Sadly, frog populations have been declining in recent years. This is a worldwide problem, the reasons for which are not well understood. In our area, probably the leading cause of this decline is the unfortunate introduction, and population explosion, of the bullfrog. This nonnative predator feeds on smaller frogs, as well as baby turtles, birds, and other unfortunate victims.

In this wet climate, reptiles are less common than amphibians. Lizards, for example, are fairly common east of the Cascades, but they are very rare in the area covered by this book. You are likely to see them only on the drier slopes on the Washington side of the Columbia River Gorge. Snakes are much more common. In and around Portland there is no need to worry about rattlesnakes, except in the eastern Columbia River Gorge. What you *will* encounter throughout this area are various species of harmless garter snakes and racers.

No list of area wildlife would be complete without mentioning one of the most famous, and strangely popular, residents of the Pacific Northwest—the lowly banana slug. Mollusks aren't generally the most beloved of organisms and, even here in the slug capital of the world, area gardeners have been in a long-standing war with the creatures (usually a *losing* battle, or so my gardening friends lament). One of the most memorable encounters you will have on a rainy day in the woods is with the banana slug. The first tell-tale sign is the famous slime trail crossing your path. Follow this sticky slime and you will soon come across the source, a surprisingly colorful, and almost frighteningly large, slug. The banana slug comes in an array of colors, mostly greenish-yellow with black spots, and can be up to 10 inches long (the average is about 6 or 7 inches). Many Northwest residents have a strong affection for the slug, which people from other parts of the country find to be evidence that all the rain up here has made Portlanders a bit addled. One town in western Washington holds an annual slug festival, and it is even possible to purchase various souvenir items featuring the banana slug.

Welcome to the Pacific "Northwet": The Local Weather

Anyone who lives in this part of the world knows that there's no getting around rain. For eight or so months of the year it rains *a lot* in Portland. But there is much more to the climate story than just precipitation. Each season has its own weather-related quirks, and all the hills, canyons, river valleys, and mountains in our area help to create numerous microclimates. Once you master these local weather idiosyncrasies, you'll stay drier and have more fun in the outdoors.

Summer in the Pacific Northwest is just about ideal. From mid-July until early October rain is unusual, despite all those stories we tell out-of-staters in an effort to keep them out. This is not to say that we never get clouds in the summer months. In fact, morning clouds are quite common. One of the best times to go hiking is when clouds cover the Willamette Valley. A large percentage of summer days in our region begins with a layer of marine air, which pushes in from the Pacific Ocean carrying low clouds with it. What far too many hikers in Portland and Vancouver fail to realize is that once you climb above about 2000 feet, you leave the clouds and fog behind and enjoy brilliant sunshine. A great aesthetic advantage of hiking in such weather is that you can climb to a viewpoint and look down on the billowy white fog covering the valleys with its delicate fingers that creep through low passes in the ridges. The fog also hides most of the clear-cuts and helps to ensure greater solitude because outdoor lovers in the socked-in Portland/Vancouver lowlands look out their windows, see the low clouds, and wrongly assume that it's too gloomy to go hiking.

Despite being farther north than Minneapolis, Portland's proximity to the Pacific Ocean keeps the winter weather relatively mild. It may rain a lot, but severe winter weather is rare. Generally we get only two or three days of snow per year, and even that usually melts away in a day or two. The mountains, of course, get lots of snow, and with several feet piling up every winter, it takes many months for all that white stuff to melt away. Precisely when trails open for travel varies from year to year, but a pretty good rule of thumb is that trails below 1000 feet remain open all year. At 2000 feet, trails begin to open by mid-March. With every 1000 feet of elevation, it takes an additional month for the snow to melt. Thus, by mid-April the snow line will be around 3000 feet; by mid-May it's 4000 feet, and that number becomes 5000 feet by mid-June. The highest trails open some time in July. Sunnier south-facing slopes melt out sooner than north-facing ones. Although true everywhere in the country, it is probably less pronounced here than elsewhere because the heavy tree cover keeps the snow well shaded, even on south-facing slopes.

Don't let yourself and your hiking boots go into hibernation just because it's winter. Despite all that famous rain, every wet season features at least some welcome sunshine and, if you are properly equipped, many trails are a joy to hike even in the rain. You can almost always rely on any trail below 1000 feet to be open all year.

Fall and spring weather is less predictable than winter and summer. There is a local joke that you can tell it's spring in Portland when the rain starts to get warmer. By the time May and June roll around, the skies are still all too often covered with clouds, and people start to get frustrated. Statistically, there are a lot more sunny days at this time than we've had in the previous six or seven months. Taking advantage of these welcome brighter days is highly rewarding. Spring hikers will be treated to a natural world positively bursting with new life that has definitely noticed the increase in life-giving sunshine.

Autumn in the Portland/Vancouver area produces weather that is best described as variable. In some years, it starts raining in September and everyone knows that it won't really let up until the following June. In at least one year in three, however, we enjoy a glorious Indian summer, with nice weather extending all the way into October. This is one of the best times to go hiking, because the temperatures are cool, the bugs are gone, and many areas feature wonderful fall colors. After Labor Day the trails are virtually deserted. On a day just after the first light dusting of snow in early October, be sure to make a trip to the high trails on Mt. Hood. The mountain really comes alive with this first covering of snow. You can also take some spectacular photographs of the snow-dusted peak, over the golden meadows framed by the red splashes of huckleberry bushes. Down in the valleys, and especially in the Columbia River Gorge, the fall colors remain excellent into mid-November. Be aware, however, that in the deep, shady canyons on the Oregon side of the Gorge, the sun goes down very early. In November, you should expect darkness by about 3 PM. Bring fast film and a tripod to take photographs in this low light, and carry plenty of warm clothing for the hike back out.

The mountains and valleys surrounding the Portland/Vancouver area cause different wind and precipitation patterns that create localized climates. One of these so-called microclimates is the small, but noticeable, rain shadow just east of the Coast Range. The downsloping hills of Yamhill and western Washington counties get noticeably less annual rainfall than do the upsloping hills in eastern Clackamas, Multnomah, and Clark counties.

The most important microclimate in our region is the Columbia River Gorge. As those familiar with it already know, the Gorge is almost always windy. The violently twisted trees and the abundance of windsurfers attest to the strength of the winds here, so hikers must come prepared for often bitter wind chills. For most of the year, the prevailing wind is from west to east. But during the winter months, the Gorge often acts as a funnel for cold air from east of the Cascade Mountains. As a result, the almost-sea-level Gorge stays much colder than anywhere else in our region. Consequently, the Gorge gets a lot more snow and freezing rain than do neighboring Portland and Vancouver. An inch of cold rain in Portland may fall as a foot or more of snow in Cascade Locks, even though Cascade Locks is only about 20 feet higher in elevation. This means that the aforementioned elevation rules for snow-free hiking generally don't apply in the Gorge. The much sunnier Washington side melts out a lot faster and, in fact, often provides the nicest early-spring hiking in our region. For photographers, and those who can stand bitterly cold temperatures, it's also fun to visit the Gorge during a mid-winter cold spell. With luck, the waterfalls will be encased in a spectacular coating of ice.

Trail Safety & Courtesy

Although generally very safe, the sport of hiking does involve a certain level of risk. In the Portland/Vancouver area the risks are relatively minor, but they are real, and good preparation is important to help minimize the potential dangers.

Preparation & Equipment

The most important preparation for a hiking trip is being in good physical condition. The trips in this book range in difficulty from quite easy to extremely strenuous. Each trip is rated as easy, moderate, difficult, or strenuous. Trips rated as "easy" are the easiest and should be enjoyable to anyone, although a small degree of conditioning is always helpful. Trips rated as "strenuous," on the other hand, are beyond the abilities of all but a handful of the best-conditioned hikers. Before selecting a hike, be honest about your physical condition. Don't overextend yourself by taking a trip that is beyond your fitness level. After all, you go hiking to enjoy yourself, not exhaust yourself, and, most important, a wilderness trail miles from your car is not the place to suddenly realize that your body is not prepared for strenuous activity. On average, about one hiker a week has to be rescued on the backcountry trails of the Portland/Vancouver area—don't let yourself become a statistic. There are plenty of hikes in this book at every ability level. Work your way up to the more difficult trips, so you can enjoy every outing comfortably and safely.

Although the weather in the Portland/Vancouver area is often cold and wet, we humans are most comfortable and perform best when we stay warm and dry. The proper clothing is the best way to resolve this discrepancy. For strenuous activities like hiking, your best bet is to wear several layers of synthetic or wool clothing. It is relatively easy to regulate your temperature by simply adding or removing layers. Years ago hikers had only two options for clothing fabrics—cotton and wool. Wool kept you warm but was scratchy and uncomfortable. Cotton was comfortable but provided no insulation when it got wet—a certain recipe for hypothermia in our rainy climate. The science of fabrics has come a long way since then. Today there is a dizzying array of synthetic fabrics and special wool blends that wick moisture away from your body, are lightweight, feel comfortable against your skin, keep you warm on cold, rainy days, and help you stay comfortably cool in hot weather. More new fabrics are developed all the time.

The first layer against your skin should be something like Capilene or Coolmax, which are warm, comfortable, and wick away your perspiration on hot summer days. The next layer depends on the season. In colder winter weather, opt for a long-sleeve wool or synthetic shirt. On warm summer days, you may go for cotton. Regardless of the season, you should carry or wear some sort of outer shell. A waterproof windbreaker is ideal. In the Columbia River Gorge, where the wind never seems to stop blowing, a windbreaker is practically indispensable. In winter, you'll also need to carry a warm coat. A fleece jacket is a good choice because it provides insulation with minimal weight.

Below the waist, forget cotton jeans and go instead for lightweight nylon pants, which stop the wind and provide insulation even when they get wet. In winter, you might consider wool pants to keep your legs warmer. Few local hikers travel in shorts, but on hot summer days you might do so, as long as you also carry long pants should the weather turn ugly or the trail turn out to have lots of brush or poison oak.

Gaiters are also nice to have along, and some hikers wear them all the time. These usually cover from your shoe tops to just below your knees. They keep your feet and lower legs dry, especially when you are traveling through brushy or grassy areas that are often covered with dew or water from the last rain shower. Gaiters also keep snow and mud from crawling over the tops of your boots and getting your feet wet and uncomfortable.

The miracle fabrics discussed above have also done wonders for socks. Today's high-tech hiking socks provide cushioning comfort while wicking moisture away from your feet to reduce the chance of blisters. I usually wear two pairs of socks. The first is a synthetic wool blend and the second is made of thick, cushy wool. With this system and comfortable boots, I haven't had a blister in almost a decade of rugged hiking.

As for footwear, the debate about hiking boots versus lightweight shoes has gotten an amazing amount of attention in recent years. For decades, the standard advice was to wear heavy leather hiking boots to keep your feet dry and your ankles supported and to protect your feet on rough wilderness trails. Proponents of super lightweight hiking, on the other hand, scoff at this advice and wouldn't hike in anything but comfortable running shoes. Luckily, you don't have to choose because there are a whole range of lightweight hiking boots that rely on synthetic fabrics instead of heavy leather to keep water out. They also provide necessary traction, with soles designed to grip the ground. A good pair of these will meet your needs for most trails. If you are backpacking or traveling on particularly rough or muddy trails, however, you will probably want to rely on a pair of tried-and-true leather boots.

Being Properly Equipped

Except when hiking on gentle trails in city parks, hikers should always carry a pack with certain essential items. The standard "Ten Essentials" have evolved from a list of individual items to functional systems that will help to keep you alive and reasonably comfortable in emergency situations.

1. Navigation: topographic map and a compass or GPS device.

2. Sun protection: sunglasses and sunscreen, especially in the mountains.

3. Insulation: extra clothing that is both waterproof and warm.

4. Illumination: a flashlight or headlamp.

5. First-aid supplies.

6. Fire: a candle or other firestarter and matches in a waterproof container.

7. Repair kit: particularly a knife for starting fires, first aid, and countless other uses.

8. Nutrition: enough extra food so you return with a little left over.

9. Hydration: extra water and a means to purify more on longer trips.

10. Emergency shelter: a tent for overnight hikers or a large trash bag, bivy sack, or emergency blanket for dayhikers.

I strongly advise adding a small plastic signaling whistle and a warm knit cap to this list.

Just carrying these items, however, doesn't make you "prepared." Unless you know things like how to apply basic first aid, how to build an emergency fire, and how to read a topographic map or use a compass, then carrying these items doesn't do you a bit of good. These skills are all fairly simple to learn and at least one member of your group should be familiar with each of them.

More important to your safety and enjoyment than any piece of equipment or clothing is exercising common sense. When you are far from civilization, a simple injury can be life-threatening. Don't take unnecessary chances. Never, for example, jump onto slippery rocks or logs or crawl out onto dangerously steep slopes in the hope of getting a better view. Fortunately, the vast majority of wilderness injuries are easily avoidable.

Some Special Hazards

Sadly, venturing out into the natural world doesn't guarantee an escape from the problems of civilized life. Car break-ins and vandalism are regular occurrences at trailheads, so hikers need to take reasonable precautions. Don't encourage the criminals by providing unnecessary temptation. Leave your shiny new car at home, and drive a beat-up older vehicle instead. Leave nothing of value in your car, especially not in plain sight. My car has been broken into three times over the years; the last two times, the thieves only took home some pairs of ratty old tennis shoes, to which they were welcome. If all trailhead vehicles held only items of similar value, the criminals would soon seek out more lucrative targets.

In general, all water in the backcountry should be considered unsafe to drink. Dayhikers can carry all the water they need. Backpackers, however, will have to purify the water. Boiling is the most effective way to kill the nasty little microorganisms that cause the problems, but the simplest purification methods are filtering and chemical treatments like iodine.

A special hazard in autumn is hunting season. Hikers need to advertise themselves with a bright red or orange cap, vest, pack, or other conspicuous article of clothing to avoid being mistaken for a suitable target. Hunting is prohibited in state and city parks and in some wildlife refuges. It is very popular, however, in state and national forests. Oregon's general deer-hunting season usually runs from the first weekend of October through early November. In Washington the season usually starts one week later and runs farther into November. In both states, the elk-hunting season is in late October or early November.

Ticks are a minor annoyance in spring and early summer, especially in grassy or brushy areas and in the Columbia River Gorge. Ticks in other parts of the country often carry serious diseases such as Rocky Mountain spotted fever and Lyme disease. Fortunately, only a handful of cases have been reported in Oregon and Washington, so ticks here are more disgusting than dangerous. Still, it's wise to check your body and clothing regularly when in tick habitat and to remove the little buggers quickly.

Also not terribly dangerous, but extremely bothersome, are mosquitoes. These annoying invertebrate vampires can be numerous enough to ruin your trip if you're not prepared with bug repellent, long pants, and a long-sleeve shirt. The flying blood suckers are most abundant around lower elevation marshes and near lakes and ponds in the Cascades. At low elevations, they are at their worst from spring to midsummer. At higher elevations, they peak for a period of about three weeks following the snowmelt at any given elevation.

Two other bits of common wisdom also deserve mention. The first is that you should never hike alone. This is probably good advice on rarely traveled wilderness trails, but I would never forego a trip just because I couldn't find a hiking partner. You can simply choose a more popular trail. These routes invariably have a fair number of other hikers around, so you're never really alone.

The second bit of advice is that you should let a responsible person know where you're going and when you expect to return. That will greatly aid in any search-and-rescue efforts, should they become necessary. If you stay on the trail and stick to popular areas, this caution may not be necessary, but it never hurts, and it's a good habit to develop.

Being a Good Neighbor

All hikers take with them a responsibility not only for their own safety, but for being good stewards of the natural environment. Be respectful of the land you are visiting, and leave it in the same condition as you found it. Common sense should make the following rules obvious: never litter; never pick wildflowers; never cut switchbacks; and never let your dog or children chase wildlife. Less obvious guidelines help not only to preserve the resource but to leave it in even better shape than before you arrived. One easy thing to do is to pick up any litter left by others. You should also do some minor trail maintenance as you hike by removing rocks, limbs, and debris from the path.

These rules are either common courtesy or carry the force of law: avoid disturbing other hikers and wildlife with shouts or any other unnatural sounds; leave all plants, mushrooms, logs, and even rocks where nature put them; do not damage or remove any item of historic or archaeological interest, such as Native American vision-quest sites or pits, old trapper cabins, pottery, or arrowheads, all of which are protected by federal law; stay on the trail and avoid trampling plants, especially delicate meadows and streamside locations that tend to draw crowds.

If you are backpacking, be especially scrupulous to follow "no-trace" principles. Camp well away from water on an established site that won't be further damaged by your tent and your activity around camp. In wilderness areas, the rules generally require that all camps be at least 200 feet from any trail or water source. Leave the site in as natural a condition as possible. Avoid building a campfire and rely instead on a small backpacking stove to cook your food. Finally, deposit human waste in a small "cat hole" about 6 inches deep and cover it.

How to Use This Book

I hope that this book will serve as both a field reference and a catalyst for dreaming about the outdoors. On those all-too-frequent dismal days of winter you can pick up this guide and read about the beautiful places you hope to enjoy as soon as the rain stops. You don't need any explanation for how to use a book for dreaming, so this section will focus on the best ways for using it as a planning tool and a field guide.

For hikers unfamiliar with our region and for outdoor veterans looking for new places to explore, I suggest that you start with the Best Hikes listing in Appendix 1. Based on thousands of miles of hiking in and around Portland, this list gives the reader my recommendations for the best walks to see waterfalls, wildflowers, great views, and other attributes popular with hikers. Armed with this information, you can rapidly narrow your options to a hike that meets your preferences. Keep in mind, however, that every trip in this book is worth hiking. Some may be better than others, but there isn't a dud in the lot, so you really can't go wrong.

After scenery, the second most important consideration of most hikers is location. This book covers only trails within a one-hour drive of the Portland/Vancouver area, so every hike is close enough for that spur-of-the-moment outing. To narrow things even further, the trips have all been organized by their general geographic region (Coast Range, Western Columbia River Gorge, Clackamas River Area, etc.). Each region begins with a brief introduction that discusses its general character, terrain, and other notable features and an overview map that shows the location of major highways, towns, and natural features. From there, individual hikes or hiking areas are covered

by detailed maps that show the particular trails described in the text. The numbers on these maps correspond to the hike numbers in the text.

Capsulized Summaries

Each hike begins with capsulized summary information that allows you to immediately see if the trip fits your current interests, your fitness level, and the time of year. Here is what each line in the summary tells you.

DISTANCE

This is the total round-trip distance of the hike to the nearest 0.1 mile. For the few hikes that are recommended as one-way trips, the mileage is labeled accordingly.

ELEVATION GAIN

This is the total (not the net) elevation gain for the round-trip hike. Once again, one-way hikes are specifically identified as such. Keep in mind that for most hikers the difficulty of a trail is determined at least as much by how far up they go as by simply how far they go.

HIKING TIME

This category lists the approximate time it will take the average hiker to complete the round-trip hike. If a trip is recommended as a one-way adventure, it is so identified, and the hiking time will correspond to the one-way distance.

OPTIONAL MAP

For many hikes, the map in this book will suffice for your trip. However, you may want to carry a contour map of the area to help pick out landmarks and to more closely follow your upward, or downward, progress. This entry identifies the best available contour map for each hike. In many areas the privately produced Green Trails maps are the best because they are specifically designed for hikers, are reasonably up-to-date, and use an ideal scale for pedestrians. When U.S. Geological Survey maps are recommended, the listed maps are in the 7.5-minute series.

USUALLY OPEN

This category tells you when the trail is typically snow-free enough for hiking.

BEST TIMES

This is my subjective judgment of the time(s) of year when a trip is at its best for hiking. In general, it will be when the flowers are at their peak, the fall colors at their best, the wildlife most abundant, and so on.

TRAIL USE

This category describes the uses for which the trail is suited, including backpacking and mountain biking, whether the trail is a good choice for kids, and whether dogs or horses are allowed on the trail.

AGENCY

This refers to the government agency that manages the area covered by the hike. It never hurts to call ahead to the appropriate agency for the latest information about trail conditions, closures, regulations, etc. See Appendix 3 for a complete list of addresses and phone numbers for each agency.

DIFFICULTY

This category lists an overall rating of how difficult this trip is relative to other hikes with the following four designations. In general, each higher level represents a doubling of difficulty level.

On average, "Moderate" trips are twice as difficult as "Easy" trips, and so on.

Easy: Relatively short hikes over gentle terrain, these trips are suitable for hikers of any age or ability.

Moderate: Most reasonably fit people should be able to take these hikes, which are of moderate length or shorter but over more difficult terrain, although they may need to take several rest breaks.

Difficult: A good workout even for fit hikers, these hikes combine longer distances with a fair amount of elevation gain.

Strenuous: Only very fit hikers should attempt these challenging hikes that are very long and/or cover rough terrain with great changes in elevation.

NOTES

Let's face it, the Portland/Vancouver area gets more than its share of gloomy, overcast days. Fortunately, you don't have to forego an enjoyable day on the trail just because the sun is hiding. Unlike viewpoint hikes, the forests, waterfalls, and other features of trips labeled in the notes field as "Good in cloudy weather" are just as good in the gloom as they are under clear skies.

Highlights & Directions

After the summary information is a short paragraph or two that is designed to give you the "flavor" of this outing by discussing its unique or special features. This section will quickly inform you if the hike has an interesting history, features great views, or has unusually abundant wildflowers or some other feature that makes it worth your time and attention.

Other Useful Information

Many hikers prefer loop trips because they allow one to sample a greater variety of scenery on the hike. All hikes that are recommended as loop trips are so named.

Every hike in this book follows either established trails or unmaintained hiking routes that are easy to navigate. The forests and thick undergrowth that cover virtually all of the Portland/Vancouver area make cross-country travel somewhere between very difficult and impossible. In general, off-trail routes should be left exclusively for very experienced travelers. The Portland/Vancouver area has more than enough worthwhile destinations that can be reached by trail. There is no need to resort to bushwhacking.

Until recently, one joyful aspect of hiking was that it was an outdoor activity you could do for free: You didn't have to buy a fishing license, pay for a lift ticket, or even get expensive lessons. You could just drive or hitch a ride to the nearest trailhead and take off. Most public land agencies now, however, require that you pay a fee of some kind to use their trails.

In national forests, all cars parked with 0.25 mile of major developed trailheads must display a trailhead parking pass. In 2007, daily permits cost $5, and an annual pass, good in all the forests of Washington and Oregon, was $30. The permits can be purchased at all ranger stations and many sporting goods stores in the Portland area. Many, but not all, state parks also require that visitors pay an entrance fee, whether or not they are hiking. Finally, on Sauvie Island, the Oregon Department of Fish and Wildlife requires a day-use pass for hikers, birdwatchers, and all other users.

If you want to avoid paying for the privilege of going for a hike, your options are more limited. To date, anyway, state forests and most national wildlife refuges in Oregon and Washington do not charge fees. In addition, all city parks in the Portland area are free. You can also visit the less popular state parks, which generally don't charge a fee.

◯ Map Legend

▰▬▰▬▰	Featured Trail		**5**	Trip Number
▬▬╳▬▬	Other Trail and Saddle		⌂	Ranger Station
••••••••	Cross-Country Route		**S**	Fee Collection Station
T	Trailhead		**?**	Information
P	Parking		⊢──⊢	Railroad
▲	Car Campground		─ ─ ─	Power Line
▲	Backcountry Campsite		⟨**5**⟩	Interstate Highway
⊞	Picnic Area		⟨**26**⟩	U.S. Highway
↶~~↳	Spring, Stream, and Falls		⟨**14**⟩	State Highway
⌐~ ⌐ ⌐	Intermittent Stream		⌒⌒	Paved Road
◖	Lake		⌒⌒	Gravel Road
ⱟ	Marsh		⌐≈⚵=⌐	Primitive Road and Gate
▲	Mountain		*2175'*	Elevation

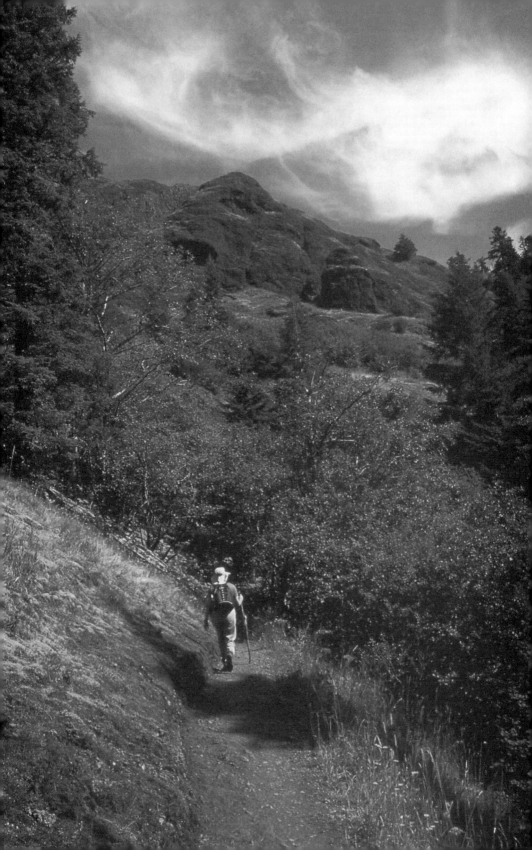

Chapter 1

Coast Range

The Oregon Coast Range, which separates the Willamette Valley from the Pacific Ocean, is a rolling sea of second-growth forests that spreads across a contorted land of gnarled hills and stream canyons. Those streams support precious runs of steelhead and salmon, while Roosevelt elk wander the hills providing sport for hunters in the fall and viewing pleasure for visitors throughout the year. Unfortunately, despite plenty of worthwhile destinations, trails through these mountains have generally been few and far between. For the most part, local hikers have ignored this interesting country, thinking of it as only a depressing sea of clear-cuts between the city and the beach. But that attitude needs to change because there is plenty here worth seeing and a rapidly expanding network of trails for pedestrians to explore.

With their mild and famously wet climate, these mountains are probably the best place in the world to grow evergreen trees. In addition, the Clatsop and Tillamook State Forests, which administer this land, have traditionally focused almost exclusively on timber harvest, in an effort to maximize state revenues and produce jobs. In fact, until recently, recreation was almost completely ignored, since managers did not see this as part of their mandate. In the last decade or so, however, some of that thinking has changed, and, at least from a hiker's perspective, all to the better.

After the monumental replanting efforts following the Tillamook Burns of the 1930s and 1940s, much of forest here is uniformly green and impressive, with just enough lingering snags to add scenic and historical interest. Those trees are now ready for harvest, however, so if you want to see this land without the scars of clear-cuts, you'd better hike the trails here soon. More important, now is the time to get involved in the efforts of the Sierra Club, the Audubon Society, and other environmental groups to save at least part of this beautiful landscape from the ravages of the chainsaw.

There are two main access roads into the northern Coast Range. From Portland, go about 20 miles northwest on U.S. Highway 26, better known as the Sunset Highway, to a road split. The main highway continues straight (northwest)

Saddle Mountain from upper viewpoint

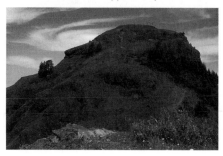

Hiking along lower Saddle Mountain Trail

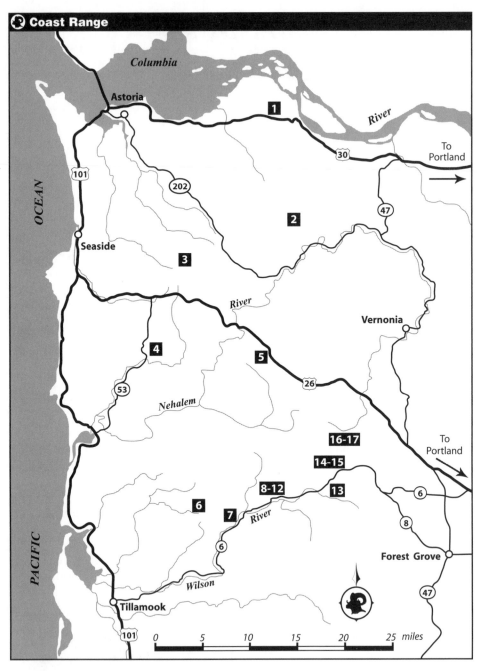

Coast Range

Columbia

Astoria

River

To Portland

30

101

202

47

2

Seaside

3

River

Vernonia

4

5

53

Nehalem

26

16-17

To Portland

14-15

8-12

13

6

6

8

7

River

6

Forest Grove

PACIFIC

Wilson

47

Tillamook

101

0   5   10   15   20   25 miles

toward the popular coastal resorts of Seaside and Cannon Beach. Along the way this highway provides access to the spectacular trail up Saddle Mountain and to several exciting new trails in the Clat-sop State Forest. Turning left (southwest) at the road split, onto State Highway 6, gains you access to the much greater number of scenic trails in the Tillamook State Forest.

TRIP 1 Gnat Creek

Distance	2.5 miles, Out-and-back
Elevation Gain	150 feet
Hiking Time	2 hours
Optional Map	USGS *Knappa, OR; Cathlamet, WA* (trail not shown)
Usually Open	All year
Best Time	Any
Trail Use	Good for kids, dogs OK, fishing
Agency	Clatsop State Forest
Difficulty	Easy
Note	Good in cloudy weather

HIGHLIGHTS This recently completed trail makes for an enjoyable and relatively easy leg-stretcher for families driving to Astoria. With the sounds of nearby traffic on U.S. Highway 30, the hike is not a wilderness experience, but the dense forest and clear stream are a beautiful and soothing change of pace. In addition, the fish hatchery at trail's end is educational and entertaining for both young and old.

DIRECTIONS Drive 76 miles north and west of Portland on U.S. Highway 30 to a junction with Gnat Creek Road shortly after milepost 78. Turn right, following signs to Gnat Creek Campground, and drive 0.1 mile on this good gravel road to the large trailhead parking area just before a bridge over Gnat Creek.

After climbing a set of wooden stairs, the trail heads west (upstream) amid a dense, moss-draped, second-growth forest of western hemlocks, Sitka spruces, and western red cedars. The winding but well-built trail remains entirely in forest with lots of mushrooms, deer and sword ferns, salmonberry bushes, and forest wildflowers to keep your interest along the way. Several huge stumps allow visitors to marvel at the size of the trees that once grew here and to mourn the loss of these ancient giants. Views are nonexistent, but the trail passes several places where hikers can look down on the clear, rippling waters of Gnat Creek, which flows about 30 feet below the trail. The only easy access to the water comes at 0.9 mile at a lovely spot on the banks of the creek that makes a perfect picnic location.

At a little more than 1.1 miles the trail crosses Highway 30. Watch carefully for

Backlit red alder

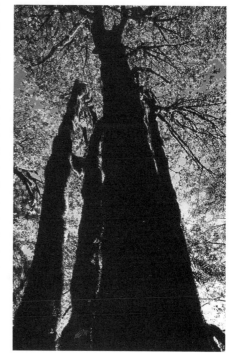

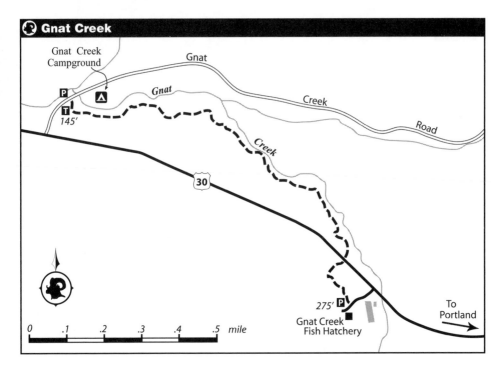

Gnat Creek

Gnat Creek Campground

Gnat

Gnat

Gnat

Creek

Creek

Road

Creek

30

145'

275' P

To Portland

Gnat Creek Fish Hatchery

0   .1   .2   .3   .4   .5 *mile*

traffic on this busy thoroughfare, the source of all those car and truck sounds you have been hearing from the start of the hike. On the other side of the highway the trail goes 0.1 mile to its end at the Gnat Creek Fish Hatchery. Spend some time touring this facility before returning the way you came.

TRIP 2 Northrup Creek Loop

Distance	8.5 miles, Loop; 3.8 miles, Out-and-back
Elevation Gain	1500 feet, Loop; 300 feet, Out-and-back
Hiking Time	2 to 5 hours
Optional Map	USGS *Nicolai Mountain* (trail not shown)
Usually Open	All year (except during winter storms)
Best Time	Any
Trail Use	Dogs OK, mountain biking, horseback riding
Agency	Clatsop State Forest
Difficulty	Moderate
Note	Good in cloudy weather

HIGHLIGHTS Built in 2005, the Northrup Creek Trail cobbles together existing logging roads, abandoned roads, and sections of new trail to form a pleasant loop through a little-known valley in the Coast Range. Although walking the road sections can be tedious, the scenery is generally quite attractive, including forested ridges, riparian areas, meadows, and a lovely creek. The trail is designed for equestrians, but is open to all nonmotorized uses and has surprisingly little of the mud so often associated with horse trails. If you do not have time to do the entire loop, then settle for a much easier out-and-back hike along Northrup Creek. This segment has the nicest scenery and involves no road walking.

DIRECTIONS Drive west on U.S. Highway 26 to the junction with State Highway 103 (the Jewell Road) near milepost 22. Go 9.2 miles north to the junction with Highway 202, turn right (east), and proceed 5.9 miles to a signed junction with Northrup Creek Road. Turn left (north), go 1.7 miles to the end of pavement, and then drive 3.3 miles on good gravel to the large day-use area and trailhead parking lot just after a bridge over Northrup Creek.

F or a clockwise circuit, which saves the best scenery for the end, turn right on the woodchip-covered trail and go 100 yards downstream beside clear Northrup Creek in a loop around the trailhead parking lot. When you come to the road,

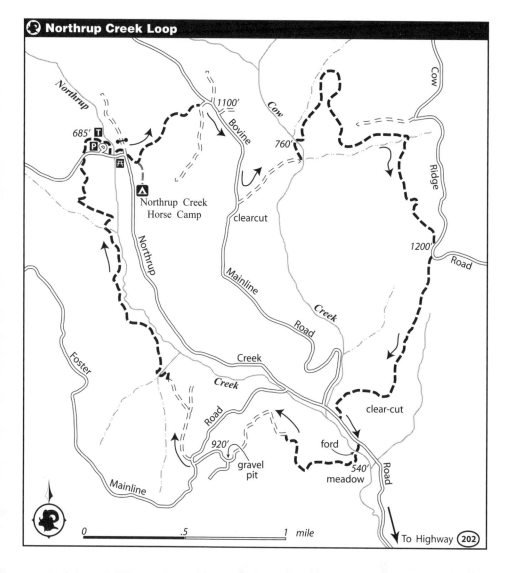

Northrup Creek Loop

Northrup

1100'

685'

Cow

Bovine

760'

Cow

Ridge

Northrup Creek Horse Camp

clearcut

1200'

Road

Northrup

Mainline

Creek

Road

Foster

Creek

Creek

Road

clear-cut

920'

gravel pit

ford

540' meadow

Road

Mainline

0   .5   1 mile

To Highway (202)

cross the creek on the road bridge, then pick up the trail again on the left as it briefly loops around a small picnic area. At 0.1 mile you cross a spur of Northrup Creek Road and then begin climbing in a lush second-growth forest of Douglas firs. Just 100 yards later, you go left at a junction with a spur trail to Northrup Creek Horse Camp.

Now on a long abandoned road, you hike uphill for 0.2 mile and then veer right onto a narrower trail that gradually ascends in a dense forest of young trees. There are no views, but the setting is pleasant and shady. So shady, in fact, that very few understory plants survive beneath the trees. At 0.8 mile you pass an area that has been selectively logged and then come to a spur road. The trail follows this road uphill for 50 yards to a junction with gravel Bovine Mainline Road. You turn right and walk along this good gravel road over a little hill then in a long curving downhill atop a forested ridge. After 0.7 mile on the road, just as you enter a large clear-cut, you turn sharply left on a more primitive road that follows the edge of the clear-cut. This road goes gently downhill for 0.4 mile to its end beside Cow Creek. Turn left (upstream), and follow a closed road for 0.1 mile to a bridgeless crossing of the creek. There is usually a convenient

log across this small creek just upstream from the horse crossing.

After all the road walking it is a pleasure to be back on trails as you go very gradually uphill, first beside a seasonal creek and then looping to the right as you ascend a forested hillside. The alder- and fir-lined trail winds uphill all the way to a junction with Cow Ridge Road at about 4 miles. You turn right, walk along this gravel road for 0.1 mile, and then go straight on an abandoned road blocked by a berm.

This wide route goes steadily but not steeply downhill for 0.8 mile to the upper edge of a large clear-cut, where you gather the hike's only significant views of the Northrup Creek Valley and a forested ridge to the south. Instead of crossing the clear-cut, turn right and follow a trail that skirts the edge of the logging scar down to the Northrup Creek Road. You turn left, walk along this gravel road for 0.15 mile, and then turn right onto a signed foot trail.

The path goes 150 yards through a lovely, low-elevation deciduous woodland featuring dappled sunshine and tiny wildflowers to a bridgeless crossing of Northrup Creek. By midsummer you can usually rock hop across this stream, but for most of the year getting to the other side requires a chilly ford. Just 100 yards

Meadow along Northrup Creek Trail

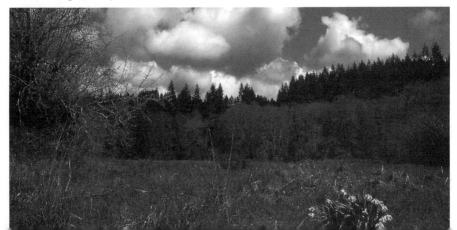

past the ford the trail reaches the edge of a large meadow that is a favorite haunt for a small herd of elk. The trail turns sharply right here, entering the forest rather than crossing the privately owned meadow, climbs rather steeply for 0.25 mile, and then levels out shortly before coming to the end of a primitive dirt road. Turn left and follow this little-used road for 0.3 mile to a gravel pit, and then walk along a better gravel road to a junction with Foster Mainline Road.

You turn right (downhill), crossing the road at an angle, and then veer left onto an unsigned primitive road. Walk gradually downhill along this tree-lined road, keeping left at a junction after 0.2 mile, all the way to the end of the road. From here, a good foot trail descends a series of short switchbacks to a hop-over crossing of a small creek.

This creek marks the start of the trail's wildest and most scenic section. For the next 1.7 miles the route remains a true trail (no road walking) as it goes up and down in the lowlands near Northrup Creek. The way alternates between dense forest, riparian areas, and tiny creekside meadows where wildlife such as deer and elk are common. The section also includes some huge moss-covered bigleaf maples that are well worth admiring. The only downsides are several muddy areas and so many elk droppings that they are hard to avoid. After 1.2 miles the trail climbs a switchback away from the creek, crosses a low ridge, and then descends to Northrup Creek Road. After crossing this gravel road, the trail curves to the right through attractive forest back to the trailhead.

TRIP 3 Saddle Mountain

Distance	6.1 miles, Out-and-back
Elevation Gain	1700 feet
Hiking Time	3½ hours
Optional Map	None needed
Usually Open	March to November
Best Time	Late May to mid-June
Trail Use	No dogs (allowed, but too rocky and rough for most dogs)
Agency	Oregon State Parks, Tillamook Region
Difficulty	Difficult

HIGHLIGHTS Saddle Mountain is undoubtedly the premier destination for pedestrians in the northern Oregon Coast Range. The open slopes near the top of this prominent landmark are home to a wide array of colorful wildflowers, including several rare species found virtually nowhere else in the world. But you don't have to be a botanist to enjoy this outing. Anyone who likes fine vistas will be thrilled with this hike because it provides the best views in this part of the state.

DIRECTIONS Follow U.S. Highway 26 to near milepost 10, about 65 miles west of downtown Portland. Turn north on the narrow paved road for Saddle Mountain State Park, and drive 7.0 miles to its end at a parking area that serves both the trailhead and a small walk-in campground.

Coast Range

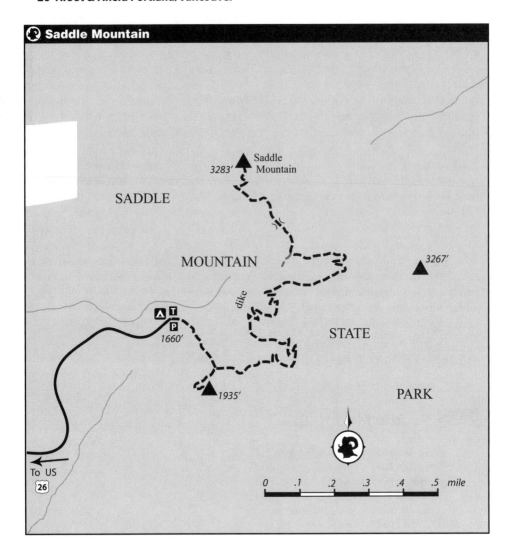

Saddle Mountain

SADDLE

MOUNTAIN

STATE

PARK

Saddle Mountain
3283'

3267'

dike

1660'

1935'

To US
26

0   .1   .2   .3   .4   .5   *mile*

The popular path up Saddle Mountain starts at the east side of the parking lot and climbs gently through a thick forest of red alder and bigleaf maple. Head-high salmonberry bushes crowd the edges of the trail, giving it something of a tunnel-like feeling. After 0.2 mile a side trail leaves the main route to your right. Take the time to do this very worthwhile side trip, as it climbs to a small knoll with terrific views of Saddle Mountain from an angle that really shows how the mountain got its name.

Back on the main trail, you climb a series of irregularly spaced switchbacks through attractive woods of mixed conifers and deciduous trees. In several places you'll notice where other hikers have cut switchbacks, causing erosion and needlessly trampled vegetation. Please stick to the official route and don't add to the problem. Geology buffs will be fascinated by a prominent basalt dike a little west of the trail at about the 1-mile point.

Continuing uphill, mostly in the shade of evergreens, you reach the wonderful

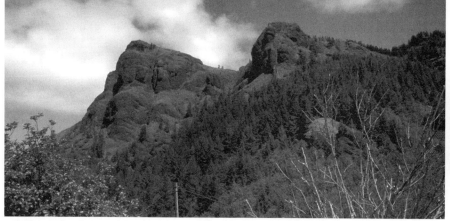

Saddle Mountain

meadows that cloak the upper slopes of the mountain. From March to September you can always enjoy at least some flowers here. The peak blooming season comes in early June, when a whole array of colors are there to enjoy, including blue larkspur and iris, red paintbrush, yellow buckwheat, and white chickweed.

Shortly before you reach the low point of Saddle Mountain's saddle, a path drops down a meadowy ridge to your left. A side trip here reveals outstanding views of the open, rounded slopes around the summit of Saddle Mountain, your next goal. To reach that goal, go across a narrow walkway through the mountain's saddle, and then climb steeply up the final 0.4 mile on a rocky trail with poor footing. You can gain greater stability by hanging onto the intermittent cable handrail on that last trail section.

The view from the often windy summit includes Cascade snow peaks as far north as Washington's Mt. Rainier, the shimmering Pacific Ocean to the west, and even (with the aid of binoculars) the 125-foot-high Astoria Column on a hill in the town of the same name to the northwest. Return the way you came.

TRIP 4 Soapstone Lake

Distance	2.4 miles, Semiloop
Elevation Gain	250 feet
Hiking Time	2 hours
Optional Map	USGS *Soapstone Lake* (trail not shown)
Usually Open	All year (except during winter storms)
Best Time	Any
Trail Use	Good for kids, backpacking option, dogs OK, fishing
Agency	Clatsop State Forest
Difficulty	Easy

HIGHLIGHTS Of the several recently completed trails in the Clatsop State Forest, this one to Soapstone Lake is the best. The hike's most noteworthy feature is its variety. While most Coast Range hikes travel exclusively through dense forest, this trail explores an attractive and relatively open second-growth forest, visits a small meadow, crosses a lovely stream, and ends at a pretty lake that would be worth the hike all by itself.

DIRECTIONS Drive west on U.S. Highway 26 to the junction with State Highway 53 near milepost 9.5. Turn left (south), drive 4.8 miles, and then turn left on a gravel road signed Soapstone Trailhead. Proceed 0.4 mile on this narrow road to the well-signed trailhead and parking area.

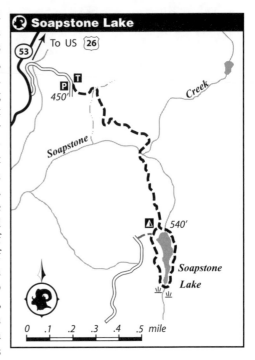

The wide, smooth, and gently graded trail travels through a second-growth forest dominated by western hemlocks towering above a thick mat of oxalis, various ferns, and thimbleberry bushes. Several huge stumps with old logging springboard holes attest that the forest here was once composed of much larger specimens. The trail crosses two often-dry creeks on wooden bridges and then at 0.3 mile gradually loses a little elevation before crossing a small grassy meadow. In late summer this meadow delights the visitor with lots of ripe blackberries and blooming goldenrods. At the far end of the meadow is a bridgeless crossing of clear Soapstone Creek. This crossing can be wet in winter but is an easy rock hop the rest of the year. After the crossing, you climb a rather steep set of wooden stairs and then wander uphill through a lovely forest of impressive old Douglas firs before coming to a T-junction near the north end of Soapstone Lake.

For a clockwise tour around the lake, turn left, cross a large bridge over the outlet creek, and pass several inviting picnic sites along the north and east shores of this alder-lined 10-acre pool. The water is 20 feet deep in places, but the shore is often muddy and has lots of logs, so it's difficult to reach the bank. If you can get to the water, it is fun to spend some time watching the lake's thousands of rough-skin newts or to toss in a line hoping to catch a cutthroat trout or two. Keep an eye out for wildlife, because also snacking on those trout are belted kingfishers and great blue herons. The best swimming spot is along the east shore at a small rocky beach with easy access to deeper water and relatively little mud.

The up-and-down trail goes all the way around the lake, passing through forests, beside several grassy areas, and over a skunk-cabbage bog on a board-walk spanning the inlet creek at the lake's south end. Above the northwest corner of the lake is a junction with a side trail to a nearby road. Turn right, almost immediately pass a nice campsite above the lake's north shore, and soon return to the junction near the outlet where you close the loop around the lake. Turn left and retrace your steps to the trailhead.

TRIP 5 Bloom Lake

Distance	2.7 miles, Semiloop
Elevation Gain	450 feet
Hiking Time	2 hours
Optional Map	USGS *Elsie* (trail not shown)
Usually Open	All year (except during winter storms)
Best Times	April and May
Trail Use	Good for kids, backpacking option, dogs OK, fishing
Agency	Clatsop State Forest
Difficulty	Moderate
Note	Good in cloudy weather

HIGHLIGHTS Until recently, the Clatsop State Forest, a major public landholder in northwest Oregon, had no maintained hiking trails. In 2004, however, the forest managers belatedly embraced the idea of "multiple use," which necessarily includes nonmotorized recreation, and constructed several fine paths for local pedestrians to explore. The most easily accessible of these routes is this trail to shallow but very pleasant Bloom Lake.

DIRECTIONS Drive west on U.S. Highway 26 to milepost 24.5 (exactly 4.2 miles west of the Sunset Rest Area), and park in the large gravel pull-out on the south side of the road.

The trail starts by crossing a wooden hiker's bridge over South Fork Quartz Creek, whose waters are banked by stands of red alder and a low-growing assortment of ferns, mosses, coltsfoot, horsetails, bleeding heart, and various other water-loving plants. The moderately to steeply graded trail then leads uphill past several old stumps and through a second-growth forest filled with vine maples, salmonberries, and April-blooming wildflowers such as trillium, wood violet, and oxalis. Winter wrens, varied thrushes, and chestnut-backed chickadees bring music to your stroll, helping to drown out the sounds of traffic on Highway 26.

Bloom Lake

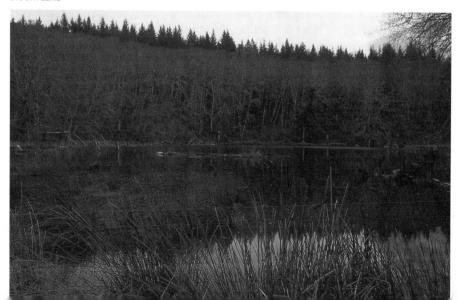

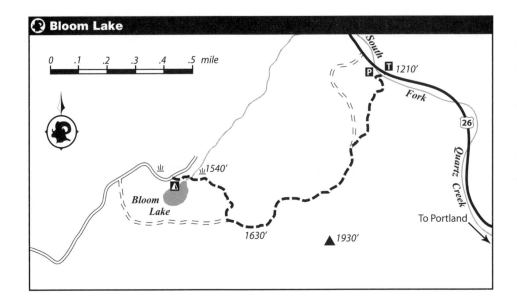

At 0.3 mile the path meets and follows a long-abandoned logging skid road, which now serves as a wide trail. Although the surrounding woods contain a few western hemlocks and Douglas firs, deciduous trees dominate, giving this area a pleasant open feeling, especially in winter and early spring. At 0.8 mile, the trail levels off for 0.1 mile and then comes to a junction marked with a small brown plastic post.

The old road goes straight here (a possible return route), but you turn right on a winding trail that goes downhill under the shade of large vine maples. After 0.25 mile you reach the outlet of shallow, 4-acre Bloom Lake. Although not wildly scenic, this pond makes a very pleasant lunch spot, surrounded as it is by white-barked alders and marshy areas that support a profusion of skunk cabbage, which blooms in March and April. The lake is popular with anglers, looking to snag some of the water's small cutthroat trout. Wildlife enthusiasts will enjoy looking at the old beaver dam on the outlet creek just below the lake.

You can make a semiloop out of this adventure by crossing Bloom Lake's outlet creek on a log and then picking up a sketchy path above a campsite on the west shore of the lake. Follow this path for 150 yards to a junction with a gravel road. Turn left on this road, walk uphill for 0.2 mile, and then turn sharply left on an old logging skid road. After 0.4 mile this up-and-down road reaches the junction with the trail you turned onto to reach Bloom Lake. Go straight and return the way you came.

TRIP 6 Cedar Butte

Distance	2.6 miles, Out-and-back
Elevation Gain	800 feet
Hiking Time	1½ hours
Optional Map	*Tillamook State Forest*
Usually Open	Late March to November
Best Time	Late May to mid-June
Trail Use	Dogs OK
Agency	Tillamook District, Tillamook State Forest
Difficulty	Moderate

HIGHLIGHTS In its continuing (and much appreciated) efforts to build more hiking trails, the Tillamook State Forest recently replaced the old boot path up Cedar Butte with a new, well-engineered trail. As a result, this old fire lookout site, which features grand views over a little-known section of the Coast Range, is much easier to access. The drive to the trailhead remains long and confusing, but once you get there the hike is a real treat.

DIRECTIONS Drive west on State Highway 6 toward Tillamook to a junction with Cedar Butte Road just past milepost 18. Turn right on this narrow, but relatively smooth gravel road and climb steeply for 2.2 miles to a fork. Bear right, proceed 2.9 miles to another fork, and then bear left. The road is now quite rough and has lots of sharp gravel (good tires are important), but it remains passable. Go 0.5 mile, and then park at a saddle in the middle of a large clear-cut where a rough dirt road goes left (uphill).

The possibly unsigned trail starts 60 yards up the dirt road at a fence stile on the right. The stile was installed to exclude ATVs from using this hiker-only route.

The trail climbs gradually through an ugly clear-cut above a logging road for 0.3 mile and then enters a much more pleasant forest environment of young Douglas firs. The ground cover, typical of mid-elevations in the Coast Range, is a mix of Oregon grape, sword fern, and salal. After steadily climbing a series of short switchbacks, the trail becomes increasingly steep and winds up a forested ridge toward the summit. Occasional openings in the tree cover provide partially obstructed views, and rocky areas support plenty of wildflowers in May and June. Look for wood sorrel, beargrass, and cliff penstemon. Just below the top of the butte the trail peters out, but it is easy

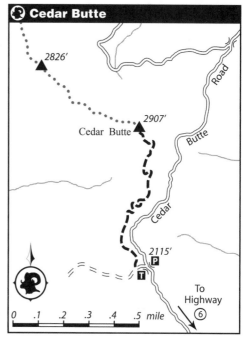

to negotiate the last 30 yards to the open summit. The small meadowy flat spot at the top is littered with shards of glass (the remains of the old fire lookout), so be careful where you sit.

The view from the summit is expansive, including the rugged outcroppings on Sawtooth Ridge and Mutt Peak to the west and northwest, the roadless canyon of Little South Fork Kilchis River to the north, and countless other ridges summits and canyons that are unfamiliar to most Oregon hikers. Bring a *Tillamook State Forest* map to help identify the convoluted assortment of jagged peaks and ridges.

Dedicated scramblers can continue northwest from Cedar Butte, traveling cross-country along a mostly open but very rugged ridge past a string of high viewpoints and rock gardens. Solitude is virtually guaranteed. After about 2 miles you reach a deep little pass beyond which reasonable travel becomes impossible.

TRIP 7 Wilson Falls

Distance	2.9 miles, Out-and-back
Elevation Gain	350 feet
Hiking Time	1½ hours
Optional Map	*Tillamook State Forest*
Usually Open	All year
Best Time	Mid-April to early June
Trail Use	Good for kids, dogs OK, mountain biking
Agency	Forest Grove District, Tillamook State Forest
Difficulty	Moderate
Note	Good in cloudy weather

HIGHLIGHTS This relatively short outing makes either a great leg-stretcher while traveling to the coast or a worthwhile destination in its own right. The tranquil forest setting and beautiful Wilson Falls are both top-notch, and if they aren't enough to justify the drive, several other nearby attractions are of both scenic and historical interest.

DIRECTIONS Drive west on State Highway 6 toward Tillamook and park at gravel pull-outs on either side of the road just after you pass milepost 20.

The trail goes 80 yards west along the highway shoulder and then descends a flight of moss-covered stone stairs to a large wooden bridge over a rocky gorge on the Wilson River. Once across the bridge, the trail crosses a small flood-damaged area and then climbs 150 yards to an unsigned junction with the Wilson River Trail.

You turn right (upstream) and wander gradually uphill through a lovely woodland dominated by red alder and vine maple. Although you can hear the sounds of traffic on nearby Highway 6, the landscape feels and looks like a remote wilderness. This is particularly true in the spring and summer when the deciduous trees have all their leaves and effectively block any view of the road. Another advantage of a visit in spring or early summer is that the forest is alive with the songs of warblers, flycatchers, thrushes, wrens, and other birds.

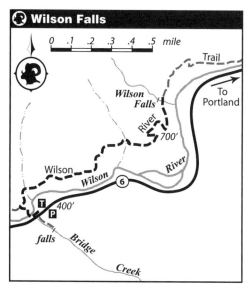

Wilson Falls

0 .1 .2 .3 .4 .5 mile

Trail

Wilson Falls

To Portland

River

700'

Wilson

River

Wilson

6

400'

falls

Bridge

Creek

cascades down a very steep cliff creating a veil-like appearance that is quite beautiful. Maidenhair ferns, devil's clubs, yellow monkeyflowers, bleeding hearts, and other water-loving plants complete the scene. The falls is most attractive in the spring when the plants are bright green and the creek is full of water. Although the Wilson River Trail continues beyond the falls, most of the next few miles are near the road and are not recommended.

Since this is a fairly short hike, you might consider extending your stay by visiting other nearby attractions. First and foremost, don't miss the short hike to Bridge Creek Falls. Starting from the same trailhead as the main hike, walk 40 yards west along the south side of Highway 6, and then turn left up a short flight of stone stairs into the canyon of Bridge Creek. The narrow trail climbs for 0.1 mile to the base of this tall waterfall, which cascades down a dark cliff face. Two unnatural but very interesting nearby attractions are also worth your time. Smith Homestead and the Tillamook Forest Center both offer human and natural history displays and information. They are located about 2 miles east (back toward Portland) on Highway 6.

You soon cross a seasonal side creek on a log bridge and then wander up and down through a lush and attractive forest. After crossing a second seasonal creek at 0.8 mile, the trail climbs two switchbacks and comes to the top of a minor ridge. Here the path makes a sharp left turn and then goes mostly downhill for 0.2 mile to the base of Wilson Falls, which is on an unnamed side creek. Instead of dropping in a single spectacular fall, Wilson Falls

Wilson River below Footbridge Trailhead

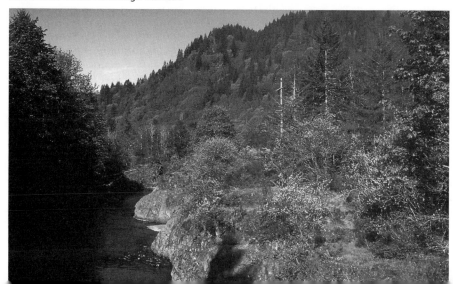

TRIP 8 Lester Creek Pinnacles

Distance	6.2 miles, Out-and-back
Elevation Gain	1350 feet
Hiking Time	3 to 4 hours
Optional Map	*Tillamook State Forest* (trail not shown)
Usually Open	Mid-March to November
Best Times	May and June
Trail Use	Dogs OK, mountain biking
Agency	Forest Grove District, Tillamook State Forest
Difficulty	Difficult

HIGHLIGHTS For most of its 21-mile length, the Wilson River Trail stays close to both State Highway 6 and the river that gave the trail its name. At times, however, private property forces the trail away from the river and onto higher ground. By far the most scenic of these detours is the section that takes you high on the western slopes of Kings Mountain into the drainage of Lester Creek. The views here are tremendous, and since few hikers have discovered this relatively new trail, there is a good chance you will have the scenery all to yourself.

DIRECTIONS Drive west from Portland on State Highway 6 toward Tillamook. Near milepost 22.6, turn right on gravel North Fork Road. Cross a bridge, go 0.3 mile to a junction, and then turn right, following signs to Diamond Mill Off-Highway Vehicle site. After 1.3 miles turn right into the huge parking area for the off-highway vehicle (OHV) site, and park as far from the noisy machines as possible, preferably at the north end of the lot.

The trail, which is closed to motorized vehicles despite the fumes, noise, and ugliness of the trailhead, starts from the northeast corner of the parking lot and descends for 50 yards to a junction with Wilson River Trail just before a gracefully arcing wooden bridge over North Fork Wilson River. Before crossing the bridge, consider taking a quick side trip to the right (south) on the Wilson River Trail. After 0.1 mile this trail takes you past a viewpoint of Lester Creek Falls, a two-tiered 15-foot drop where Lester Creek tumbles into the river. After visiting this lovely falls, return to the bridge and cross to the east side of the clear river.

The trail climbs a switchback away from the bridge and then ascends into a lovely second-growth forest mostly comprised of Douglas firs. The grade remains gentle using long switchbacks and winding traverses to accomplish its ascent. You soon climb past a small, wet meadow choked with red alders and then resume hiking in coniferous woods with only occasional views of craggy Kings

Pinnacle along Wilson River Trail

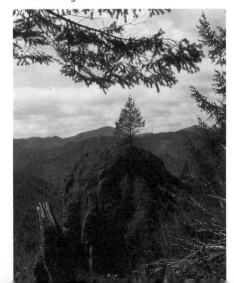

Mountain to the east and Kings Mountain Junior to the southeast. Although the trail twice crosses traces of ancient logging tracks, signs of human activity are otherwise rare. Signs of elk, however, are abundant, especially in the form of frequent piles of droppings, so watch your step. More uphill switchbacks and traverses take you over a side ridge and then high into the rugged drainage of Lester Creek. The views become more frequent as you climb, becoming truly exceptional at a little past 2 miles when you cross an open slope with an unobstructed look at the west face of Kings Mountain.

Once on the mountain's flanks, the trail makes an extremely scenic up-and-down traverse, crossing several small feeder streams of Lester Creek. The real attractions here, however, are a large basalt outcropping and a pinnacle next to the trail at 3 and 3.1 miles, respectively. These both feature terrific views to the west and make great lunch spots.

The pinnacles are the logical place to turn around, but if you have more energy, continue on the Wilson River Trail as it crosses the main stem of small Lester Creek and then traverses to an unsigned junction on a ridgetop at about 4 miles. The steep spur trail to the left goes to the top of Kings Mountain Junior, a good alternate destination for athletic types (see Trip 9). If you have a second car and want to make this a one-way adventure, you can continue 1.6 miles down the Wilson River Trail to the Kings Mountain Trailhead (see Trip 9).

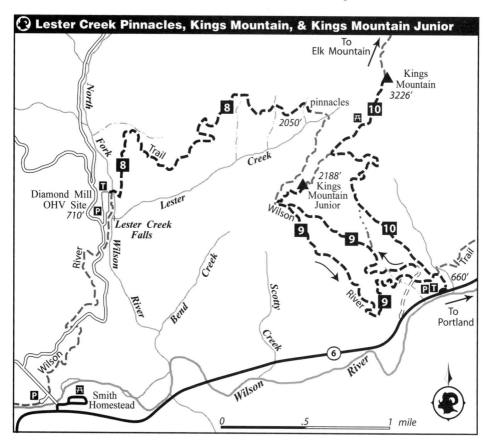

Lester Creek Pinnacles, Kings Mountain, & Kings Mountain Junior

TRIP 9 Kings Mountain Junior Loop

Distance	4.6 miles, Loop
Elevation Gain	2100 feet
Hiking Time	3 to 4 hours
Optional Map	*Tillamook State Forest* (trail not shown)
Usually Open	March to November
Best Times	May and June
Trail Use	No dogs (allowed, but too rocky and rough for most dogs)
Agency	Forest Grove District, Tillamook State Forest
Difficulty	Difficult

see map on p.35

HIGHLIGHTS Here is your opportunity to find both solitude and fine scenery on an excellent loop just west of popular Kings Mountain. The goal is a first-rate viewpoint from which you can enjoy sweeping vistas of the vast Tillamook Forest, including a particularly interesting perspective of the rugged west face of Kings Mountain.

DIRECTIONS Drive west from Portland on State Highway 6 toward Tillamook. Near milepost 25, turn right into the signed parking lot for the Kings Mountain Trailhead.

The hike starts with a gradual ascent of 0.1 mile on the well-traveled Kings Mountain Trail to a junction with the Wilson River Trail. About 20 feet past the signed junction with the eastbound Wilson River Trail, you turn left on the westbound section of that path and gradually climb through dense forest. After just 0.2 mile the trail crosses an old jeep road. The recommended loop returns on the Wilson River Trail, but, for now, turn sharply right onto the jeep road.

The abandoned jeep track soon makes a sweeping turn to the left as it steadily climbs through a forest dominated by red alders and bigleaf maples. Soon after this turn the route narrows to become a foot trail. Although blowdown is sometimes a problem, this unmaintained trail remains easy to follow. As always, do your part to keep this path open by removing limbs, rocks, and debris as you hike. More sweeping turns take you to a short but welcome level stretch at about 0.8 mile. Expect to hear tiny winter wrens here belting out their remarkably loud songs.

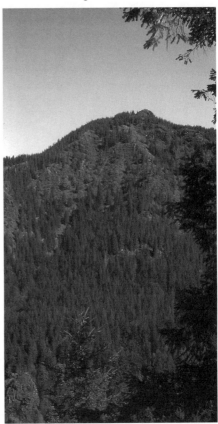

View east from Kings Mountain Junior

After the level stretch, the trail ascends in a sweeping left turn and comes to a potentially confusing junction with an old trail that angles off to the right. You bear left on the main trail, climb for 0.4 mile, and then reach another junction, this time with a sketchy trail that crosses your route and which may be marked with red plastic tape on the trees.

Go straight, still on the main trail, and cross a slope where two small rock slides have tumbled over the trail making the surface a bit uneven. Despite the rocks, the route remains obvious as you push forward and catch your first glimpses of Kings Mountain to the northeast. At 1.7 miles you come to a small opening on a ridgetop. Ignoring a game trail that goes steeply uphill to the right, you go straight and contour across a steep hillside for 150 yards to an unsigned junction with the well-maintained Wilson River Trail, which angles in from the left. This is the return route of the recommended loop.

To reach Kings Mountain Junior, go straight on the Wilson River Trail and follow it for 100 yards to an unsigned junction on a ridgecrest. The main trail goes straight here, on its way to Lester Creek (see Trip 8). You turn right, however, onto a very steep hiker's route. Watch your step on this section, especially on the way back down, because loose gravel here makes for poor footing. After 0.2 mile the very steep uphill abates, as you snake along the top of a narrow ridge. The views are excellent, but hikers who are particularly afraid of heights may get a bit squeamish. When you reach the 2188-foot summit of Kings Mountain Junior the views are partially obstructed but still good, especially of the impressively rugged west face of Kings Mountain to the northeast.

One possible return route is to go northeast on a sketchy and overgrown path that goes steeply downhill then back up for 0.3 mile to an unsigned ridgetop junction at a switchback in the well-maintained Kings Mountain Trail. From here, you turn right and descend 1.9 miles to your car. (See Trip 10 for a description of this trail.)

For the recommended loop, however, backtrack downhill to the ridgetop junction with the Wilson River Trail. Turn left (back the way you came), walk 100 yards to the junction with the trail you came in on, and then bear right, going downhill on the Wilson River Trail. This maintained trail has a much gentler grade than the way you came up, so it is easier on the knees. The trail winds down lazy switchbacks and long traverses always in the forest but with occasional views through the trees of Kings Mountain. After about 1.3 miles the trail crosses a small seasonal creek on a bridge a little above an unseen waterfall and, shortly thereafter, reaches the junction with the jeep road you turned onto on the way up. Cross the jeep road and retrace your steps to the Kings Mountain Trailhead.

TRIP 10 Kings Mountain

Distance	5.5 miles, Out-and-back
Elevation Gain	2800 feet
Hiking Time	3 hours
Optional Map	*Tillamook State Forest*
Usually Open	Late March to November
Best Time	Mid-May to mid-June
Trail Use	Dogs are allowed, but it's too rocky and rough for most.
Agency	Forest Grove District, Tillamook State Forest
Difficulty	Difficult

see map on p.35

HIGHLIGHTS If you take only one hike in the upper Wilson River drainage, make it the trail up Kings Mountain. The peak is one of the highest in the northern Oregon Coast Range, and the views from the open meadows atop its 3226-foot summit are terrific. On a clear day you can see, not only the extensive green hills of the Coast Range, but also the Pacific Ocean and even distant snow peaks in the Cascades, including Mounts Hood and Jefferson. The advantage of this hike over neighboring Elk Mountain is that while the total elevation gain is greater, the grade, while still steep, is less exhausting and the trail is better maintained. Finally, the flowers are more abundant in the large meadows atop this peak, so you can luxuriate in views and in the smell and color of the blossoms.

DIRECTIONS Drive west from Portland on State Highway 6 toward Tillamook. Near milepost 25, look for the brown sign with a hiking figure on it, and the small trailhead parking lot for the Kings Mountain Trailhead on the right.

Like so many other paths in western Oregon, this trail begins in a lush forest of Douglas fir, western hemlock, and red alder whose branches are draped with mosses. The forest floor is covered with sword fern and a low carpet of oxalis and candyflower, both of which feature small white flowers in spring. Just 0.1 mile from the start is a junction with the eastbound Wilson River Trail, which forks off to the right (Trip 11). Go left, then, 20 feet later, go right where the westbound Wilson River Trail departs.

From here, the Kings Mountain Trail makes an irregular but usually gentle climb through attractive woods. At first there are small creeks in the gullies on either side of the trail, but afterward the trail is entirely dry. About 1 mile from the trailhead the forest gets drier and

View north from atop Kings Mountain

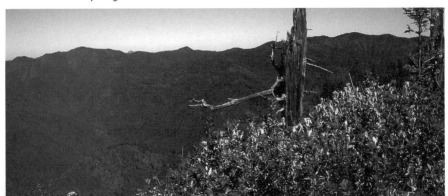

the slopes steeper as you begin to tackle the worst of the climb. As with all paths in this area, you will notice blue paint markings on the trees along the route. These aren't really necessary, as the trail is obvious throughout. The uphill climb is uneventful (and unrelenting) except near the 2000-foot level. There you'll find two places where the path stays nearly level for a couple hundred yards as it follows sections of very old roads that seem to come from nowhere and end for no apparent reason.

Fairly steep climbing eventually leads you to a picnic table right beside the trail, just 0.3 mile from the top. You can stop here for a rest, but save your longer lunch break for the very top, where the view is far superior. The final climb to the summit is quite steep in some sections, with loose gravel that can be a little dangerous on the way back down. On the plus side, most of the final 0.2 mile is a joyous route through open meadows that are ablaze with wildflowers in early June.

Very adventurous hikers can continue this hike over the rugged path that connects Kings Mountain with Elk Mountain to the east. For a description of this difficult route, see Trip 12.

TRIP 11 Upper Wilson River Trail

Distance	3.4 miles, Point-to-point
Elevation Gain	700 feet
Hiking Time	1½ hours
Optional Map	*Tillamook State Forest*
Usually Open	All year (except during winter storms)
Best Times	April to June and mid- to late October
Trail Use	Dogs OK, mountain biking
Agency	Forest Grove District, Tillamook State Forest
Difficulty	Moderate
Note	Good in cloudy weather

HIGHLIGHTS This path provides a welcome link allowing hikers to make a challenging loop hike that connects Kings and Elk mountains (Trips 10 and 12). As a separate hike, this lower-elevation trail is a pleasant leg-stretcher with attractive forests, several splashing creeks, and some nice viewpoints. Since it is at such a low elevation, this trail provides a nice alternative for hikers looking for a scenic place to walk in early spring or even mid-winter, although the path will be muddy then.

To do this hike as a one-way trip, it is better to begin from Elk Creek, as that involves a total elevation loss of about 400 feet. As part of the Kings and Elk mountains loop trip, however, it is more likely that you will do this trail from the Kings Mountain end, so that is the way it is described here.

DIRECTIONS Drive west on State Highway 6 toward Tillamook. Near milepost 25, look for the brown sign with the hiker on it and the parking lot for the Kings Mountain Trailhead on the right. For the upper trailhead at Elk Creek, turn north off Highway 6 near milepost 28 and drive the gravel access road to Elk Creek Campground for 0.3 mile to its end just beyond a bridge over Elk Creek.

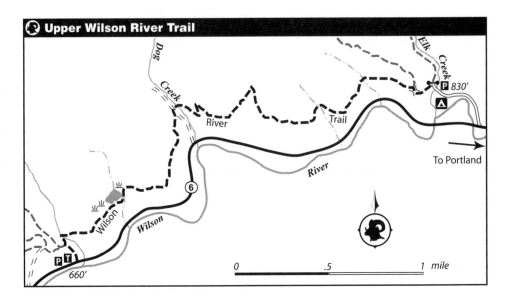

The Kings Mountain Trail begins in a lush forest of Douglas fir, western hemlock, and red alder most of whose branches are covered with hanging mosses. Just 0.1 mile from the start is a junction. The Kings Mountain Trail veers off to the left, while the Wilson River Trail goes to the right.

The trail almost immediately hops over a small creek and then begins the gentle ascent that will dominate the entire route. An abundance of vine maple in the understory makes this section particularly attractive in mid- to late October. The path goes around the south side of a small pond and marshy area and then crosses the outlet creek for the marsh.

As you hike you will probably see the knobby tire tracks of mountain bikes and the paired crescents of deer hooves. You may also see the makers of these tracks, the former more common on weekends, the latter on quiet weekdays. As for sounds, in addition to birds and wind in the trees, you will often hear traffic on Highway 6 to the right, but the noise is never terribly intrusive.

Beyond the pond you make an extended contour of a forested hillside above the road and then dip into a canyon to cross a jeep road and rock hop across good-sized Dog Creek. Two switchbacks and more climbing now lead you to a rocky, open hillside above the highway. As you hike, keep an eye out for large, old stumps, many still showing that loggers cut slots for springboards. The daring woodsmen then stood on the precarious springboards so they could cut higher on the tree trunk.

The rest of this easy trail alternates between forested hillsides overlooking the road and small side canyons with trickling creeks that provide opportunities to cool off by dunking your head. The trail ends with a short climb to a saddle where there is a poorly marked junction with the Elk Mountain Trail. You continue straight and drop a few hundred yards to the Elk Creek Trailhead.

TRIP 12 Elk Mountain Loop

Distance	8.5 miles, Out-and-back
Elevation Gain	2500 feet
Hiking Time	4 to 5 hours
Optional Map	*Tillamook State Forest*
Usually Open	Late March to November
Best Time	Mid-May to mid-June
Trail Use	Dogs are allowed, but it's too rocky and rough for most.
Agency	Forest Grove District, Tillamook State Forest
Difficulty	Difficult

HIGHLIGHTS All your hard work on that stair-climber at home will come in handy on this thigh buster. The trail up Elk Mountain is short, but it's brutally steep. Fortunately, the flower show is excellent, and inviting views stretch over hundreds of square miles of hills and valleys. Be aware that this trail can be treacherous, especially downhill, because of loose gravel and extremely slippery mud. Boots with good traction are a necessity. There is no drinking water along the route, and since you will do a lot of sweating, you'll need to carry at least two quarts of water per person on a hot day.

DIRECTIONS Drive west on State Highway 6 toward Tillamook. Near milepost 28, turn right on the well-marked gravel access road to Elk Creek Campground. The trailhead is at the end of this 0.3-mile road, just after you cross a bridge over Elk Creek.

The trail starts with a moderately steep climb of 0.1 mile in mixed coniferous and deciduous forest to a junction at a saddle. The path going straight is the Wilson River Trail (Trip 11). For Elk Mountain you turn right on a trail marked with a large blue dot painted on a tree. The path climbs steeply, sometimes through red-alder and Douglas-fir forests, but mostly up open, rocky areas on the spine of a narrow ridge. The views are frequent and superb, especially looking down the Wilson River Canyon and up to the ramparts of Elk Mountain. Flowers are numerous in May and June. Look for starflower, salal, paintbrush, lomatium, wild rose, thimbleberry, and a host of others.

At several points this ridgetop route loses elevation, but it is quickly regained. Steep climbs are the hike's dominant feature. The terrain is very wild, although

View of Kings Mountain from north ridge of Elk Mountain

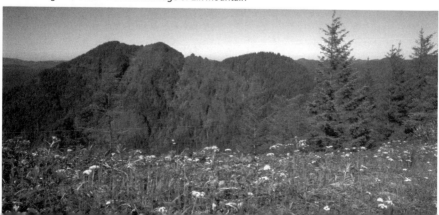

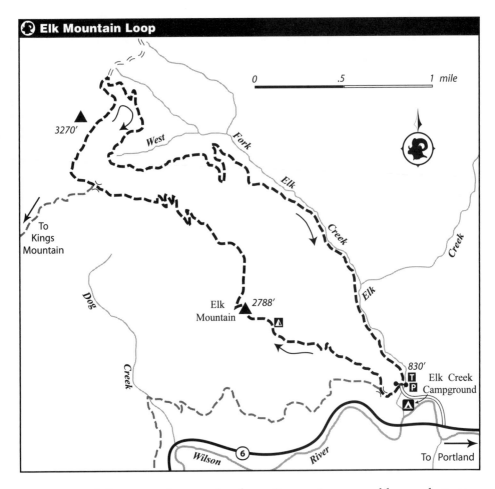

you never fully escape the sounds of well-traveled Highway 6, almost directly below.

The route continues to resemble going the wrong way on a very steep downhill ski run, until the 2500-foot level. Here you level off a little, pass a small, waterless camp, and then traverse the west side of a rocky spine. Another series of steep uphills and open ridgetop viewpoints finally take you to a small open spot atop 2788-foot Elk Mountain. As expected, the views are terrific; look west to craggy Kings Mountain for the most photogenic. In early June wildflowers abound, including penstemon, lupine, arnica, beargrass, paintbrush, and Washington lily.

You can turn around here and return the way you came, but if you aren't exhausted from the climb, there are two loop options you might consider. Both loops begin by dropping very steeply down a trail on the northwest side of Elk Mountain. This path, appropriately marked with signs stating CAUTION—STEEP AREAS, is narrow, challenging, and rugged. Subtlety was clearly not the goal of the trail builders, as they scornfully bypassed obvious opportunities for gentle sidehill traverses, opting instead for dangerous routes along the up-and-down, knife-edge ridge. Fortunately, these difficulties end within a mile, as you hit an old road that wanders pleasantly through shady forests.

This overgrown road is also well-traveled by wildlife, as frequent elk droppings and piles of bear scat attest. You make several short and gentle uphill switchbacks and then follow a view-packed ridge crest to a saddle and an unmarked T-junction with another closed road.

For the recommended shorter loop, turn right at the saddle, and in 0.5 mile you reach a junction with the road leading back down to Elk Creek Campground. This old logging road often runs near Elk Creek, whose clear, cascading waters are a nice diversion from the otherwise rather monotonous red-alder forest. The total length of this shorter loop is about 8.5 miles.

More athletic hikers looking for a real challenge can turn left at the T-junction and head west to Kings Mountain. This longer loop initially follows a closed road, which soon turns to trail and gets fairly nasty. You must negotiate about 1 mile of very steep ups and downs as you skirt the north side of some sheer cliffs and rock pinnacles. Expect to use your hands and probably your backside from time to time, to safely negotiate this section. As compensation for your efforts, exceptional views to the north are frequent and flowers are abundant. In addition to the previously mentioned species, look for wallflower, phlox, larkspur, clover, stonecrop, bunchberry, and dandelion. Finally, the rough scramble eases off, as you enter the gorgeous open meadows atop Kings Mountain.

From here, the loop follows the trail down from Kings Mountain (Trip 10) and returns to Elk Creek Campground via the Wilson River Trail (Trip 11). The total length of this very difficult loop is 12.0 miles. Since there are no reasonable campsites along the way, the loop must be completed in one day.

TRIP 13 University Falls

Distance	5.0 miles, Out-and-back
Elevation Gain	400 feet
Hiking Time	3 hours
Optional Map	*Tillamook State Forest*
Usually Open	March to November
Best Time	April to June
Trail Use	Good for kids, dogs OK, mountain biking, horseback riding
Agency	Forest Grove District, Tillamook State Forest
Difficulty	Moderate
Note	Good in cloudy weather

HIGHLIGHTS In a part of the Tillamook State Forest that is generally overrun by all-terrain vehicles (ATVs), the newly rerouted Gravelle Brothers Trail provides a welcome respite from the machines. While it never completely escapes the motorcycles' noise, this route is nonetheless a pleasant adventure on a nonmotorized trail with a destination that is a real eye-popper. University Falls is justifiably one of the most photographed spots in Tillamook State Forest, and when you catch sight of this 80-foot cascade you will no doubt want to take a few snapshots of your own.

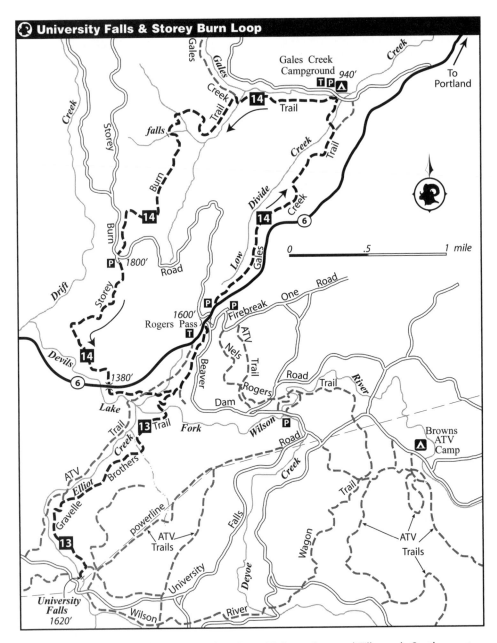

University Falls & Storey Burn Loop

DIRECTIONS Drive west from Portland on State Highway 6 toward Tillamook. On the west side of Rogers Pass, near milepost 33, turn left (south) on a gravel road signed Rogers Camp Trailhead. Go 0.1 mile to a junction, turn left, and proceed another 0.1 mile to the large trailhead parking lot.

Start by walking the road almost all the way back to Highway 6. Just 50 feet before the highway, turn left at a trail sign and follow the outside of a barrier that loops around a highway department gravel yard and storage building. At the west end of the facility, turn left on Gravelle Brothers Trail, which goes downhill following an abandoned jeep road. At 0.3 mile veer right onto a narrow foot trail and walk 120 yards to a possibly unsigned junction with the Storey Burn Trail. You go straight, still on the Gravelle Brothers Trail, and make a short switchbacking descent to a log bridge over clear-flowing Devils Lake Fork Wilson River. This is a lovely spot at any time of year but especially in mid-spring and late fall when the red alders that fill this area are either coming out in full greenery or putting on an impressive display of muted yellow.

The trail climbs slowly away from the river through a second-growth forest of Douglas firs and red alders. Although viewless, the scenery is very attractive especially around the several small intermittent creeks that cross your path. You may hear the occasional truck on increasingly distant Highway 6 or perhaps be disturbed by the noise of ATVs on a paralleling trail on your right, but the dominant sounds are the songs of winter wrens and kinglets in the forest. After a short up-and-down traverse, you curve to the south and follow a hillside well above often unseen Elliot Creek.

At 1.7 miles is a junction with a spur trail to the paralleling ATV trail. You go straight and then climb rather steeply over a small ridge, before dropping to a junction and horse-hitching area. Turn right on the hiker-only University Falls Trail, and go 130 yards to the base of this lovely fall, which cascades over a rocky terrace. On a hot summer day the spray at the base of this falls provides a cool retreat and a great place for lunch.

It is possible to make an 8-mile loop out of this hike by turning left (uphill) at the University Falls junction and following the Wilson River Wagon Trail and Nels Rogers Trail back to Rogers Pass. This is not recommended, however, because of countless confusing ATV trail junctions and the abundant noise from all the machines. Returning the way you came is much more pleasant.

University Falls

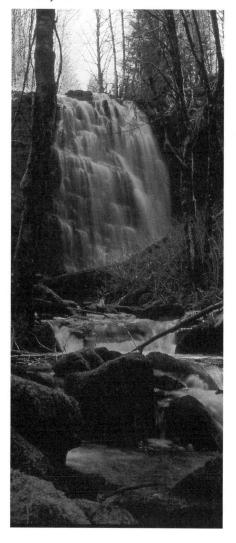

TRIP *14* Storey Burn Loop

see map on p.44

Distance	8.1 miles, Loop
Elevation Gain	1500 feet
Hiking Time	4 hours
Optional Map	*Tillamook State Forest*
Usually Open	March to December
Best Times	May and June
Trail Use	Dogs OK, mountain biking
Agency	Forest Grove District, Tillamook State Forest
Difficulty	Difficult
Note	Good in cloudy weather

HIGHLIGHTS This accessible hike is a welcome addition to the rapidly developing system of hiking and biking trails in Tillamook State Forest. Although less attractive than the route along Gales Creek (Trip 15), which starts from the same trailhead, this circuit gives you a better workout and views from the wooded ridges north of Rogers Pass.

DIRECTIONS Drive west on State Highway 6 toward Tillamook. Just before you reach mile-post 35, turn right on the well-signed gravel road to Gales Creek Campground. After about 1 mile, pull into the day-use parking lot on the left just before the road crosses a bridge over Gales Creek. This campground is closed from November to May when a gate blocks the access road from Highway 6. If you are hiking in the off-season, start at the busier Summit Trailhead on the east side of Rogers Pass another 2 miles up Highway 6 from the Gales Creek turnoff.

For a counterclockwise loop, take the Gales Creek Trail to the right (northwest) from the parking area and begin a slow steady climb. After traversing the woodsy hillside above Gales Creek for 0.8 mile, a narrow log bridge takes you over an unnamed side creek. You immediately reach a junction with the Storey Burn Trail.

Turn left (uphill) and begin a steady climb that keeps pace with the small cascading creek on your left. You travel through second-growth forests composed of the usual Coast Range mix of Douglas fir, western hemlock, western red cedar, bigleaf maple, and red alder. Although the forest canopy is quite dense in places, it allows ample sunshine to reach the forest floor in order to support a thick growth of sword fern and Oregon grape. About 1 mile after starting on the Storey Burn Trail, you splash across a small creek right beside a pretty, stair-step waterfall—a great place for a leisurely rest stop. Above this point the trail slowly winds uphill through a partially logged area to a junction with the gravel Storey Burn Road.

To relocate the trail, find a dirt jeep track directly opposite where you hit the road; walk 80 yards up this track to the large gravel parking lot for the little-used Storey Burn Trailhead. Your signed trail loop continues on the west side of this parking lot.

The Storey Burn Trail now travels gently up and down for 0.5 mile taking you past forest openings offering good views of heavily forested Larch Mountain to the north and the upper reaches of the Wilson River Canyon to the west. Past these openings the well-graded trail

Coast Range

winds down through attractive woods to Highway 6. You avoid the traffic by crossing under a tall road bridge. About 0.2 mile later is a signed junction with an all-terrain vehicle trail.

Go straight. For the next 0.3 mile you cross the flats beside Devils Lake Fork Wilson River. These often muddy flats are covered with a tangle of mixed deciduous trees. Look for the tracks of elk, deer, raccoons, and black bears. After leaving the flats, the trail climbs a hillside for 0.1 mile to a junction with the Gravelle Brothers Trail (Trip 13). Turn left (uphill) and walk 120 yards to a junction with an old jeep road. Go left again (uphill) and walk 0.3 mile on this road to a large highway department facility at Rogers Pass. After you hike around the highway facility, go 300 yards east along the shoulder of the busy highway to a large gravel pull-out signed as the SUMMIT TRAILHEAD.

The trail angles down from this pull-out and drops fairly steeply for 0.4 mile through relatively dense woods. When the reddish-orange clay becomes wet—a depressingly high percentage of the time in this rain forest—it is difficult for hikers to maintain their dignity on the slippery surface. After the steep section ends, the trail goes up and down (mostly down) beside small Low Divide Creek for another 1.3 miles to a signed junction. Either direction will take you back to Gales Creek Forest Camp; the most direct route is the one on the left. This trail soon crosses a wooden bridge over Low Divide Creek and then continues another 200 yards back to the day-use parking lot and your car.

Falls along Storey Burn Trail

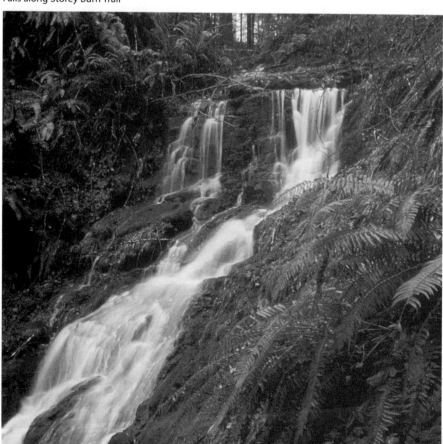

TRIP 15 Central Gales Creek Trail

Distance	10.1 miles, Out-and-back
Elevation Gain	1200 feet
Hiking Time	4 to 6 hours
Optional Map	*Tillamook State Forest*
Usually Open	All year (except during and shortly after winter storms)
Best Time	April to June
Trail Use	Good for kids, dogs OK, backpacking option, horseback riding, fishing
Agency	Forest Grove District, Tillamook State Forest
Difficulty	Moderate
Note	Good in cloudy weather

HIGHLIGHTS This new trail is not yet known to most Portland area hikers, but it's bound to draw more admirers as word spreads about this attractive and relatively easy creekside ramble through the second-growth forests of the Tillamook State Forest. Despite heavy rainfall, this is a good winter hike, because the tread drains well and remains in good shape with relatively few mud problems.

DIRECTIONS Drive west on State Highway 6 toward Tillamook. Just before you reach milepost 35, turn right on the well-signed gravel road to Gales Creek Campground. After about 1 mile, pull into the day-use parking area on the left just before the road crosses a bridge over Gales Creek. This campground is closed from November to May when a gate blocks the access road from Highway 6. The gate is sometimes open during the off-season, but even if it is, do not drive through it—it may close at any time without warning.

Take the Gales Creek Trail to the right (northwest) from the parking area and begin a slow steady climb. For the next 0.7 mile you travel across a hillside about 50 feet above Gales Creek generally staying near the transition line between the second-growth coniferous forests on the slopes above you and the alder woodlands near the stream. The forest floor beneath these trees is covered with a dense mat of sword fern, which grows so profusely it forces out nearly all other understory species.

After 0.8 mile you take a narrow log bridge over an unnamed side creek and then immediately reach a junction with the Storey Burn Trail (Trip 14). Turn right and travel up and down on a trail that alternately hugs 15-foot-wide Gales Creek or traverses the woodsy hillside above the water. Much of the time the

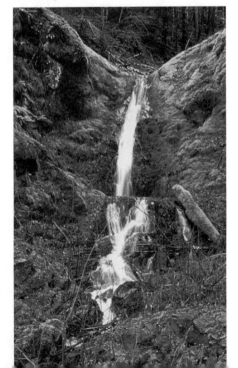

Falls along Gales Creek Trail

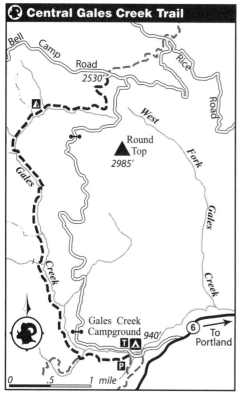

Central Gales Creek Trail

Bell

Camp

Road

2530'

Rice

Road

West

Fork

Round

Top

2985'

Gales

Gales

Creek

Creek

Creek

Gales Creek
Campground 940'

6 To
Portland

0 .5 1 mile

trail follows an old road, long since abandoned and now just a wide, well-graded trail. A little more than 1 mile from the Storey Burn junction, the trail crosses a small side creek. Look left to see a 20-foot-tall, sliding waterfall. In winter or early spring when the water runs high and the waterfall is not obscured by foliage, it's at its best.

The forest scenery remains unchanged as you continue up the canyon of Gales Creek for another mile to a sturdy log bridge that takes you over the creek. After another 0.5 mile, you come to a second log bridge and cross the flow again. As it slowly gains elevation, the trail goes over several side creeks. Quaint wooden bridges sometimes convey you, but more often you simply hop over. Although these side creeks are small, they make up a large percentage of Gales Creek's volume, so the main stream gets noticeably smaller as you continue up the canyon.

Near the 4.5-mile point, you pass a nice campsite after which the creek and

The author on a log bridge over Gales Creek

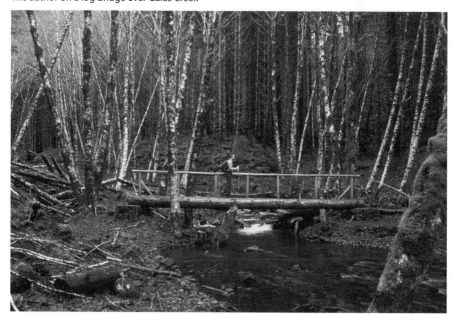

accompanying trail curve to the east and the canyon narrows. The ascent now gets more strenuous as the grade becomes moderately steep. Just beyond the 5-mile point, Gales Creek has diminished to the point where it barely deserves to be called a creek. Here the trail pulls away from the water to ascend a woodsy hillside.

Most hikers will want to turn around here because the scenery is less interesting away from the creek. If you prefer to make this a longer one-way hike, however, stay on the trail as it climbs another mile to a wide, forested ridgeline where it crosses remote Bell Camp Road. From there the trail is described in Trip 16.

TRIP 16 Northern Gales Creek Trail

Distance	6.8 miles to Bell Camp Road, Out-and-back
Elevation Gain	1500 feet
Hiking Time	3 to 4 hours
Optional Map	*Tillamook State Forest*
Usually Open	February to November
Best Time	April to June
Trail Use	Dogs OK, backpacking option, mountain biking, horseback riding
Agency	Forest Grove District, Tillamook State Forest
Difficulty	Difficult
Note	Good in cloudy weather

HIGHLIGHTS Starting beside a lovely stream, this trail climbs through second-growth woods to a road atop a high ridgetop. The route has no spectacular scenery, but it provides good exercise and is fun to hike. Beware, however, that parts of this trail, especially in its upper reaches, are rather unattractive, with some logged areas and many new logging roads. Even so, it is a pleasant hike, and provides relatively quick access to the upper reaches of Gales Creek, where there are some excellent options for both anglers and overnight backpackers.

DIRECTIONS Drive U.S. Highway 26 west from Portland to a junction a little past milepost 38. Turn left (south) on Timber Road, drive 3.1 miles, and then turn right on Cochran Road, which starts as pavement but soon changes to good gravel. At 2.5 miles from Timber Road and 0.1 mile past the turnoff for Reehers Campground, turn left into the signed parking area for the Reehers Campground Trailhead and day-use area.

From the east side of the parking lot, pick up the Gales Creek Trail as it curves downhill and to the west to a meeting with the clear waters of the small Nehalem River. From here the trail meanders upstream, through a bottomland ecosystem of deciduous trees and some surprisingly large specimens of western red cedars. The understory is a tangle of thimbleberry and other thorny shrubs, which effectively discourage any off-trail travel. At about 0.4 mile you reach the road, where you turn left and cross the river on the road bridge. Just 20 yards after this crossing, bear left onto an unsigned road, walk 10 yards, and then turn left onto an obvious foot trail.

This winding path gradually makes its way uphill through a tangled forest with numerous large, moss-draped vine maples overhanging the trail. In late October the fall colors from these maples are a real treat. At about 0.8 mile the trail crosses the tracks of the Tillamook Railroad and then twists and turns in a slow ascent of the forested hillside. Look here for numerous ancient stumps with old logging springboard holes and fire scars from the massive Tillamook Burns of the 1930s and 1940s. The trees planted after those fires are now large enough to harvest, so don't be surprised if you hear chainsaws (especially on weekdays) and encounter brand new (usually unmapped) logging roads crossing the trail. As of early 2007 there

were two such new roads that you must cross in the next mile, but more can be expected in the future.

At about 2 miles you cross gravel Round Top Road and then wind uphill along the edge of a recently thinned area that still shows many logging scars. The remaining forest is an open mix of Douglas firs and western hemlocks with an understory featuring the Coast Range's usual "Big Three," Oregon grape, sword fern, and salal. Although the uphill grade is sometimes moderate, it is rarely too steep. About 0.5 mile above Round Top Road you cross a rarely used logging spur and then switchback uphill through another selectively cut area. Near the top of this logging scar you cross the end of another logging spur road, walk 0.2 mile,

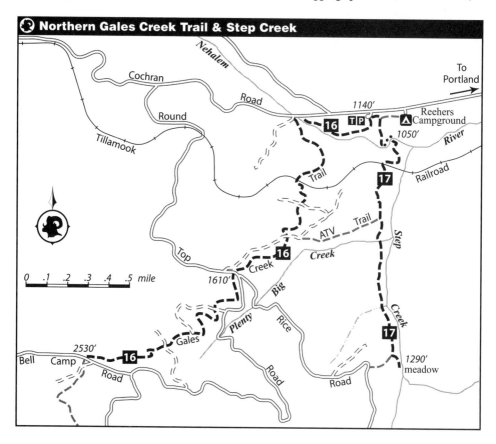

Northern Gales Creek Trail & Step Creek

and then cross a final logging road. This entire section is rather unattractive, but the scenery will improve in the future as time heals the logging scars. A final 0.6 mile of uphill hiking through partially cut timber takes you to a ridgetop junction with Bell Camp Road, 3.4 miles from the trailhead.

From Bell Camp Road you can either return the way you came or stay on the Gales Creek Trail as it descends the south side of the ridge and soon picks up the headwaters of its namesake stream. From Bells Camp Road it is 6 miles of downhill hiking to Gales Creek Campground (see Trip 15). If you have access to two cars, a one-way 9.4-mile hike between the two trailheads makes for a fun dayhike or weekend backpacking trip.

TRIP 17 Step Creek

Distance	3.0 miles, Out-and-back
Elevation Gain	400 feet
Hiking Time	2 hours
Optional Map	*Tillamook State Forest* (trail not shown)
Usually Open	All year (except during winter storms)
Best Time	Any
Trail Use	Dogs OK, horseback riding
Agency	Forest Grove District, Tillamook State Forest
Difficulty	Moderate
Note	Good in cloudy weather

see map on p.51

HIGHLIGHTS Although unsigned and unofficial, the path up Step Creek is a fun and relatively easy hike that is well worth finding. The lovely forest and creek setting is reason enough to visit, but for those who want a more identifiable destination, a good stopping point is a small meadow where quiet hikers stand a good chance of seeing elk.

DIRECTIONS Drive U.S. Highway 26 west from Portland to a junction a little past milepost 38. Turn left (south) on Timber Road, drive 3.1 miles, and then turn right on Cochran Road, which starts as pavement but soon changes to good gravel. At 2.5 miles from Timber Road and 0.1 mile past the turnoff for Reehers Campground, turn left into the signed parking area for the Reehers Campground Trailhead and day-use area.

From the east side of the trailhead parking lot, ignore the main Gales Creek Trail, which curves downhill to the west (see Trip 16), and follow instead a trail that goes east toward Reehers Campground. After 100 yards, turn right (downhill) on the signed Nehalem River Access Trail. This path descends 0.15 mile to the banks of the beautiful and clear Nehalem River, which here is really just a creek. Walk downstream along the trailless bank for about 0.1 mile, crossing the flow on any of several possible logs. When the river makes a fairly sharp turn to the right, take a jeep track that goes up the south bank.

Follow this jeep track uphill for 0.2 mile to a crossing of the Tillamook Railroad, and then pick up the trail angling to the southeast (slightly left) on the other side of the tracks. The trail is now wide and easy to follow, as it travels through a very attractive second-growth forest of Douglas firs with the usual tangle of sword fern and Oregon grape carpeting the forest floor. About 0.3 mile from the railroad tracks the trail begins to cross a hillside above the rollicking waters of unseen Step Creek on your left.

At 0.7 mile is a junction. An all-terrain vehicle trail angles to the right, but you take the left fork and soon hop across (greatly overstated) Plenty Big Creek. Beyond here the gently graded route continues south, mostly in a relatively open deciduous woodland where you can see down to joyfully cascading Step Creek. At about 1.1 miles you cross a trickling side creek, and then at 1.4 miles the trail curves uphill to the right away from Step Creek. Instead of taking this route, leave the trail here, and follow a use path that goes downhill to the left. In about 100 yards this route leads to a beautiful marshy meadow. Enter the meadow quietly and you may spot elk, whose tracks and droppings are everywhere, or beavers, whose activity is quite noticeable on the creek. This is the recommended turnaround point.

Chapter 2
Southwest Washington

With countless streams, forested ridges, waterfalls, and rocky viewpoints, southwest Washington has all of the same attributes possessed by other favored hiking areas near Portland. Due to misguided state pride, however, hikers living south of the Columbia River rarely cross the bridge and explore the many scenic trails in the Evergreen State. Vancouver residents appreciate the solitude, but if you are one of those overly provincial Beaver Staters, it is time to take a look at what you're missing.

Siouxon (pronounced *soo-son*) Creek features easy trails through a lovely old-growth forest in that rarest of local ecosystems, an unlogged low-elevation watershed. Without the erosion associated with logging, the stream is remarkably clear, splashing through gentle riffles, pausing in quiet eddies, dropping over scenic waterfalls, and sliding through slot canyons. All of this adds up to an enchanting hiking experience. Meanwhile the nearby ridges provide fine viewpoints and trails that challenge the most athletic hiker.

In the region around Three-Corner Rock, you'll discover an attractive landscape of second-growth forests, view-

Looking north from the northern ridge of Silver Star Mountain

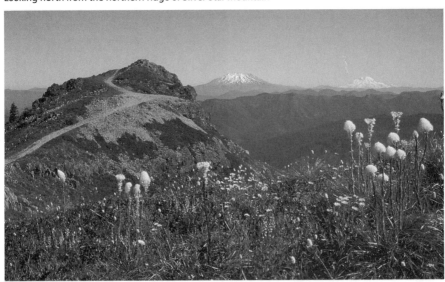

packed ridges, stream canyons, lush vegetation, and little-known trails. The road access is rough and confusing, but once the driving difficulties are surmounted the scenery is something to savor.

For spectacular views and flowers, however, southwest Washington's "star" attraction is undoubtedly Silver Star Mountain. Seen from Portland, Silver Star is that long ridge to the northeast that blocks the view of Mt. Adams. Once atop this mountain's scenic ridges, however, there is nothing to block the breathtaking views, not only of Adams, but of pretty much every other landmark within 50 or more miles. In addition, the peak boasts acres of open meadows filled with subalpine wildflowers, numerous rock formations, and some interesting Native American history. A wonderful network of surprisingly little-traveled trails invite the wanderer, who will no doubt want to return again and again to enjoy everything this mountain has to offer.

Most of the public land in southwest Washington is administered by either the Yacolt State Forest or the Gifford Pinchot National Forest. Be sure to obtain the most updated maps available from these agencies, so you can negotiate this region's often poorly marked roads with greater safety and confidence.

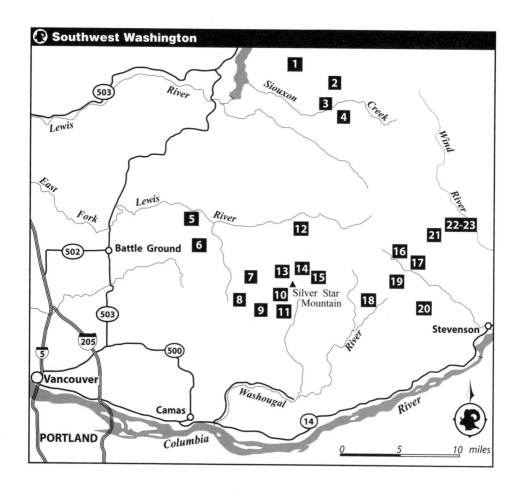

Southwest Washington

TRIP **1** North Siouxon Creek

Distance	9.4 miles, Out-and-back
Elevation Gain	1300 feet
Hiking Time	5 hours
Optional Map	USGS *Mount Mitchell, Siouxon Peak, Yale Dam* (part of trail not shown)
Usually Open	Mid-March to November
Best Times	April and May
Trail Use	Dogs OK, horseback riding
Agency	Yacolt State Forest
Difficulty	Difficult
Note	Good in cloudy weather

HIGHLIGHTS Although similar to the much better known trail on the main branch of Siouxon Creek (Trip 3), the trail up North Siouxon Creek has two important differences. While both hikes feature fine forest scenery and a lovely creek, North Siouxon Creek has much more difficult road access, so solitude is virtually guaranteed. And while its six waterfalls make the trail along Siouxon Creek more scenic, the North Siouxon Creek Trail is no slouch in the scenery department and the one waterfall along the way is absolutely first rate. Also, since this trail has almost no people, wildlife is much more common, especially elk, which quiet hikers have a good chance of seeing.

DIRECTIONS From the intersection of State Highways 502 and 503 in Battleground, drive 12 miles north on Highway 503 to a junction at the north end of Amboy. Turn right, still on Highway 503, and proceed 5.2 miles to a junction just 0.1 mile past the Mt. St. Helens National Volcanic Monument headquarters. Turn right on Healy Road, which becomes Forest Road 54, and drive 5.2 miles to a major fork. Bear left on gravel Road S 1000, which is often rough and muddy, go 0.4 mile, and then bear right at a second fork, still on S 1000. Stay on the main road for 4.7 miles, passing several minor intersections, until you come to the next major fork. Bear left (downhill), drive 1.4 miles, and then park at an unsigned pull-out where an old logging road goes right (south).

The unsigned but obvious trail goes sharply down the embankment on the southeast side of the pull-out, descends four quick switchbacks, and then skirts the edge of a clear-cut. Once reentering forest, the path settles into a pattern of ups and downs that will continue for the remainder of the hike and add significantly to the total elevation gain of the trip. The abundantly green vegetation is the usual mix of western hemlock and Douglas fir draped with mosses and ferns. Although the trail stays well above cascading North Siouxon Creek, you can always hear this rollicking stream in the canyon on the right.

At 1.6 miles, just as the trail reaches creek level, you cross a good-sized but

Black Hole Falls, North Siouxon Creek

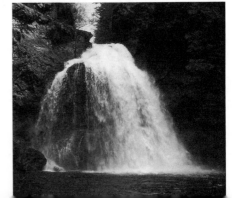

unnamed side creek. In early spring this crossing can be a bit intimidating, so look for a log just downstream. After the creek crossing, the trail makes a couple of uphill switchbacks and then descends near the base of an old clear-cut before resuming its up-and-down pattern. At 3 miles you make a sometimes tricky crossing of another good-sized side creek, this time in the middle of a steep, sliding cascade that doesn't quite merit the title "waterfall."

More uneventful but attractive forest hiking takes you to 4.5 miles, where you turn right onto a spur trail signed BLACK HOLE. This path switchbacks downhill for 0.2 mile to the base of Black Hole Falls,

easily the scenic highlight of the trip. Thundering over a basalt cliff and filling a terrific (but *cold*) swimming hole at its base, this 55-foot waterfall is an impressive sight. In the spring, when the water is high, the spray from the falls fills the rocky amphitheater here providing constant moisture for the mosses and ferns that cling to the rock face. Expect to see dippers, chunky little gray birds that live along mountain streams, feeding in the creek and tending a nest behind the falls. This waterfall is an ideal lunch spot. Unfortunately, there is no adequate campsite in the area, so hikers must make this a day trip.

Southwest Washington

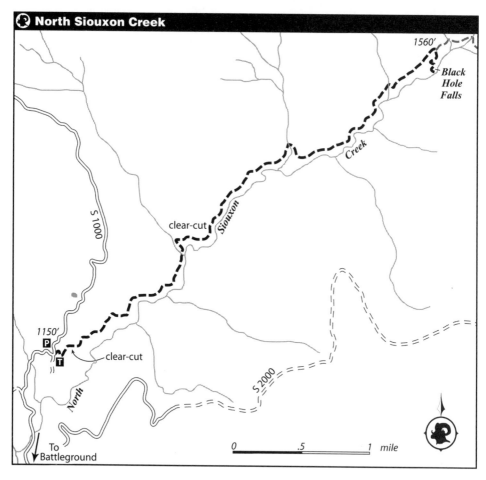

TRIP 2 Huffman Peak Loop

Distance	14.5 miles, Loop
Elevation Gain	3000 feet
Hiking Time	7 to 8 hours
Optional Map	Green Trails *Lookout Mountain*
Usually Open	May to October
Best Time	Mid-June
Trail Use	Dogs OK (but ford may be dangerous), horseback riding
Agency	Mt. St. Helens National Volcanic Monument, Gifford Pinchot National Forest
Difficulty	Difficult

HIGHLIGHTS So you've come to the Siouxon Creek area and you feel that the Siouxon Creek Trail (Trip 3), while beautiful, just doesn't provide enough exercise. Well, there's another worthy option here for athletic hikers looking to pump up that heart rate. The climb to Huffman Peak will satisfy the cardiovascular needs of the most avid hiker and has the added benefit of providing a first-rate view of Mt. St. Helens.

By making a loop out of the trip and returning on the Siouxon Creek Trail, you won't even miss the waterfalls and forests that are the area's main attraction. In addition to strong lungs and thighs, this hike requires an unusual piece of equipment—a pair of wading shoes. You'll need them to make the bridgeless lower crossing of Siouxon Creek.

DIRECTIONS Begin by driving to Battleground, either by going north on State Highway 503 from Interstate 205, or by going east on State Highway 502 from Exit 9 off Interstate 5. From the intersection of the two state highways in the middle of Battleground, proceed north on Highway 503 for 16.8 miles, and turn right on N.E. Healy Road just after you pass the Mt. St. Helens National Volcanic Monument headquarters.

After 9.2 miles on N.E. Healey Road, bear left at a poorly signed junction and travel on single-lane, paved Forest Road 57. Drive another 1.3 miles, and then turn sharply left on often unsigned Forest Road 5701. Follow this rough, paved road for 3.7 miles to its end at a trailhead parking lot.

The trail departs near a large signboard about 100 yards west of the parking area. You hike just 50 feet and turn left (west) at a signed junction. For the next couple of miles you follow an easy trail that parallels the road, staying some distance below it in a lovely western-hemlock forest. Along the way you splash across three small side creeks that won't even get the tops of your boots wet, but which provide enough water to satisfy an array of riparian plants like devil's club and maidenhair fern.

After 1.9 miles the trail splits, and you go right on a path that winds steadily downhill for 0.2 mile to a good camp beside a ford of Siouxon Creek. This is where you need to break out the wading shoes. The stream is about 30 feet wide and calf- to thigh-deep, depending on the season. The ford isn't particularly dangerous, but until late summer you can expect it to be chilly.

Pick up the trail above a little gravel bar on the opposite bank and quickly climb away from the water. The trail uses several short switchbacks and a couple of fairly steep traverses to reach the rounded crest of a forested ridge.

This forest is a good example of the succession process that takes place at low elevations of the western Cascades. The high canopy of the forest is made up of tall Douglas firs, while beneath this canopy grow shade-tolerant western hemlocks. If this forest manages to avoid logging or fires for the next couple centuries, the firs will die and the hemlocks will take over as the climax species. But since you don't have time to wait for this process to take place, pick up your pack and push on northeast up the ridge.

For almost a mile the going is very easy as you stay level or gradually climb in a dense forest, and then the uphill grade picks up a little as you climb near the southern edge of the rim. Along the way you often come to open areas where you have to push through thickets of Oregon grape and salal, but which give you frequent views over the deep, green depths of the Siouxon Creek drainage. The trail gets steeper as it works away from the rim and traverses the heavily wooded north side of the ridge. This steeper grade lasts for almost 1 mile before you level off and contour across the ridge's south side. As you go higher, wildflowers become more common, especially lupine, beargrass, bunchberry, and white anemone. When the uphill finally ends, the trail curves to the left and crosses a partly forested slope with lots of huckleberries and good views east to Huffman Peak, and then you come to a saddle and a junction with the North Siouxon Trail.

If you are up for a cross-country scramble, take the time to visit the top of Huffman Peak from this saddle. The

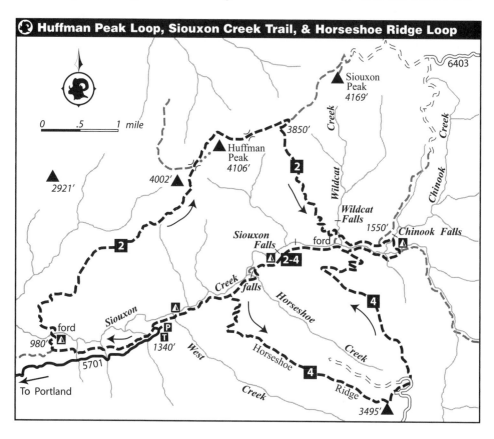

Huffman Peak Loop, Siouxon Creek Trail, & Horseshoe Ridge Loop

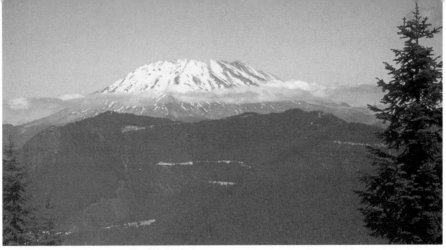
View of Mt. St. Helens from Huffman Peak

climb initially goes through forests and then up an open rocky slope. The way is often steep and requires some rock scrambling, but it is not dangerous. The reward for this effort comes in the form of extensive views from the rocky summit. Several roads and clear-cuts spoil things a little, but the fine views of massive Mt. Rainier, truncated Mt. St. Helens, and bulky Mt. Adams more than make up for it.

After returning to the main trail at the saddle, you turn east and traverse the steep slopes on the shady north side of Huffman Peak. The trail goes through the saddle east of the peak and then stays level or goes gradually downhill for a little less than a mile before reaching a small brown sign marking the junction with Wildcat Trail 156.

The recommended loop turns sharply back to the right here, climbing very steeply for a few hundred yards to the top of a viewless knoll and then descending a little ridge to the south. The downhill along this ridge is gentle for most of the first 0.5 mile, but as the little ridge peters out, the pace of the descent quickens. A few miniature switchbacks help somewhat, but generally you steeply descend the forested hillside. For a short time the pace lessens as the ridge reappears, but this respite is followed by nine very steep switchbacks. You know you are near the bottom when you start to hear the sound of crashing Wildcat Falls, in the canyon on your left, and come to a rocky overlook above the falls. From this viewpoint the trail descends six more switchbacks to a stunning viewpoint near the base of the falls' 100-foot sheer drop. From here the trail follows the creek downstream for 0.2 mile to a junction just above Siouxon Creek.

The trail to the right goes down 50 yards to a knee-deep ford of Siouxon Creek. Since you still have those wading shoes, this ford should be no problem. A short distance up the south bank is a campsite and a junction with the Siouxon Creek Trail. If you want to extend the trip a bit, bear left at the junction on the north side of Siouxon Creek, hop across Wildcat Creek, and then climb upstream for 0.5 mile through lovely forests to a junction with the Chinook Trail. Bear right (downhill) and drop to a rock-hop crossing just below 50-foot-high Chinook Falls. To close out the loop, walk downstream past a couple of campsites and across a wooden bridge over Siouxon Creek. Turn right at a junction on the opposite side of the bridge and walk 3.7 miles along the scenic Siouxon Creek Trail back to your car.

TRIP 3 Siouxon Creek Trail

Distance	7.6 miles, Out-and-back
Elevation Gain	700 feet
Hiking Time	3½ to 4 hours
Optional Map	Green Trails *Lookout Mountain*
Usually Open	March to November
Best Times	Mid-May to mid-June
Trail Use	Good for kids, dogs OK, backpacking option, mountain biking, horseback riding, fishing
Agency	Mt. St. Helens National Volcanic Monument, Gifford Pinchot National Forest
Difficulty	Moderate
Note	Good in cloudy weather

see map on p.59

Southwest Washington

HIGHLIGHTS This is the premier hike in the Siouxon Creek drainage. There are no grand viewpoints, but the glories of two Pacific Northwest trademarks, forests and streams, are nowhere on better display than here. A cloudy day is as good as a clear one because the forests and waterfalls are spectacular even in the gloom.

DIRECTIONS Begin by driving to Battleground, either by going north on State Highway 503 from Interstate 205, or by going east on State Highway 502 from Exit 9 off Interstate 5. From the intersection of the two state highways in the middle of Battleground, proceed north on Highway 503 for 16.8 miles and turn right on N.E. Healy Road just after you pass the Mt. St. Helens National Volcanic Monument headquarters.

After 9.2 miles on N.E. Healey Road, bear left at a poorly signed junction and travel on single-lane, paved Forest Road 57. Drive another 1.3 miles, and then turn sharply left on often unsigned Forest Road 5701. Follow this rough, paved road for 3.7 miles to its end at a trailhead parking lot.

The trail departs from the north side of the lot and drops 50 feet to an intersection with the Siouxon Creek Trail. You turn right and descend through a lovely forest composed predominantly of western hemlocks. On the forest floor are lots of downed nurse logs, mosses, sword fern, and oxalis. After 0.1 mile of downhill, you reach the creek bottom and cross West Creek on a flat-topped log bridge. The walls of the lush side canyon holding this creek are draped with mosses and ferns. Immediately after the bridge, you pass the first of many excellent creekside campsites. After this camp, the trail travels in small ups and downs, gradually making its way uphill but staying about 50 feet above the clear waters of Siouxon

Creek. About 0.9 mile from the trailhead is the signed junction with the Horseshoe Ridge Trail (Trip 4).

The Siouxon Creek Trail goes straight and does a series of small ups and downs, alternating between creek-level flats covered with a tangle of junglelike vegetation, and hillsides sprouting tall cedars, firs, and hemlocks. Several tiny tributary creeks cross the trail, providing ample water for plants like devil's club and salmonberry. You cross Horseshoe Creek on a plank bridge just above lacy Horseshoe Creek Falls and, about 100 yards later, come to a junction with a 180-yard spur trail to a viewpoint at the base of the falls.

About 0.2 mile after Horseshoe Creek Falls is a camp with a little wooden bench

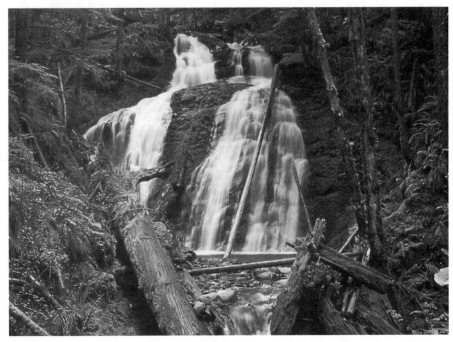

Horseshoe Creek Falls

where you can sit and enjoy a classic view of nearby Siouxon Falls, a twisting cataract with a deep swimming hole at its base. A short distance farther upstream is a smaller waterfall with an equally good but not-as-popular swimming hole. At both locations the water is very cold. As you continue hiking on this lovely path, you pass numerous unsigned side trails leading to terrific campsites and lunch spots that are perfect places for the kids to play or for adults to quietly contemplate nature.

About 0.8 mile above Siouxon Falls is the unsigned junction with the upper end of the Horseshoe Ridge Trail bearing uphill to the right. You stay straight on the lower path and walk 0.7 mile to a second junction right next to a bridge. The official Siouxon Creek Trail continues straight, reaching Forest Road 58 in about 4.5 miles. A more attractive route turns left and crosses the bridge above a deep pool of water. You then climb past two excellent camps and follow Chinook Creek upstream to the base of Chinook Falls, a 50-foot drop over a sheer cliff.

You can turn around here, but for even more scenery, you can cross Chinook Creek and traverse a hillside to a junction with the Chinook Trail. Turn left here and travel downhill for 0.5 mile to a simple crossing of Wildcat Creek, a little above where this stream joins Siouxon Creek. To visit 100-foot-high Wildcat Falls, turn right at a junction and climb 0.2 mile to a viewpoint at the base of this falls. To close out the trip, either return the way you came, or, if it is late summer and you are willing to get wet, turn left at the junction below Wildcat Falls and drop to a knee-deep ford of Siouxon Creek. Wading shoes and a walking stick may come in handy, depending on the water level. On the opposite bank, an obvious use trail climbs about 100 feet back to the Siouxon Creek Trail.

TRIP 4 Horseshoe Ridge Loop

Distance	10.4 miles, Loop
Elevation Gain	2700 feet
Hiking Time	6 to 7 hours
Optional Map	Green Trails *Lookout Mountain*
Usually Open	April to early November
Best Times	May and June
Trail Use	Dogs OK, horseback riding
Agency	Mt. St. Helens National Volcanic Monument, Gifford Pinchot National Forest
Difficulty	Difficult
Note	Good in cloudy weather

see map on p.59

Southwest Washington

HIGHLIGHTS Exercise is the principal attraction of this hike. The infrequent views are generally limited to ridges covered with clear-cuts. So this is a good hike to tackle in gloomy weather, as you won't feel like you missed anything. The relatively low elevation ensures that this trail opens earlier in the season than most others in the Cascades.

DIRECTIONS Begin by driving to Battleground, either by going north on State Highway 503 from Interstate 205, or by going east on State Highway 502 from Exit 9 off Interstate 5. From the intersection of the two state highways in the middle of Battleground, drive north on Highway 503 for 16.8 miles, and turn right on N.E. Healy Road just after you pass the Mt. St. Helens National Volcanic Monument headquarters.

After 9.2 miles on N.E. Healey Road, bear left at a poorly signed junction and travel on single-lane, paved Forest Road 57. Drive another 1.3 miles, and then turn sharply left on often unsigned Forest Road 5701. Follow this rough, paved road for 3.7 miles to its end at a trailhead parking lot.

The trail departs from the north side of the lot and drops 50 feet to an intersection with the Siouxon Creek Trail. You turn right here, drop to a bridged crossing of West Creek, and then continue another 0.8 mile through lovely creekside forests to a signed junction with the Horseshoe Ridge Trail.

You turn right here and climb away from the creek on a grade that starts off fairly steep but soon becomes very steep. More than 20 switchbacks of varying length help to lessen the grade slightly, but at other times the trail simply goes directly up the extremely steep slopes. The trail is also quite narrow, so watch your step. After about 1.5 miles you reach a minor ridge crest, after which things get a lot easier.

The trail turns left to follow the ridge, sometimes climbing in steep sections and sometimes going along at a welcome level grade. Most of the trees are either western hemlock or Douglas fir, while salal, beargrass, and Oregon grape cover the ground. You pass a small rocky overlook with a decent view to the west and then travel on or near the narrow crest of woodsy Horseshoe Ridge.

The gentle path along this ridge does some short ups and downs to avoid rock outcrops but mostly stays level. Along the way you leave the forest three times and go through small, sloping meadows with lots of ground-hugging juniper bushes and a few scattered wildflowers.

After a long, very gradual climb you eventually make a couple of small switchbacks just before the ridge widens and the trail curves to the left. From here the path gradually loses about 200 feet and comes to the end of a dirt road where there is a small hunter's camp. Pick up the trail on the opposite side of the camp and follow it over a low rise and then down a short distance to a second isolated gravel road.

To resume the trail, turn left on the road and 25 yards later bear right onto a signed foot trail. Staying on the east side of the ridgeline, this generally level route

goes along a viewless ridge with lots of beargrass. After about 1 mile you begin to descend very steeply for 0.6 mile. Once you reach the first of four long switchbacks, the trail is much better graded and remains so all the way down the densely forested slopes to an unsigned junction with Siouxon Creek Trail.

To return to your car, turn left and walk this easy and very scenic route for 2.1 miles, as it passes Siouxon and Horseshoe Creek falls back to the lower junction with the Horseshoe Ridge Trail.

TRIP 5 Moulton Falls Trails

Distance	2.5 miles, Point-to-point
Elevation Gain	100 feet
Hiking Time	Up to 2 hours
Optional Map	USGS *Yacolt* (trail not shown)
Usually Open	All year (except during winter storms)
Best Time	Any
Trail Use	Good for kids, dogs OK, wheelchair accessible, mountain biking, horseback riding, fishing
Agency	Clark County Parks
Difficulty	Easy
Note	Good in cloudy weather

HIGHLIGHTS Although the trails in Moulton Falls County Park barely qualify as "wild," the excellent scenery makes this trip worth including. The star attraction is the crystal clear East Fork Lewis River, with its rocky benches, sandy beaches, cascading waterfalls, and great swimming holes. But the hike also features a small wildlife-rich lake, impressive rocky cliffs, a varied and interesting forest, and, for those willing to make a quick side trip, a lovely waterfall on a tributary stream. All in all this county park offers a fun hiking experience that is suitable for the entire family.

DIRECTIONS From the intersection of State Highways 502 and 503 in Battleground, drive 5.7 miles north on Highway 503. Turn right on N.E. Rock Creek Road, which soon becomes Lucia Falls Road, and proceed 5.4 miles to the junction with Hantwick Road. If you are leaving a car at the lower trailhead, turn right on Hantwick Road, drive 0.6 mile, and then turn left into the large trailhead parking lot.

To reach the starting point, return to Lucia Falls Road, continue east another 3 miles, and then turn right into the small, signed parking lot for Moulton Falls County Park.

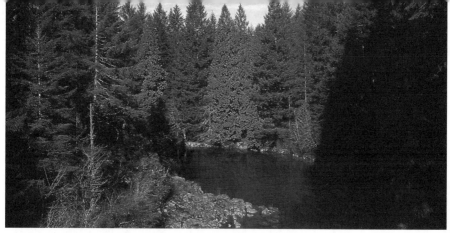

East Fork Lewis River from trail bridge in Moulton Falls County Park

You start by walking east on a gravel path that goes 80 yards along the right (south) shoulder of Lucia Falls Road. Just before the bridge across Big Tree Creek, a marked crosswalk goes across the road to a trail going north. This very worthwhile side trip goes upstream through the forest along Big Tree Creek for 0.15 mile, passing an inviting picnic area along the way, to an overlook of a very attractive waterfall. Stone steps take you down to a bridge just below the falls. This bridge provides access to a loop trail that takes you across the road and then south to the main part of Moulton Falls County Park. Unfortunately, the bridge is closed in winter, so off-season hikers must backtrack from the falls, recross the road to the main trail, and cross Big

Tree Creek on a wooden trail bridge that parallels the road bridge.

By either route, you now enter the developed part of Moulton Falls County Park. To find the continuation of this trail, loop to the south through a picnic area and past a popular summer swimming hole and then pick up a wide gravel trail that climbs slightly to a tall arching bridge spanning the East Fork Lewis River, fully three stories above the green-tinged waters.

After crossing the river, the 10-foot-wide, virtually level, and wheelchair-accessible trail heads downstream through a forest of Douglas firs, western red cedars, bigleaf maples, and red alders towering over an understory dominated by ferns and thimbleberries. Although well above the river, the trail remains close enough

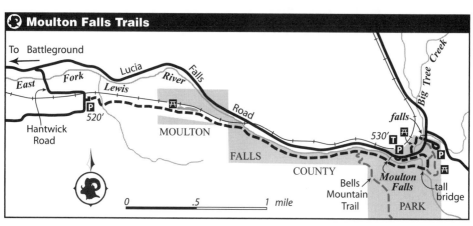

Moulton Falls Trails

To Battleground

East Fork Lewis

Lucia Falls River Road

Hantwick Road

520'

MOULTON

FALLS

COUNTY

Bells Mountain Trail

falls

530'

Moulton Falls

PARK

tall bridge

Big Tree Creek

0   .5   1 mile

to allow hikers to look down into the stream's lovely waters. The path soon passes Moulton Falls, really just a rocky cascade, and then, at 0.35 mile from the arched bridge, comes to a junction.

The narrow trail that goes left (uphill) is the Bells Mountain Trail (Trip 6). For this hike you continue straight on the wide gravel path. As you walk (calling it "hiking" would give the impression that the trail is much more challenging than it really is) you will frequently see homes and cars on the other side of the river. From spring through fall, however, leaves on the deciduous trees hide most of these unnatural sights, while in winter, traffic on the road is less frequent and not too intrusive. In fact winter is a particularly nice time to visit because several seasonal side creeks are filled with rainwater then and cascade over small waterfalls into the river. Unfortunately this canyon gets almost no sun during the winter months, so it can be dark and chilly.

At about 1.5 miles a railroad track crosses the river and parallels the trail. A nice highlight comes at 1.9 miles when you reach a lovely unnamed lake on the north side of the trail. Here you can look for wildlife such as deer and a variety of birds or eat lunch on a small bench and picnic table at the lake's west end. The trail's last 0.5 mile are paved and include a bridge over a small but very attractive side creek just before trail's end at the Hantwick Road Trailhead.

While in the area, take the time to check out Lucia Falls, in a small county park 0.3 mile west of the Hantwick Road turnoff. Swimming is not allowed here to protect the fish, but the cascading falls is picturesque and well worth a visit.

TRIP 6 Bells Mountain Trail

Distance	4.2 miles, Out-and-back; 7.5 miles, Point-to-point
Elevation Gain	1100 feet, Out-and-back; 1800 feet, Point-to-point
Hiking Time	2 to 8 hours
Optional Map	USGS Dole, Yacolt (trail not shown)
Usually Open	February to November
Best Time	February to November
Trail Use	Dogs OK, mountain biking, horseback riding
Agency	Yacolt State Forest
Difficulty	Moderate to Difficult

HIGHLIGHTS The relatively new Bells Mountain Trail serves as a useful link between the trails in Moulton Falls County Park and the extensive network of trails around Silver Star Mountain. Although not wildly scenic, the trail is fun because it is hikeable nearly all year, includes some nice views and creekside scenery, and gives you a good workout. On the downside, the middle section of the trail is unattractive since it passes through several clear-cuts and illegal all-terrain vehicles (ATVs) have badly damaged the tread. At either end, however, the trail is quite lovely and fun to explore.

DIRECTIONS From the intersection of State Highways 502 and 503 in Battleground, drive 5.7 miles north on Highway 503. Turn right on N.E. Rock Creek Road, which soon becomes Lucia Falls Road, and proceed 8.4 miles to the small parking lot for Moulton Falls County Park on the right.

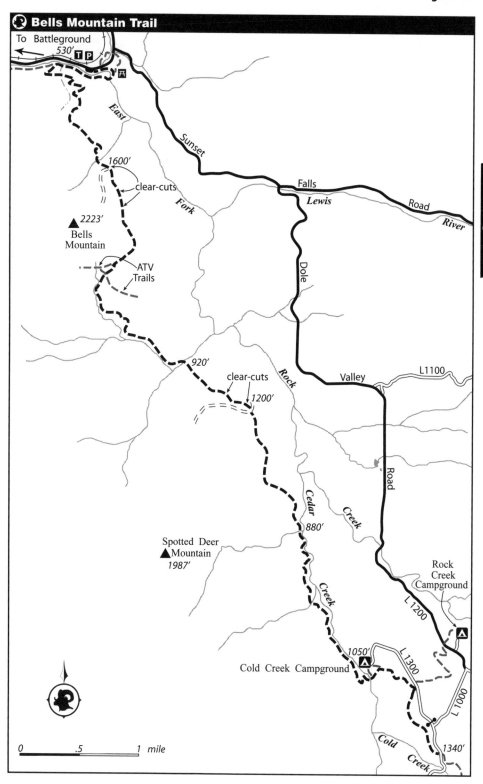

Bells Mountain Trail

To Battleground
530'
T P

East

Sunset

Fork

1600'
clear-cuts

▲ 2223'
Bells
Mountain

ATV
Trails

Falls

Lewis

Road

River

Dole

920'

clear-cuts
1200'

Rock

Valley

L1100

Road

Cedar

880'

Creek

Spotted Deer
▲ Mountain
1987'

Creek

Rock
Creek
Campground

L 1200

L 1300

1050'
Cold Creek Campground

L 1000

Cold

Creek

1340'

0   .5   1 mile

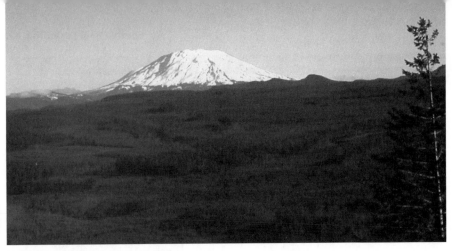

Mt. St. Helens from Bells Mountain Trail

Walk the gravel path that goes east along the road's shoulder and cross rushing Big Tree Creek on a wooden bridge that parallels the road bridge. From here you walk through the developed area of Moulton Falls County Park, generally looping to the south through a picnic area and past an outstanding swimming hole that is very popular in summer. Pulling away from the picnic area, the wide gravel trail climbs to an impressively tall arching bridge that spans the East Fork Lewis River.

After crossing the river, the 10-foot-wide gravel trail heads downstream through a forest of Douglas firs, western red cedars, bigleaf maples, and red alders towering over an understory dominated by ferns and thimbleberries. At 0.5 mile, shortly after passing the roaring cascades of Moulton Falls, is a junction.

Turn left (uphill) on the narrow Bells Mountain Trail, and begin exercising those thighs as you tackle a solid uphill grade. In the next 1.6 miles the trail gains about 1000 feet in an uneven but often moderately steep ascent with numerous switchbacks and twisting turns. Several gullies and seasonal creeks along the way are spanned by wooden plank bridges, which help to keep things interesting. The forest is also attractive, although not particularly varied being dominated by sec-ond-growth Douglas firs and red alders. Sword fern is so abundant on the forest floor it crowds out virtually all other plants. At 2.1 miles the main climbing ends where you hit the end of a logging spur road at a small clear-cut. Although the surroundings are a bit unsightly, the opening provides excellent views to the north over the East Fork Lewis River valley to Mt. St. Helens, mantled in snow for most of the year. This viewpoint is a reasonable turnaround point for those seeking a shorter hike.

Those continuing south on the Bells Mountain Trail will find the next section of gentle ups and downs to be easy walking. Sadly, it is not very attractive, because the area is dominated by clear-cuts. Seemingly every tree is either already cut or assigned for harvest in the near future. On the plus side the clear-cuts provide nice southeasterly views of Silver Star Mountain. When you reenter the forest, you soon encounter a second problem, ATVs. Although officially prohibited on the Bells Mountain Trail, the riders of these noisy intruders either haven't gotten the message or simply don't care. One of the many problems the machines cause is confusion, as unmarked bike trails sprout up and lead off to various unknown destinations. At the first of these junctions you should veer left, and then just 0.15

mile later go straight where another ATV trail cuts directly across your path. Don't be surprised if more of these unmarked ATV trails spring up in the future. There would be much less confusion if it were easy to distinguish your foot trail from those made by ATVs. Unfortunately, the ATVs muck up the works even more by riding on the Bells Mountain Trail itself. The result is not just confusion but a sloppy mess of muddy trails, erosion, and torn up tread.

The ATV damage is especially sad because, apart from the machine-caused eyesores, the surroundings are quite attractive, especially as you descend along an unnamed but pretty creek that rapidly increases in volume. At about 4 miles you cross the creek on a sturdy metal bridge and then gradually climb to another group of clear-cuts. In the midst of this logging activity, at about 5 miles, the trail comes to another primitive logging road. To relocate the trail, you need to cross the road at an angle going slightly to the right and a little uphill.

After this extended unattractive section, you are finally rewarded with some of the trail's nicest scenery. Back in forest, the trail descends to Cedar Creek and follows this clear, rollicking gem upstream for about 2 miles to a sturdy metal bridge. Immediately on the other side of the bridge is a junction with a gravel, wheelchair-accessible trail to Cold Creek Campground. You cannot leave a car at this permit-only site, so to reach a legal trailhead, go right (uphill), still on the Bells Mountain Trail, and continue through pretty forest for 0.5 mile to another trail junction. This junction comes immediately before the main trail crosses the gravel access road to Cold Creek Campground. To reach the nearest legal parking area, go right and in about 0.6 mile of gradual climbing through second-growth forest come to the Cold Creek Trailhead on Road L 1000 (see Trip 8 for directions).

TRIP 7 Tarbell Trail to Hidden Falls

Distance	10.0 miles, Out-and-back
Elevation Gain	1100 feet
Hiking Time	5 hours
Optional Map	USGS *Dole*
Usually Open	Mid-March to November
Best Time	April to June
Trail Use	Dogs OK, mountain biking, horseback riding
Agency	Yacolt State Forest
Difficulty	Moderate
Note	Good in cloudy weather

HIGHLIGHTS More than 100 years ago, a man named George Tarbell lived alone in the roadless forests northwest of Silver Star Mountain. He made a living by farming and mining for gold. His isolated cabin was connected to the outside world only by a narrow 6-mile-long trail that led to the nearest wagon road. Today that trail has been reopened and you can walk in the hermit's footsteps. They lead you to a spectacular waterfall that remains nearly as unknown today as it was in Tarbell's time.

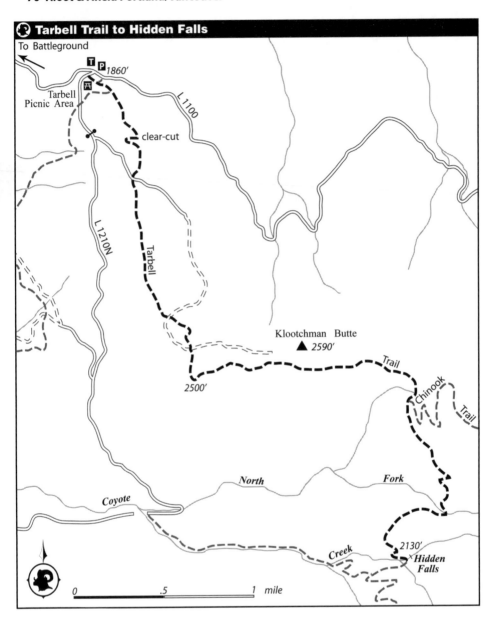

Tarbell Trail to Hidden Falls

To Battleground

1860'

Tarbell
Picnic Area

L 1100

clear-cut

L 1210N

Tarbell

Klootchman Butte
▲ 2590'

Trail

2500'

Chinook

Trail

North   Fork

Coyote

Creek   2130'
×Hidden
Falls

0   .5   1 mile

DIRECTIONS Begin by driving to Battleground, either by going north on State Highway 503
from Interstate 205, or by going east on State Highway 502 from Exit 9 off Interstate 5.
The two state highways intersect in the middle of Battleground. From here drive north
5.7 miles on Highway 503. Turn right on N.E. Rock Creek Road, which soon becomes Lucia
Falls Road. After 8.5 miles turn right on N.E. Sunset Falls Road. Go another 2.0 miles on this
road, then turn right again onto N.E. Dole Valley Road. Exactly 2.4 miles farther on turn left
onto gravel Road L 1100, which is marked with a small brown sign for the Tarbell Picnic
Area. After 2.2 miles, turn right at a junction. Fifty feet later, park in the signed lot on the
left side of the road.

You begin by a sign saying that Hidden Falls is 4.75 miles away. Walk through a pleasantly rustic picnic area, and then turn right at an unsigned junction. Soon thereafter you come to a second junction—this one with the Tarbell Trail, which is heavily used by horses. The sign here says that Hidden Falls is now 5.8 miles away. Apparently the falls is not only hidden, it is also a moving target! Actually neither sign is correct. Hidden Falls is actually 4.9 miles away.

Turn left onto the Tarbell Trail, which wanders gradually uphill in a typical, second-growth, Douglas-fir forest. With just over a century of growth since the 1902 Yacolt Burn, most of the trees are little more than 1 foot thick, but a few are as much as 3 feet thick and nearly 100 feet tall. Vegetation covers almost every square inch of the forest floor, especially Oregon grape, oxalis, thimbleberry, salal, false lily-of-the-valley, and sword and bracken fern. There are also lots of vine maples, whose leaves turn scarlet and orange in late October.

Two switchbacks climb past the edge of a clear-cut and take you up to a crossing of a narrow gravel road. The small seam of sunlight created by this road is just enough for June-blooming iris to thrive. Continuing past this junction, you make a series of gentle climbs and level walks through dense foliage that creates a sort of living tunnel. In places horse hooves have churned the tread into a muddy mess, so wear boots rather than tennis shoes.

After topping a low rise, you turn east and cross a very isolated old road in the middle of an equally old clear-cut. Trailside thimbleberry and the enormous spreading fronds of bracken fern are racing to capture as much light as possible before the rapidly regrowing Douglas firs cover them with a shady canopy. Shortly after reentering an older forest, you cross a rarely used motorcycle track and then wander along the south side of low and rounded Klootchman Butte. Several openings in the forest provide room for flowers like vetch, iris, golden pea, dandelion, beargrass, and wild rose. There are also some partially obstructed views of Silver Star Mountain to the southeast and Larch Mountain to the south. The trail loses some elevation among the trees and crosses more partially forested slopes before making a long, looping contour into a densely forested valley on the northwest side of Silver Star Mountain.

You should eventually come to a junction with a newly constructed route that

Hidden Falls along Tarbell Trail

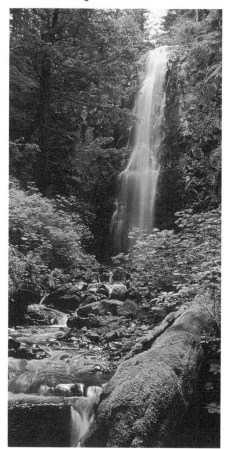

is part of the planned Chinook Trail, which will one day be a loop route along both sides of the Columbia River Gorge. This section of it leaves the Tarbell Trail and goes to the left on its way to Silver Star Mountain. The signs here give distances to various destinations, but like the signs at the trailhead, these are not to be trusted. One sign claims that it is only 2 miles back to the Tarbell Picnic Area where you started. The actual distance is close to 3.5 miles.

In any case, the trail stays level for a short distance before it descends six quick switchbacks and makes a bridged crossing of North Fork Coyote Creek. After this, it contours around a forested ridge and switchbacks downhill to take you into the next creek canyon. This canyon holds South Fork Coyote Creek and 92-foot-high Hidden Falls, just above a log bridge.

A wooden bench at the base of this lacy falls makes an ideal lunch spot and turnaround point. Beyond the falls, the trail makes a tough switchbacking climb onto a shoulder of Silver Star Mountain. Since you can reach this area more easily from Grouse Vista (Trip 10), be satisfied with the falls and return to your car the way you came.

TRIP 8 Cold Creek Trail to Larch Mountain

Distance	12.8 miles, Out-and-back
Elevation Gain	2400 feet
Hiking Time	6 to 7 hours
Optional Map	USGS *Dole, Larch Mountain*
Usually Open	May to early November
Best Time	Mid-May to June
Trail Use	Dogs OK, mountain biking, horseback riding
Agency	Yacolt State Forest
Difficulty	Difficult

HIGHLIGHTS Located a little to the southwest of Silver Star Mountain, Larch Mountain is lower in elevation, but it features many of the same attributes of its larger neighbor: open wildflower meadows, good views, and wildlife. There are two good trails to this high point, the more interesting of which is the long climb up the valley of scenic Cold Creek.

The trails here are used mostly by mountain bikers and equestrians, but why should they have all the fun? Hikers are also welcome, and it's high time we came to see what everybody else has kept secret. As always, be sure to give horses the right of way by stepping off the trail on the downhill side to let them pass. Motor vehicles are prohibited from most of the recommended trails, although you will cross several motorcycle tracks. Many riders seem to view the official trail restrictions as merely optional and routinely ignore the rules, so you can expect the quiet of your wilderness experience to be rudely broken by the noise of motorbikes, especially on weekends.

DIRECTIONS Begin by driving to Battleground, either by going north on State Highway 503 from Interstate 205, or by going east on State Highway 502 from Exit 9 off Interstate 5. The two state highways intersect in the middle of Battleground. From here drive north 5.7 miles on Highway 503. Turn right on N.E. Rock Creek Road, which soon becomes Lucia

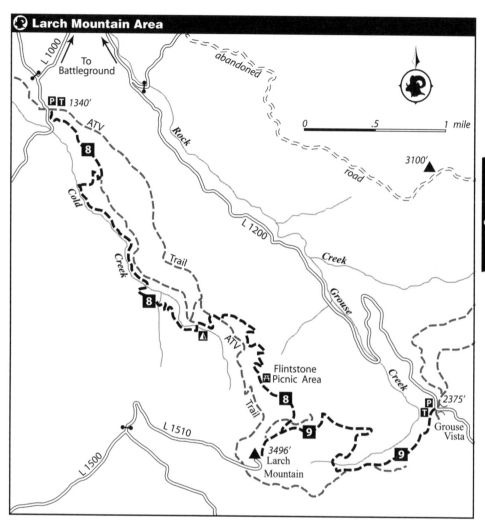

Larch Mountain Area

To Battleground

L 1000

P T 1340'

ATV

8

Rock

abandoned

road

3100'

0   .5   1 mile

L 1200

Cold

Creek

Creek

Trail

8

Grouse

A

ATV

Creek

Flintstone
Picnic Area

8

Trail

P T 2375'

Grouse
Vista

L 1510

9

9

L 1500

3496'
Larch
Mountain

Falls Road. After 8.5 miles turn right on N.E. Sunset Falls Road. Go another 2.0 miles on this road, and then turn right again onto N.E. Dole Valley Road. Stay on this road for 5.2 miles to a junction and the end of pavement. Veer right on Road L 1000, following signs for the Larch Corrections Center, and drive exactly 0.8 mile before parking in a pull-out on the left. A large sign here gives trail mileages to various destinations.

The recently rerouted trail parallels Road L 1000 for about 100 yards through a logged area, turns left, and then enters a dense second-growth Douglas-fir forest. For the next 0.7 mile the trail works its way slowly uphill, before turning left and switchbacking down to reach Cold Creek.

The trail now goes upstream closely following the splashing creek. The forest floor is almost completely covered with bracken and sword fern, bleeding heart, oxalis, salmonberry, thimbleberry, and other common species in various shades of green. The "river music" of cascading water and the songs of birds, especially those of the ever-present American robin and winter wren, provide audio stimulation and enjoyment. The trail does lots of small ups and downs but gradually gains elevation. At about 1.9 miles you go straight across an unsigned junction where an unofficial mountain bike trail comes in from the left. Shortly thereafter, you cross Cold Creek on a plank bridge. A horse-hitching post and two wooden benches make this a good rest stop.

Continue hiking amid increasing numbers of lovely, droopy-limbed western hemlocks. You briefly pull away from the creek and switchback up a heavily forested hillside. After this you make bridged crossings of two branches of Cold Creek about 0.4 mile apart. At the second crossing are a decent campsite and an unsigned trail heading downstream. You go straight on the main trail and switchback uphill, gradually leaving behind the sounds of "river music."

About 0.4 mile after the last creek crossing, you pass diagonally through a confusing and unsigned junction with a motorbike track and then switchback to the right on top of a wide, forested ridge. More climbing takes you up to and around a small rockslide and cliff where red paintbrush, purple penstemon, white beargrass, and yellow golden pea grow profusely.

After climbing a little more in forest, you come to a lovely open slope of shale rock with lots of June-blooming lupine, lomatium, and beargrass. There are also fine views here, especially northeast to bulky Silver Star Mountain and north to Mounts Rainier and St. Helens. Several roads and clear-cuts mar the scene somewhat, but it is still very attractive. A lone picnic table just below the trail is signed as the FLINTSTONE PICNIC AREA. It provides Fred and Wilma, or any other

visitors, a first-rate lunch spot, although this exposed location is often windy.

Above the rocky slope you enter open, mid-elevation forests of Douglas fir and Pacific silver fir, with lots of star-flowered smilacina and bunchberry covering the ground. Go straight through an unsigned four-way junction and 100 yards later you will come to a signed fork in the trail. The path to the left goes down to Grouse Vista (see Trip 9), but your route turns right and climbs 0.2 mile to a junction with another motorcycle track.

The only sign here says HORSE TRAILS, and it points to the trail you came in on. To reach the top of Larch Mountain, bear left and walk uphill on the motorcycle track past a large beargrass meadow on your right and through nice forests to the rather disappointing summit. There is a nice view southwest to Vancouver and Portland, but most of the scene is despoiled by a clear-cut right at the top, as well as by a gravel road and microwave and cellular-phone towers—the modern plague of so many mountain tops. To enjoy your lunch where the views are better, go back to the meadows you passed near the junction below the summit.

Cold Creek Trail

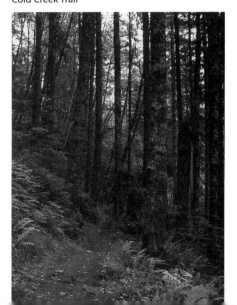

TRIP 9 Larch Mountain from Grouse Vista

Distance	6.0 miles, Out-and-back
Elevation Gain	1200 feet
Hiking Time	3 hours
Optional Map	USGS *Larch Mountain*
Usually Open	May to early November
Best Time	Mid-May to June
Trail Use	Dogs OK, mountain biking, horseback riding
Agency	Yacolt State Forest
Difficulty	Moderate

see map on p.73

HIGHLIGHTS For a shorter approach to the meadows and the views on Larch Mountain, try this route from Grouse Vista. The distance and elevation gain are only about half as much as the Cold Creek Trail (Trip 8), and the views from the meadows near the top are just as spectacular.

Neither this Larch Mountain nor the more famous one in Oregon have any larch trees growing on them. The western larch grows only east of the Cascade Divide. The name comes from early loggers who used the term *larch* to refer to the noble fir. The two species actually have little in common.

DIRECTIONS Begin by driving to Battleground, either by going north on State Highway 503 from Interstate 205, or by going east on State Highway 502 from Exit 9 off Interstate 5. The two state highways intersect in the middle of Battleground. From here drive north 5.7 miles on Highway 503. Turn right on N.E. Rock Creek Road, which soon becomes Lucia Falls Road. After 8.5 miles you turn right on N.E. Sunset Falls Road. Go another 2.0 miles on this road, then turn right again onto N.E. Dole Valley Road. Stay on this road for 5.2 miles to a junction and the end of pavement. Turn left on Road L 1200 and climb for 5.2 miles to the pass at Grouse Vista. The best parking is on the right.

Three routes leave from the right (west) side of the pass. The two southernmost are motorcycle tracks, which are nothing but an annoyance for hikers. Instead, take the northernmost of the three routes and very soon you will come to a brown sign giving distances to various points along the trail. After an all-too-brief warm up, the trail starts to climb steeply on a wide, rocky tread. While you climb, the rocks and boulders on the trail are merely a nuisance, but on the way back down they can easily twist your ankle, so be extra careful on the return trip.

Views here are generally obstructed by trees, mostly short Douglas fir, grand fir, and western hemlock. As you climb,

the sounds of rushing water from Grouse Creek in the canyon on your right gradually grow louder as the creek gets closer.

After a little more than 1 mile, the trail is joined by an unsigned motorbike track coming in from the left. But 0.2 mile later this track splits off again. Shortly after this, you pass an active beaver pond and large dam on your right. If you arrive here in the early morning, take some time to scan the pond for the busy builders of this impressive construction project.

Above the pond, you make a bridged crossing of Grouse Creek, loop back to the right, and traverse up the increasingly open hillside. When the trail tops a ridge, the views improve greatly, as most of the trees disappear and you stand in an open meadow. Bulky Silver Star Mountain lies to the northeast, but the best views look to the distant snow peaks of Oregon's Mt. Hood and decapitated Mt. St. Helens in Washington. You can also see the region's better known Larch Mountain, on the Oregon side of the Columbia River.

The trail turns west and follows the ridge up through more meadows and strips of trees. Wildflowers abound here, including such colorful favorites as beargrass, lupine, iris, queen's cup, and golden pea. This is the most attractive part of the hike, although the trail is a bit rocky and deeply gouged by motorcycles.

About 2.5 miles from the trailhead is a junction with the trail coming up from Cold Creek (Trip 8). To reach the top of Larch Mountain, you bear left here and climb 0.5 mile past a beargrass meadow and through several confusing junctions with motorcycle routes. The mountain-top is rather ugly, however, with a clear-cut and electrical towers, so for better views return to the meadows below.

With a car shuttle you can make a long one-way trip by going down the Cold Creek Trail (see Trip 8 for details).

TRIP 10 Silver Star Mountain: Grouse Vista Loop

Distance	7.5 miles, Loop
Elevation Gain	2300 feet
Hiking Time	4 hours
Optional Map	USGS *Bobs Mountain, Dole, Gumboot Mountain, Larch Mountain*
Usually Open	Mid-May to October
Best Time	Mid-May to June
Trail Use	Dogs OK, mountain biking, horseback riding, backpacking option
Agency	Yacolt State Forest & Mt Adams Ranger District, Gifford Pinchot National Forest
Difficulty	Difficult

HIGHLIGHTS This is the most popular route to the top of Silver Star Mountain, perhaps because it has the easiest road access and lends itself perfectly to a loop. Although the hike is very attractive, it is neither as scenic nor as abundant in wildflowers as either the northern loop (Trip 13) or the Bluff Mountain Trail (Trip 15). Nonetheless, it is an enjoyable hike with glimpses of a towering waterfall to go along with the extensive views from the top.

DIRECTIONS Begin by driving to Battleground, either by going north on State Highway 503 from Interstate 205, or by going east on State Highway 502 from Exit 9 off Interstate 5. The two state highways intersect in the middle of Battleground. From here drive north 5.7 miles on Highway 503. Turn right on N.E. Rock Creek Road, which soon becomes Lucia Falls Road. After 8.5 miles turn right on N.E. Sunset Falls Road. Go another 2.0 miles on this road, and then turn right again onto N.E. Dole Valley Road. Stay on this road for 5.2 miles and a junction to the end of pavement. Turn left on Road L 1200 and climb 5.2 miles to the pass at Grouse Vista. The best parking is on the right.

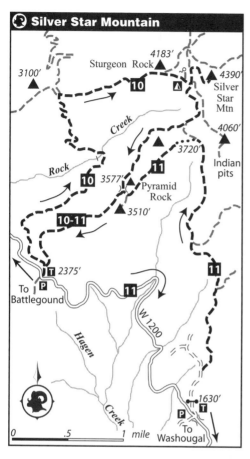

Silver Star Mountain

3100'

Sturgeon Rock 4183'

10

4390'
Silver
Star
Mtn

Creek

4060'

3720'

11

Indian
pits

Rock

10

3577'

Pyramid
Rock

10-11

3510'

T 2375'

To P
Battlegound

11

11

W 1200

Hagen

Creek

1630'
P T

0   .5   1 mile
To
Washougal

The trail on the east side of the pass starts as an old jeep track blocked by berms intended to keep motor vehicles out. After about 0.1 mile, there is a junction with the Tarbell Trail, a narrow foot trail that bears off to the left. Take this pleasant little trail that goes up and down through woods that come alive in May with small pink blossoms of bleeding heart.

After rounding a ridge, you contour across intermittently open slopes on the walls of a huge forested canyon. As you get close to the head of the canyon, you will be able to glimpse a towering 100-foot waterfall on Rock Creek to your left. Unfortunately, you never get a really good look at the falls from the trail, and there is no easy scramble to a better viewpoint. Cross the wooden bridge over Rock Creek and begin your climb out of the canyon at a moderate grade. A mix of eight switchbacks and long traverses eventually leads up heavily wooded slopes to a junction with an old road near a saddle in the ridge.

Turn right on this bumpy and rocky track and climb steeply through viewless

Sturgeon Rock

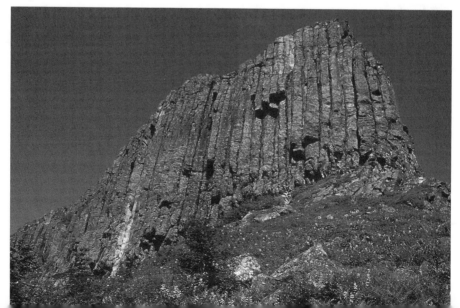

forests on the south side of the ridge. After a little over a mile, check carefully on the left for a look at the sheer columnar basalt cliffs of Sturgeon Rock. For a better look, you can scramble off the trail to some excellent viewpoints at the base of the cliffs, where you can sometimes see climbers inching their way up the rock face.

An unsigned footpath veers off to the left near the east end of Sturgeon Rock, but you should stay on the road, as the uphill grade lessens somewhat for the final 0.3 mile to the junction. About 80 feet before you reach this junction, an unsigned trail goes left for about 100 feet to a piped spring with refreshingly cool water.

The return route to Grouse Vista goes right at this junction, but you can take a scenic side trip to the summit by turning left. After 20 feet, a foot trail cuts sharply right on its way out to some Native American rock pits (see description in Trip 13). For the summit, you go straight and climb to a little saddle where there is a final junction. Turn right (uphill) and

climb for 0.2 mile on a rock-strewn old jeep road to the saddle between the two summits of Silver Star Mountain. Both summits have terrific views and are well worth visiting. Views extend for hundreds of miles over large parts of two states, but some of the most interesting views are of the nearby ridges and canyons of Silver Star Mountain itself. Flowers are also abundant, including paintbrush, beargrass, pink heather, and avalanche lilies near the top.

To return to your car, go back to the road junction near the spring, and follow the old jeep track downhill to the southwest. This fairly steep route travels through extensive meadows with good views and lots of flowers. The tread is very rocky, so watch your step to avoid turning an ankle. At a little saddle about halfway down, there is a junction with an abandoned track that goes left. It's worth exploring this track for a short distance to check out the cliffs of prominent Pyramid Rock. Once you've had your fill, return to the main trail and drop down the ridge to the trailhead.

TRIP 11 Silver Star Mountain: South Ridge Loop

Distance	7.5 miles, Loop (including 3.3-mile road walk)
Elevation Gain	2200 feet
Hiking Time	4 hours
Optional Map	USGS *Bobs Mountain, Larch Mountain*
Usually Open	Mid-April to November
Best Times	May and June
Trail Use	Dogs OK, mountain biking, horseback riding
Agency	Mount Adams Ranger District, Gifford Pinchot National Forest
Difficulty	Difficult

HIGHLIGHTS Silver Star Mountain was "love at first hike" for me. Every one of the many trails here is a joy, with great views, wildflowers, and relatively few people. For the dedicated hiker, it is simply impossible not to love this place. Of the five approach trails described in this book, this hike up the south ridge is the first to clear of snow and provides some of the best views.

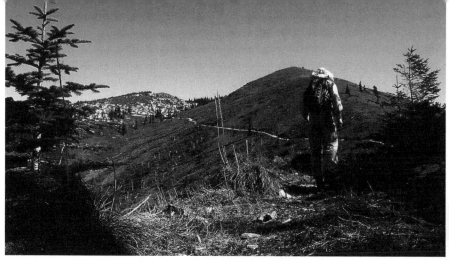

Approaching Silver Star Mountain from south ridge trail

DIRECTIONS From Washougal, 10 miles east on State Highway 14 from its intersection with Interstate 205, turn left (north) at a traffic light onto 15th Street. Go straight, through two traffic lights, as the road's name changes first to 17th Street and then to Washougal River Road. After 6.9 miles, turn left (uphill) on Northeast Hughes Road and proceed 3.2 miles to a junction. Turn left on 412nd Avenue, which soon becomes Skamania Mines Road. After 1.4 miles this road turns to gravel and then continues another 1.4 miles to a junction. Keep left, go 0.1 mile, and then bear left again at a fork onto Road W 1200. This gravel road has lots of potholes and some rocks, but it is fine for passenger cars if you drive slowly. Exactly 2.5 miles from the last fork is an unsigned junction in a minor saddle. Park here.

Walk up the side road that goes north (uphill) from the junction and soon go through a gate that may or may not be open. After 0.3 mile, look for an abandoned jeep track blocked by a berm going to the right. A small sign states that this route is closed to motor vehicles.

You turn onto the jeep track, which has been abandoned for so many years it is now just a wide trail, and ascend at a moderately steep grade, initially in a second-growth Douglas-fir forest with little in the way of views. At 1.1 miles is an unsigned junction. Go straight, and after a brief respite on level trail, resume going uphill. At 1.7 miles is another unsigned junction. You go straight again and soon notice a change in your surroundings. The lower-elevation forest thins rapidly and is replaced with brushy clearings and a scattering of perky higher-elevation Pacific silver firs. Views to the south of Oregon's Larch Mountain and Mount Hood become more frequent. Another sign that you are gaining elevation is the presence of beargrass, a local harbinger of the 3000-foot elevation line.

The rocky trail continues going uphill, often rather steeply, as it makes its way up the west side of Silver Star Mountain's southern ridge. Here the terrain becomes extremely scenic, as the trail crosses huge open slopes of talus fields, grasses, and scattered wildflowers. The views are superb and unobstructed. Most noteworthy are the colorful open slopes of Silver Star Mountain to the north and the ridge containing Pyramid Rock to the west. Bring binoculars to scan the open slopes in this area for deer, elk, and maybe even a black bear. The trail remains rocky but becomes less steep as it rounds the head of an impressive high basin.

About 0.15 mile before the trail tops a side ridge coming in from the southwest, you face a choice. To reach the top of Silver Star Mountain, go straight, climb over the ridge, and soon intersect the trail coming up from Grouse Vista. Follow this route to the top (see Trip 10 for a description). Early-season hikers, however, will discover that even though the trail to this point has been free of snow, much of the rest of the way to the top remains snowbound until early June.

If you prefer to explore a different and less snowy route, veer left (slightly downhill) and make a short scramble on game paths down to a long-abandoned jeep trail. This wildly scenic route cuts across the southeast face of a ridge traversing an open slope carpeted with beargrass. In early to mid-June of favorable years the beargrass puts on a wonderful display of tall white blossoms. After about 0.8 mile the trail loops around the base of craggy Pyramid Rock and then cuts through a saddle in the ridge to an unsigned junction with the trail coming up from Grouse Vista.

To make a loop out of this hike, turn left, descend 1 mile on the steep, rocky trail to Grouse Vista, and then walk 3.3 miles down Road W 1200 to your car.

TRIP **12** Snass Creek Loop

Distance	4.8 miles, Semiloop
Elevation Gain	1200 feet
Hiking Time	2 to 3 hours
Optional Map	Green Trails *Lookout Mountain* (part of route not shown)
Usually Open	Mid-March to November
Best Times	April and May
Trail Use	Dogs OK
Agency	Mount Adams Ranger District, Gifford Pinchot National Forest
Difficulty	Moderate

HIGHLIGHTS The Snass Creek Trail is something of an outcast. The trail is not connected to any of the more popular hiking routes in the Silver Star Mountain area. The trailhead is hard to find. And once you find it, there is no convenient place to park. It's not surprising then that this trail sees very few visitors. So why go? Well, the forest is attractive, the solitude is inspiring, and you gain unusual views of some of the least known but most impressive summits in southwest Washington. If those aren't reasons enough, then you probably shouldn't be reading a hiking guidebook at all.

DIRECTIONS From the intersection of State Highways 502 and 503 in downtown Battleground, drive 5.7 miles north on Highway 503. Turn right on N.E. Rock Creek Road, which soon becomes Lucia Falls Road, and proceed 8.6 miles to a junction. Turn right on Sunset Falls Road and drive 7.4 miles to a junction at the entrance to Sunset Campground. Turn right on gravel Forest Road 41 and almost immediately cross a bridge to an unsigned junction where you go left. Proceed exactly 1.0 mile, and then look for a small sign on a tree on the left saying Summit Spring Trail. There is no room to park at the trailhead, so drive another 0.1 mile to a sharp turn in the road where there is room for 2 or 3 cars to park.

Walk back down the road to the trailhead, and follow the path as it descends briefly to cross a seasonal creek. From here the trail contours for 0.15 mile to a bridgeless crossing of somewhat larger and permanently flowing Snass Creek. The vegetation in this area is quite lush and attractive, with a profusion of ferns and mosses clinging to a canopy of second-growth western hemlocks, red alders, and Douglas firs.

After crossing Snass Creek the trail pulls away from the water, climbing rapidly to the top of a wide, forested ridge. This area features an incredible abundance of Oregon grape, which covers the forest floor with yellow blossoms in the latter part of April. The trail sticks with the ridgetop making an unrelenting but rarely steep ascent. Loggers have selectively thinned the forests here, allowing in more light and letting the remaining trees grow more rapidly.

At 0.9 mile the trail crosses a closed dirt road. If you make the recommended loop, you will hike back along this road—make a careful note of this unsigned crossing so you can relocate the path on the way back. To find the next segment of trail, turn right on the road, walk about 20 yards, and pick up the trail as it angles uphill to the left. From here the trail remains relatively level for about 0.2 mile before resuming its uphill direction. Since this trail receives only irregular maintenance the path is faint in places, but the proper course is always easy to determine.

At just short of 2 miles the trail levels out again along an old road that has been abandoned for so many decades it is now barely recognizable. At 2.2 miles you come to the indistinct top of a small side ridge where there is an unsigned and easy-to-miss junction. The main trail goes right, on its way to a remote logging road. A better option is to turn left (downhill) on a rather obscure trail that winds down to the top of a very old clear-cut. This old logging scar is now filled with perky

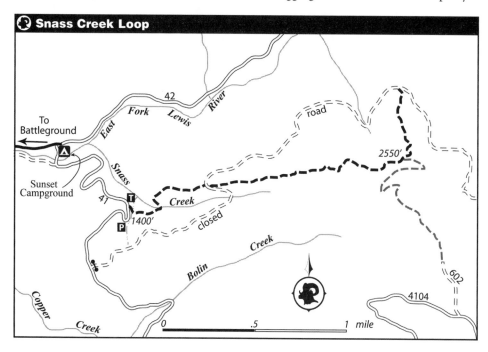

☉ Snass Creek Loop

little Pacific silver fir trees. The opening provides an excellent view to the north of an impressive grouping of peaks known as the Tatoosh Hills as well as a rock pinnacle atop Saturday Rock.

To complete the recommended loop continue downhill on the sketchy route, sometimes on overgrown trail and sometimes on an old logging skid road. The path is not difficult to follow, but it is often brushy, so hikers should wear long pants. About 0.6 mile from where it left the main trail, this route intersects the closed dirt road you crossed earlier in the hike. Turn left and make a pleasant, mostly downhill 1.1-mile walk back to the Snass Creek Trail. Turn right and return to your car.

TRIP 13 North Silver Star Mountain Loop

Distance	5.0 miles, Loop
Elevation Gain	1700 feet
Hiking Time	3 hours
Optional Map	Green Trails *Lookout Mountain, Bridal Veil* (some trails not shown)
Usually Open	Mid-May to October
Best Time	Mid-June to mid-July
Trail Use	Dogs OK (but may be difficult for them in places), backpacking option
Agency	Mount Adams Ranger District, Gifford Pinchot National Forest
Difficulty	Moderate

HIGHLIGHTS No matter how you get to the top of Silver Star Mountain, you will enjoy expansive views and abundant wildflowers. The easiest of the direct hiking routes to the summit is from the north along either an abandoned road or a wildly scenic new trail, which passes a series of jagged rock formations and goes through some of the best wildflower meadows in this book. The two routes can be easily combined into a spectacular, relatively easy, and surprisingly little-traveled loop.

DIRECTIONS From the intersection of State Highways 502 and 503 in downtown Battleground, drive 5.7 miles north on Highway 503. Turn right on N.E. Rock Creek Road, which soon becomes Lucia Falls Road, and proceed 8.6 miles to a junction. Turn right on Sunset Falls Road and drive 7.4 miles to a junction at the entrance to Sunset Campground. Turn right on gravel Forest Road 41 and almost immediately cross a bridge to an unsigned junction where you go left. Proceed 3.5 miles on this pothole-filled road, and then turn sharply right (downhill) on Road 4109. Stay on this sometimes rough road for 1.5 miles to a multiway junction. Turn left and go 2.7 steep, bumpy, uphill miles to the road-end turnaround.

There is no trail sign visible from the trailhead, and several old roads and trails look equally promising. The proper route leaves from the west end of the parking area and goes about 25 yards to a trail sign identifying this as Silver Star Trail 180. If you don't see this sign very soon after starting to hike, go back and try again. The Silver Star Trail switchbacks four times up a slope covered with brushy vine maple and then comes to a junction with a closed jeep road. Bear right (uphill) and walk about 150 yards to a large gravel turnaround in the road.

The scenery here, and for some time to come, is truly outstanding. The entire area is surrounded by huge sloping meadows that are carpeted with wildflowers in late June and early July. There are dozens of varieties, but the most common kinds are beargrass, lupine, wild carrot, paintbrush, iris, yarrow, valerian, tiger lily, and golden pea. Scattered about the open slopes are perky little noble fir trees, which look for all the world like Christmas trees, a popular use for this evergreen.

In addition to the flowers and trees, there are terrific views. Most impressive are Mt. St. Helens and Mt. Rainier, peeking over forested ridges to the north, and Mt. Adams to the east. Southward, Mt. Hood makes an almost perfectly framed

appearance in a low point in the ridge east of Silver Star Mountain.

To hike the new scenic trail, leave the road at this turnaround and bear left at a sign identifying ED'S TRAIL. This extremely scenic route is rough and narrow, and open only to hikers. The trail ascends steeply at first and then more gradually near the edge of a drop-off. The huge meadows here boast even more flowers than those you passed below. Added to the previous mix are columbine, wallflower, penstemon, fireweed, lomatium, and bistort—all looking for their place amid the other blossoms. You round a small ridge and the scenery improves yet again, as the rocky spine of Silver Star Mountain's summit ridge becomes visible directly ahead.

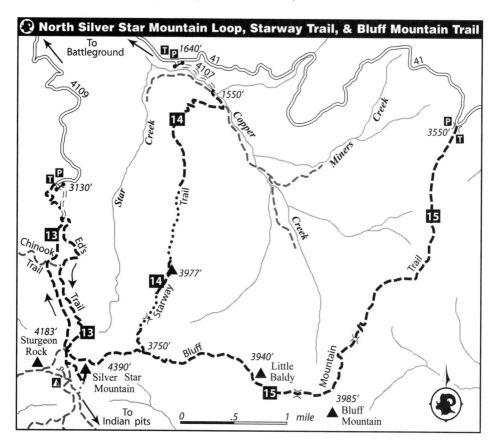

Still crossing open slopes, you climb gradually and come to the ridge crest, where you join an ancient two-rut road. Turn left and in just 100 feet you will come to a signed junction with the Chinook Trail going down the meadows to the right. Continue straight and keep climbing as the trail skirts to the left of several jagged rock outcroppings on the spine of the ridge. Along one of these detours, you will go through a natural, keyhole-shaped rock arch, before having to work your way around the base of some massive cliffs.

From here the trail goes very steeply up some improvised rock steps, climbs to a notch in the cliff, and then descends a bit through more meadows. The floral display in this higher meadow is still magnificent, with pink spiraea, yellow woolly daisy, and three kinds of light pink flowers—phlox, lewisia, and saxifrage—joining the color show. Once the trail finally leaves the meadow, it enters a forest of Pacific silver fir and soon comes to a major ridgetop junction.

The jeep road you have been paralleling meets your route here, as does the Bluff Mountain Trail (Trip 15), which angles in from the left. There is also an unsigned trail directly across the road from you, which goes southwest toward Sturgeon Rock. To reach the summit, you turn left on the jeep route and climb for 200 yards to a road junction where you should bear left. In about 0.2 mile this rock-strewn, old road works its way up to the saddle between the twin summits of Silver Star Mountain. There are trails going up to both high points. On the clearest days you can see, not only the nearby volcanic peaks already mentioned, but also Mt. Jefferson and the Three Sisters in Oregon, and the Olympic Mountains to the northwest in Washington.

Since this is the easiest route to the top of Silver Star Mountain, you might still have some extra energy to do some exploring. One of the most scenic and interesting side trips is a visit to some rock pits once used by Native American boys during their spiritual vision quests. To reach the site of these pits, take an obvious boot path from the more southern of the two summits of Silver Star Mountain and then drop very steeply down an open hillside to an unsigned junction with a better-graded official trail. Go left here and walk about 0.8 mile up and down through beargrass meadows. Watch out for a patch of thick brush here that may scratch your legs if you are wearing shorts. The rock pits are on a small talus slope near the end of the ridge. Please do not disturb this important religious and archaeological site.

Arch along Ed's Trail

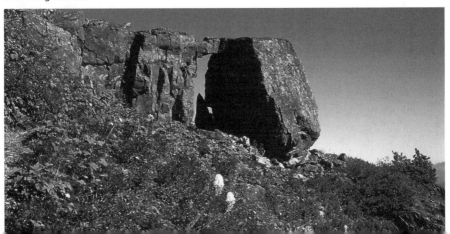

To return, walk back on the trail past the junction with the boot path up Silver Star Mountain. You will soon come to a four-way junction with a jeep road. Turn right and climb a short distance back to the junction just below the summit. Go straight and walk 200 yards down to the junction with Ed's Trail. For variety on the way back, you can stay on the old jeep road and walk this route as it gently descends for 2.0 miles through view-packed meadows back to the trailhead.

TRIP 14 Starway Trail

Distance	5.6 miles to ridge viewpoint, Out-and-back;
	10.0 miles to Silver Star Mountain, Out-and-back
Elevation Gain	2550 feet to ridge viewpoint,
	4000 feet to Silver Star Mountain
Hiking Time	3 to 6 hours
Optional Map	Green Trails *Bridal Veil, Lookout Mountain*
Usually Open	Mid-May to October
Best Time	June to early July
Trail Use	Dogs are allowed, but it's too rocky and rough for most.
Agency	Mount Adams Ranger District, Gifford Pinchot National Forest
Difficulty	Difficult to Strenuous

see map on p.83

HIGHLIGHTS With lots of steep climbing and very little trail maintenance, the Starway Trail is easily the most physically demanding of the several routes up Silver Star Mountain. Even so, it is a good choice for athletic and experienced hikers who enjoy solitude, like great views, and don't mind paying a price for these qualities. Be aware, however, that for much of its upper reaches the trail is nothing but a sketchy scramble route requiring good navigation and cross-country travel skills. The open terrain makes navigation reasonably easy, but the route is strictly for experienced hikers.

DIRECTIONS From the intersection of State Highways 502 and 503 in downtown Battleground, drive 5.7 miles north on Highway 503. Turn right on N.E. Rock Creek Road, which soon becomes Lucia Falls Road, and proceed 8.6 miles to a junction. Turn right on Sunset Falls Road and drive 7.4 miles to a junction at the entrance to Sunset Campground. Turn right on gravel Forest Road 41, and almost immediately cross a bridge to an unsigned junction where you go left. Proceed exactly 4.1 miles on this pothole-fest of a road, and park where gated Road 4107 angles downhill to the right.

Walk around the gate and go gradually downhill on Road 4107, a rough miner's road that is closed to vehicles. After 0.4 mile the road ends at Copper Creek, where the road bridge is washed out. You cross the lovely clear stream on a metal trail bridge and immediately come to an unsigned junction. Ignore the trail going sharply right, and stay on the main route as it very gradually climbs away from the creek. About 0.15 mile from the bridge is an unsigned fork.

You veer right (uphill), almost immediately switchback to the right, and then settle in for a tough climb. The wide, rocky path is typical of trails built by miners, who famously possessed a short-est-distance-between-two-points-even-if-that-is-straight-up mentality. This is fine for getting someplace quickly, but it's tough on the thighs and lungs. After a 0.3-mile traverse across mostly open terrain, the trail makes three quick switchbacks and then steeply winds its way toward the top of a long north-south trending ridge. The climb is mostly in a relatively young forest of western hemlock and Douglas fir, which offers no views but provides plenty of welcome shade.

At 1.8 miles, you finally reach the top of the wide, forested ridge, and things quickly change. To this point the path has been steep but easy to follow. Now the grade eases off considerably, but the price you pay for this respite is an increasingly faint trail plagued by blowdown. The route is relatively easy to pick out for about 0.5 mile, then it effectively disappears amid downed limbs and poorly marked junctions with sketchy dead-end routes leading to mining claims. For those confident in their off-trail navigation skills, however, the trail's best scenery is only a short distance away. To find it, make your way uphill through mostly open woods, following red plastic flags or bits of tread when available, and in 0.2 mile break out of the trees when you enter the first of several large ridgetop meadows. Flowers are everywhere and the views are superb. Although you can see all the usual snow-covered peaks (Mounts Adams, St. Helens, and Hood), the best views are of the rugged and much closer ridges radiating from Silver Star Mountain. Especially noteworthy are the views to the southeast of the dramatic north faces of Little Baldy and Bluff Mountain.

For the best views, continue uphill toward a bald-topped 3977-foot high point in the ridge. The trail is hard to find and very brushy, making travel effectively cross-country. Fortunately, the goal is frequently in sight, so it is easy to stay on course. Your tough scrambling is rewarded at the top, where the previous views are improved by greater altitude and joined by a nice look at Silver Star Mountain itself, which was previously hidden behind the ridge.

If you are determined to continue beyond this point, go south on the intermittent-at-best trail, descending to a prominent saddle after about 0.5 mile. You then steeply climb short segments of trail, generally staying on the west side of the ridgeline, and eventually reach a signed junction with the well-maintained Bluff Mountain Trail at 3.8 miles. From here you turn right and make the relatively easy 1.2-mile hike to the top of Silver Star Mountain. See Trip 15 for details.

North ridge of Silver Star Mountain from the Starway Trail

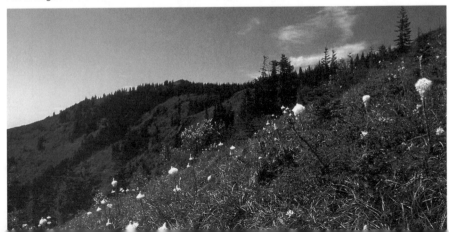

TRIP **15** Bluff Mountain Trail

Distance	13.2 miles, Out-and-back
Elevation Gain	2600 feet
Hiking Time	6 to 7 hours
Optional Map	Green Trails *Bridal Veil, Lookout Mountain*
Usually Open	Mid-May to early November
Best Times	Mid- to late June
Trail Use	Dogs OK, mountain biking, horseback riding, backpacking option
Agency	Mount Adams Ranger District, Gifford Pinchot National Forest
Difficulty	Difficult

see map on p.83

HIGHLIGHTS The summit of Silver Star Mountain is a worthwhile destination by any route, but for great scenery nothing can compare to the approach from the east along the Bluff Mountain Trail. The drive here is fairly long. In fact, at almost 1½ hours from Portland the drive is longer than the rule for inclusion in this book allows—it's included because it is one of my favorites. The well-graded trail is rarely crowded and has fine wildflower displays and almost nonstop fabulous views. On a clear day, and you should definitely save this outstanding hike for a clear day, views extend from Oregon's Three Sisters to Washington's Mt. Rainier, and even down to the skyline of downtown Portland (usually hidden beneath a haze of pollution). Carry an extra quart of water, as the route is dry and exposed to the sun over its entire length.

DIRECTIONS Begin by driving to Battleground, either by going north on State Highway 503 from Interstate 205, or by going east on State Highway 502 from Exit 9 off Interstate 5. The two state highways intersect in the middle of Battleground. From here drive north 5.7 miles on Highway 503. Turn right on N.E. Rock Creek Road, which soon becomes Lucia Falls Road.

After 8.5 miles turn right on N.E. Sunset Falls Road, and follow this route about 7.4 miles to Sunset Campground. Turn right and drive through the camp to a bridge over the East Fork Lewis River. Immediately on the other side of the bridge turn left onto gravel, pothole-filled Forest Road 41. Stay on this narrow route as it climbs 9 miles to a saddle. The trailhead parking area is on the right.

The Bluff Mountain Trail starts as an old jeep road, now closed to motor vehicles. The old road undulates along a scenic ridgetop, where in the century since the 1902 Yacolt Burn only scattered Pacific silver firs have grown back and the tallest have yet to attain a height of 20 feet. As a result, you can enjoy extensive views, not only of the region's recognizable snow peaks, but also of Little Baldy and distant Silver Star Mountain along a rugged ridge to the southwest. The open ridge is carpeted with a mix of huckle-berry, beargrass, and serviceberry bushes, along with a wide array of wildflowers.

After 2 up-and-down miles, you descend about 350 feet to a small saddle where the road ends and the trail veers off to the right. The path loses 150 feet in one long switchback to another, more prominent saddle. It then cuts across the north side of Bluff Mountain. Along this traverse, you cross one strip of larger trees where in early summer you may encounter lingering snow patches and small runoff creeks.

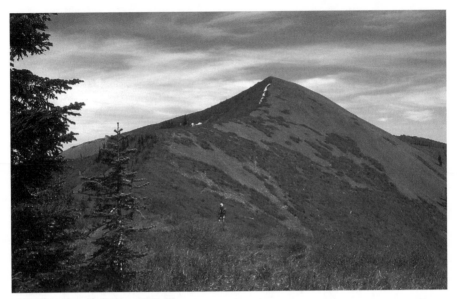

Little Baldy along Bluff Mountain Trail

Initially, this section provides excellent views west to the open talus slopes of pointed Little Baldy. Later, you can look north for views of the truncated summit of Mt. St. Helens and part of Mt. Rainier. Wildflowers on this cool slope include yellow glacier lily and wood violet, pink bleeding heart, and white false Solomon's seal and avalanche lily.

The trail now climbs to and crosses another saddle, this one in dense timber, and then traverses the open, view-packed talus slopes on the south and west sides of Little Baldy. Here you get great looks at the impressive crags of your destination, Silver Star Mountain. Still traveling west toward that goal, the well-graded trail uses a couple of short switchbacks to work its way gradually up an open ridge with lots of beargrass. You go straight at the signed junction with the rarely-maintained Starway Trail (Trip 14) before you make the final push to the mountain.

The last section snakes up the ridge and then cuts into the trees on the north side of the peak, where snowdrifts usually remain into late June. The trail ends at an intersection where a closed jeep road and several foot trails all meet. To reach the summit, turn left on the jeep road and 200 yards later bear left (uphill) at another road junction. The final 0.2 mile is a climb on a rock-strewn road to the high saddle between the dual summits of Silver Star Mountain, both of which are easily accessible.

Once you reach the top, sit back and enjoy the view. To the north and east are the great volcanic snow peaks of Washington (St. Helens, Adams, and Rainier), while to the south are the more dainty but equally impressive peaks of Oregon (Hood and Jefferson). In the distance to the south, some 125 miles away, are the Three Sisters. People familiar with this area will also be able to spot lesser landmarks such as Three-Corner Rock, Larch Mountain, Tanner Butte, the Goat Rocks, and Mt. Defiance, to name just a few. Although this is usually a dayhike, those willing to spend the night here will be rewarded with spectacular sunsets and views down to the city lights of Portland.

TRIP 16 Snag Creek Trail

Distance	4.6 miles, Out-and-back
Elevation Gain	1300 feet
Hiking Time	2 to 3 hours
Optional Map	Green Trails *Lookout Mountain* (trail not shown)
Usually Open	Mid-March to early December
Best Time	Mid-April to May
Trail Use	Dogs OK
Agency	Yacolt State Forest
Difficulty	Moderate

HIGHLIGHTS This fun trail was originally built by the Civilian Conservation Corps in the 1930s, but was abandoned for several decades and fell into disrepair. Then in 1981 an industrious Boy Scout troop in Washougal took on the project of reopening the old trail. They have done an admirable job, so today this rarely traveled route provides a nice outdoor experience and deserves more attention from hikers.

DIRECTIONS Go 1.5 miles east of Bridge of the Gods on State Highway 14, and turn left on Rock Creek Drive. After about 0.4 mile you pass the turnoff to Skamania Lodge. Immediately thereafter, turn left on Foster Creek Road. Drive 0.9 mile to a set of power lines and turn left again on paved Red Bluff Road. In just 0.4 mile the road turns to gravel at a fork. Here you bear right on Road CG 2000. After another 2.1 miles go left at another fork to continue on Road CG 2000, which gets narrower and a little bumpy with lots of potholes.

About 3.3 miles later, at a bridge over Rock Creek, take a moment to admire Steep Creek Falls, a lovely cascade on a tributary stream that tumbles directly into Rock Creek. To reach the Snag Creek Trailhead, keep driving another 2.4 miles, and then turn right on dirt Road CG 2070. After 0.4 mile, park on the very narrow shoulder of this rough road at the signed crossing of the Pacific Crest Trail (PCT).

Sedum Ridge from Snag Creek Trail

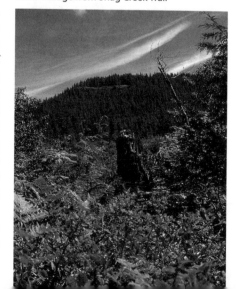

You begin the hike by veering left off the road onto the southbound PCT. The trail contours across a brushy hillside above Rock Creek in a second-growth forest of small Douglas firs and bigleaf maples. This area was logged in 1973 and replanted in 1975, which gives you a chance to see the rate at which the land recovers from logging activity. After 0.2 mile you cross cascading Snag Creek on a wide plank bridge and enter older and more attractive woods. Just 150 yards after the bridge is a junction with Snag Creek Trail, where you turn right.

Just above the PCT, the trail passes a nice campsite and then climbs

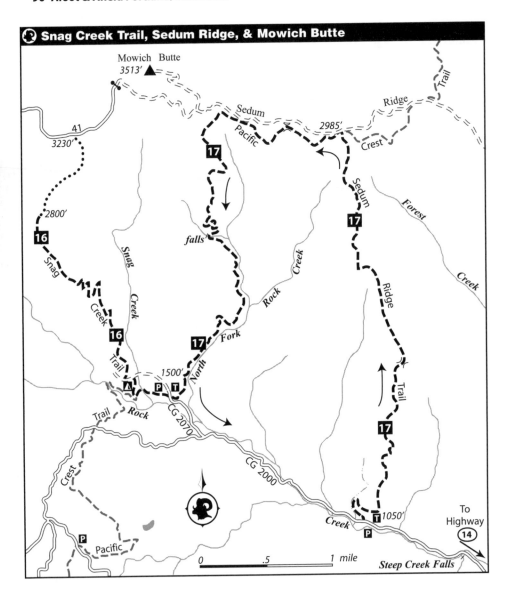

moderately steeply through a pleasant western-hemlock and Douglas-fir forest. The wide path is so lightly traveled that it is now being invaded by bracken fern. Based on the amount of elk droppings on the trail, the route seems to be used more by hoofed creatures than booted ones. For the first 0.1 mile you follow splashing Snag Creek. When you come to a junction with a washed-out jeep road, turn left on this road and walk uphill about 150 yards. Then switchback to the right at a brown sign for the Snag Creek Trail.

The trail now ascends a ridge under the shade of tall hemlock trees before coming to the edge of a clear-cut, which is a little unsightly but provides nice views up to Mowich Butte and Sedum Ridge. You climb steeply past this logging scar and then make one long switchback, followed by seven short ones, to the top of a ridge. At this point there is a break in the trees that provides an unusually good perspective of the rocky pinnacle and microwave tower on Three-Corner Rock to the southwest. You can also see a portion of Mt. Hood and several high points in the Columbia River Gorge. Two wooden benches here allow you to enjoy the view in comfort.

Just 0.1 mile past this view the trail leaves Yacolt State Forest land and enters the national forest. After this change in stewardship, the trail deteriorates rapidly. The path formerly extended for another 1.3 miles to Mowich Camp on Forest Road 41, but it is now too rough a bushwhack to be recommended. So be satisfied with the viewpoint and return the way you came.

TRIP 17 Sedum Ridge & Mowich Butte Loop

Distance	11.3 miles, Loop
Elevation Gain	2700 feet
Hiking Time	5 to 7 hours
Optional Map	Green Trails *Lookout Mountain, Wind River* (part of route not shown)
Usually Open	Late April to November
Best Time	Mid-May to June
Trail Use	Dogs OK
Agency	Yacolt State Forest & Mount Adams Ranger District, Gifford Pinchot National Forest
Difficulty	Difficult

HIGHLIGHTS The old Sedum Ridge Trail climbs a woodsy ridge that would, by itself, be a pleasant if unremarkable hike, but when you combine it into a loop with the Pacific Crest Trail you have a full day of scenic hiking. To make the trip even better, add a side trip to Mowich Butte, a viewpoint with far-ranging vistas across forested hills and valleys and to distant volcanic snow peaks.

DIRECTIONS Go 1.5 miles east of Bridge of the Gods on State Highway 14, and turn left on Rock Creek Drive. After about 0.4 mile you pass the turnoff to Skamania Lodge. Immediately thereafter, turn left on Foster Creek Road. Drive 0.9 mile to a set of power lines and turn left again on paved Red Bluff Road. In just 0.4 mile the road turns to gravel at a fork. Here you bear right on Road CG 2000. After another 2.1 miles go left at another fork to continue on Road CG 2000, which gets narrower and a little bumpy with lots of potholes.

About 3.3 miles later, at a bridge over Rock Creek, take a moment to admire Steep Creek Falls, a lovely cascade on a tributary stream that tumbles directly into Rock Creek. To reach the Sedum Ridge Trailhead, keep driving for exactly 0.9 mile, and park in a large, unsigned pull-out on the left.

The trail starts beside an inconspicuous brown sign on the north side of the road. You begin climbing almost immediately on a slope covered with dense forests of Douglas fir and western hemlock. After a few hundred yards, the path ducks into a little gully with a seasonal trickle of water, then leaves it, and traverses a hillside to the east.

When the trail turns left, the effort of the climb really picks up as you ascend a wide, steep, woodsy ridge. Views are generally blocked by trees, but you get occasional looks at the Rock Creek Valley, which drops farther and farther below you as you hike. The trail receives only intermittent maintenance but remains reasonably easy to follow without excessive blowdown to hamper your progress. After almost 2 miles the trail levels off a little, goes around the east side of a high point on the ridge, and then drops slightly into a wide saddle.

Above this saddle, the uphill resumes as you make a fairly steep traverse of the west side of a ridge. You then go through an almost imperceptible saddle on a side ridge, after which the steep uphill is over. From here you go up and down (mostly up) along the west side of the narrowing ridge and end with a mostly level section to a possibly unsigned junction with the Pacific Crest Trail (PCT). A few feet above you is the closed, dirt Forest Road 41, which hugs the crest of Sedum Ridge.

You turn left on the PCT and parallel Road 41 through a forest of small Douglas fir, Pacific silver fir, and western hemlock. After a short distance, you come to the base of a basalt cliff where you gain good views to the south toward the Rock Creek Valley and several highpoints in the Columbia River Gorge. From here you walk west to a saddle and work around the south side of a knob in the ridge. Then you will drop a bit to cross some steep slopes just below a saddle and Road 41.

To make the recommended side trip to Mowich Butte, find a place to scramble up to Road 41, noting carefully for the return trip where you'll need to turn off the road, and follow the road uphill for about 0.4 mile to a junction. Turn right and walk up a narrow dirt road to the top of Mowich Butte. A lookout once stood atop this 3513-foot peak, so, not surprisingly, the views are excellent.

To the northeast are the Wind River Valley and distant Mt. Adams. To the northwest is the recently active Mt. St. Helens. To the west is Silver Star Mountain, and to the south is distinctive Three-Corner Rock, with Mt. Hood in the distance. Fast-growing trees will eventually block this view. Although the road is closed to cars, it is often used by mountain bikers, so you may have some company. Given all the hoof tracks in the road and trail, it should come as no surprise that *mowich* is the Chinook word for "deer."

To make the return leg of the loop, return to the PCT and hike southward. The trail is well graded, as most sections of this famous trail are, so the downhill will be easier on your knees than the relatively steep Sedum Ridge Trail. First, this wide trail wanders almost due south, and then it rounds a ridgeline and turns west. You cross a usually dry gully, where there are dense thickets of salmonberry, ferns, and devil's club, and then continue downhill. You descend by four switchbacks to cross a usually flowing little creek beside a small falls. Follow the slopes about 80 feet above this creek to its confluence with North Fork Rock Creek.

Now in lower-elevation forests of large hemlocks and firs, you stay on woodsy slopes above North Fork Rock Creek for a little less than 1 mile, then veer away and cross a partially open hillside to a trailhead on Road CG 2070.

To get back to your car, turn left and walk 0.4 mile along this rough gravel road over a bridge on Rock Creek and up to a junction with Road CG 2000. Turn left and walk this pothole-filled road for 1.5 miles back to your car.

TRIP 18 Three-Corner Rock via Stebbins Creek

Distance	4.2 or 18.4 miles, Out-and-back
Elevation Gain	3800 feet
Hiking Time	2 or 10 hours
Optional Map	Green Trails *Bridal Veil*
Usually Open	April to November
Best Times	Mid-May
Trail Use	Dogs OK, backpacking option, horseback riding, mountain biking
Agency	Yacolt State Forest
Difficulty	Moderate or Difficult

HIGHLIGHTS This hike gives you the choice between a long, tiring approach on a quiet trail and a relatively short walk from a higher trailhead. Either route ends at the views and flowers around Three-Corner Rock, which by themselves justify any amount of effort. The short route is fun and scenic but somehow feels like cheating. After all, reaching the destination isn't the only reason people go hiking. Perhaps more than any other activity, hiking is about the journey itself.

DIRECTIONS Drive 10 miles east on State Highway 14 from its intersection with Interstate 205, and then turn left at the traffic light onto 15th Street in Washougal. Go straight through two traffic lights in town. The road's name changes, first to 17th Street and then to Washougal River Road. Stay on this good paved road for 17.8 miles past several intersections to a bridge over the river and the end of the pavement. Take a moment to stop here for a look at Dougan Falls, a popular swimming hole in summer.

After the bridge, turn right on pothole-filled, gravel Road W 2000, and drive a final 3.4 miles to a large trailhead parking lot on the left. This is the lower trailhead for those wishing to take the long hike.

To reach the upper trailhead, continue driving for 7.2 miles on Road W 2000, staying on the main road through several intersections and following signs, where existing, for Rock Creek Pass. At the pass is a four-way junction. Take the first right turn onto Road CG 1440, and drive on this rough road for exactly 2.3 miles. Park just after a small sign saying TRAIL CROSSING and before the road crosses a gully.

From the lower trailhead, the trail leaves from the southwest corner of the lot and drops past an outhouse to a plank bridge over a trickling creek. From here it parallels the road for a few hundred yards on river-level flats covered with red alder and Douglas fir. You cross the access road and pick up the trail on the opposite side as it goes up a wide gravel path that was once a road.

Climb this old road for about 50 yards and then turn off on a foot trail to the right that ascends six quick switchbacks to a ridge crest. The trail rounds this ridge and works its way along the hillside above Stebbins Creek in the canyon on your right. For the next 3 miles the trail makes a series of frustrating ups and downs, most of which would have been unnecessary had the trail been better engineered.

Fortunately, the scenery is pleasant as you walk through attractive second-growth forests of Douglas fir, western hemlock, bigleaf maple, and red alder. The route begins to go slightly downhill for about 0.2 mile, crosses a seasonal

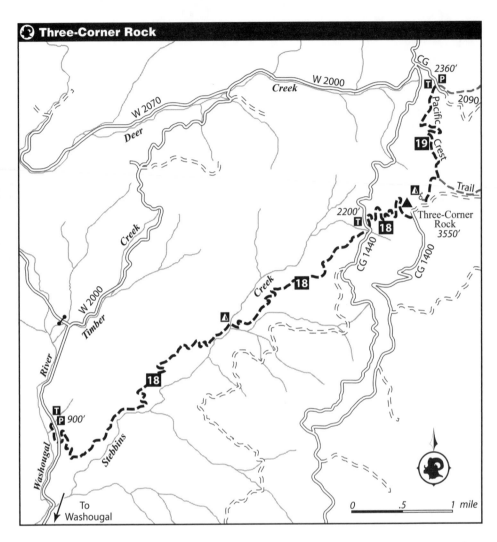

Three-Corner Rock

creek, and makes a series of traverses and short uphill switchbacks. After crossing beneath a bouldery rockslide, you ascend six switchbacks and then immediately lose most of this hard-won elevation. You make a downhill traverse to a nice viewpoint of Three-Corner Rock and the Stebbins Creek Valley and then descend five rough switchbacks to a camp next to a bridge over Stebbins Creek.

Now that the ups and downs are over, the trail crosses the bridge and then ducks into and climbs out of a side canyon on eight switchbacks that lead to the crest of a small ridge. For the next couple of miles the trail follows this ridge, rather steeply uphill at first and then more gently. Spur trails lead to decent viewpoints that make good rest stops, although the views don't compare to those from Three-Corner Rock. Eventually you make a final fairly steep uphill push and come to a rough road. This is the upper trailhead described earlier.

The trail resumes just north of a little gully and makes 18 fairly long switchbacks through increasingly interesting and open country. There are several small rockslides and brushy areas on this slope, and the partially obstructed views improve as you climb. Finally, you top the ridge in a flowery meadow and meet a small road near a microwave tower. To reach the top of the rock pile at the summit, simply walk over to its base and scramble up the boulders to the old lookout site. Beyond the microwave towers, views extend to Mounts Adams, Hood, and St. Helens and include countless forested ridges and valleys in all directions.

TRIP 19 Three-Corner Rock via the Pacific Crest Trail

Distance	4.8 miles, Out-and-back
Elevation Gain	1200 feet
Hiking Time	2 to 3 hours
Optional Map	Green Trails *Bridal Veil*
Usually Open	Mid-April to November
Best Time	Mid-May
Trail Use	Dogs OK, backpacking option, horseback riding
Agency	Yacolt State Forest
Difficulty	Moderate

see map on p.94

HIGHLIGHTS If the long trail to Three-Corner Rock from Stebbins Creek (Trip 18) is more than you want to tackle, you'll be glad to know that there is a much easier alternative. The driving access is a little tricky, but the trail is easy and the views from the destination are always spectacular.

DIRECTIONS Drive 10 miles east on State Highway 14 from its intersection with Interstate 205, and then turn left at the traffic light onto 15th Street in Washougal. Go straight through two traffic lights in town as the road's name changes, first to 17th Street and then to Washougal River Road. Stay on this good paved road for 17.8 miles past several intersections to a bridge over the river and the end of the pavement. Take a moment to stop here for a look at Dougan Falls, a popular swimming hole in summer.

After the bridge, turn right on pothole-filled, gravel Road W 2000. After 3.4 miles you pass the lower Three-Corner Rock Trailhead. Continue driving for 7.2 miles, staying on the main road past several intersections, and follow signs where existing for Rock Creek Pass. At the pass is a four-way junction. To reach the Pacific Crest Trail, take the second right, onto Road CG 2090, and drive up this rocky route for 0.3 mile to a saddle and the unsigned trail crossing. There is room here for about three cars to park beside the road.

The southbound trail heads to the right (southwest) and begins a well-graded climb in dense mountain-hemlock and Pacific-silver-fir forests. The route is unremarkable as you gradually ascend near a woodsy ridge on three irregularly spaced switchbacks, the highlights being a couple of decent viewpoints where you can see parts of Mounts Adams, Hood, and St. Helens. After 1.7 miles there is a junction with the spur trail to Three-Corner Rock. The sign for this junction may be missing, but the trail is obvious.

Turn right and wander very gradually uphill on a rocky trail through an open meadow with decent views and lots of colorful wildflowers. Blue lupine and white beargrass are the dominant

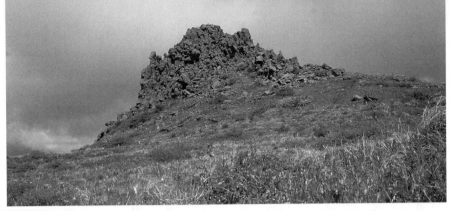
Three-Corner Rock

species, with some red paintbrush, yellow lomatium, and orange tiger lily offering a smattering of other colors. After 0.3 mile, and just 50 yards before you join a jeep road, look for a spur trail going to the right, which goes about 100 feet to a small spring with a possible campsite and a watering trough for horses.

After this spur trail, you follow the road for about 0.2 mile to a four-way junction. To your right is the large rock pile at the summit of Three-Corner Rock. Take the time to scramble to the top of this rock pile to enjoy unrestricted views of all the major snow peaks in the region,

as well as most of the major high points in the Columbia River Gorge. You can even see a small portion of the shimmering Columbia River. The extensive view explains why this location was once the site of a fire-lookout building, but all that remains of that historic structure are some concrete foundations. In modern times, mountaintops that formerly featured picturesque old wooden lookout buildings now sprout unsightly metal microwave and cellular-phone towers. Unfortunately, one of these structures is just a few hundred yards to the south.

TRIP 20 Table Mountain from the North

Distance	11.0 miles, Out-and-back
Elevation Gain	1800 feet
Hiking Time	6 to 7 hours
Optional Map	Green Trails *Bonneville Dam, Bridal Veil*
Usually Open	Mid-April to November
Best Time	Mid-May to mid-June
Trail Use	Dogs OK, backpacking option, horseback riding
Agency	Columbia River Gorge National Scenic Area
Difficulty	Difficult

HIGHLIGHTS Except for Beacon Rock, Table Mountain is the most recognizable landmark in the Columbia River Gorge. Thousands of hikers climb this peak, starting from the river in a long, tough ascent (see Trip 7 in the Western Columbia River Gorge section for details). Very few people, however, hike the more remote trails that approach this mountain from the north. This is an unfortunate oversight because although this trail passes several unsightly clear-cuts, it also includes one of the best ridge walks in the area

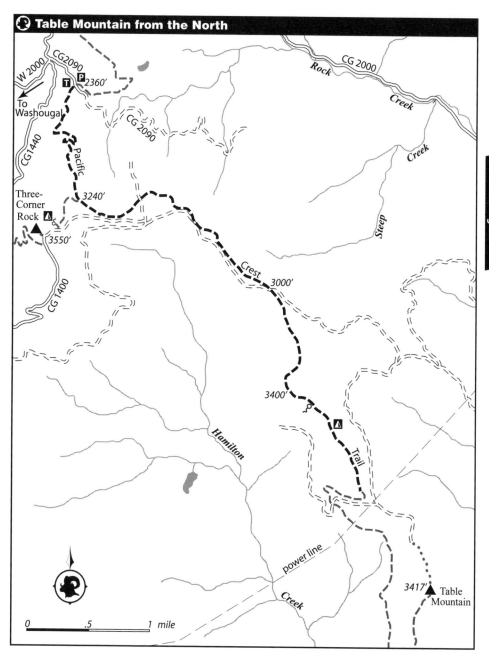

with outstanding views and fine wildflowers. If you are up for a long car shuttle, you can make this into a terrific overnight adventure to the trailhead for the Pacific Crest Trail at Bonneville. Since reaching the top of Table Mountain in a single day is both long and challenging, the recommended goal for dayhikers is actually short of the mountain along the very scenic ridge to the north.

DIRECTIONS Drive to Washougal, 10 miles east on State Highway 14 from its intersection with Interstate 205, and then turn left (north) at a traffic light onto 15th Street. Go straight, through two traffic lights, as the road's name changes, first to 17th Street and then to Washougal River Road. Stay on this good paved road for 17.8 miles to a bridge over the river and the end of pavement.

After the bridge, turn right on pothole-filled, gravel Road W 2000. Continue on the main road for 10.6 miles through several intersections, following intermittent signs to Rock Creek Pass. At the pass is a four-way junction. Take the second right, onto Road CG 2090, and ascend this rocky route for 0.3 mile to a saddle and the unsigned trail crossing. There is room here to park about three cars.

Take the southbound Pacific Crest Trail (PCT) as it makes a well-graded climb in dense mountain-hemlock and Pacific-silver-fir forests. After 1.7 miles of climbing, mostly in dense forest but with a couple decent viewpoints along the way, you come to a possibly unsigned junction with the trail to Three-Corner Rock.

Go left (south) on the PCT, which for the next couple of miles goes down, up, and then down again. Most of the way is in dense forest, but you also pass two large clear-cuts. Although these logging scars are unsightly, they open up exciting views of the forested Rock Creek Valley to the northeast and of distant snow-covered peaks such as Mounts Adams, St. Helens, Rainier, Hood, and even the very tip of Jefferson far to the south. Another unnatural feature along this ridge is the presence of several logging roads that the trail either approaches, touches, or crosses at various points along the way.

After 3 miles the scenery remains natural and continuously wonderful as you break out of the forest into a series of sloping meadows with outstanding views and abundant wildflowers. In addition to some of the usual suspects (paintbrush, valerian, and lomatium), look for phlox, anemones, strawberries, serviceberry bushes, chocolate lilies, and dozens of other less common but lovely blossoms. At about 5 miles you come to a trickling seasonal spring that is usually reliable

until sometime in July and that represents the only potential source of water on this hike. About 0.4 mile later look on the left for a tiny but wildly scenic ridgetop campsite. There is only room for one tent, but the views are excellent and the sunset-observing opportunities are outstanding. Perhaps the best views are of Mt. Adams to the east-northeast. The site is sheltered from the incessant Gorge winds by a small patch of fir trees. Unfortunately, the only water is 0.4 mile back at the seasonal spring.

If you want to reach Table Mountain, continue beyond this campsite following the PCT down to a power line access road. From there you leave the trail, walk south on a dead-end jeep road to its end, and then scramble cross-country to the view-filled top of Table Mountain.

If you have a full weekend (and can arrange a rather long car shuttle), you can turn this into a 16.4-mile one-way hike by exiting at the PCT trailhead near Bonneville Dam. (See Trip 9 in the section on the Western Columbia River Gorge for driving directions.)

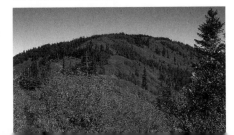

Along the Pacific Crest Trail near a ridgetop camp north of Table Mountain

TRIP 21 Sedum Ridge from Trout Creek via the Pacific Crest Trail

Distance	2.6 miles to lower viewpoint, Out-and-back; 10.8 miles, Loop
Elevation Gain	450 feet to lower viewpoint, 1950 feet as a loop
Hiking Time	1½ to 6 hours
Optional Map	Green Trails *Wind River*
Usually Open	Late April to November
Best Time	Any
Trail Use	Dogs OK, horseback riding
Agency	Mount Adams Ranger District, Gifford Pinchot National Forest
Difficulty	Moderate to Difficult
Note	Good in cloudy weather

HIGHLIGHTS This trip explores a little traveled section of the Pacific Crest Trail (PCT) as it travels amid the forested ridges between the Columbia River and the Wind River Valley. The trail is mostly in dense forest, but it includes a lovely creek, one excellent viewpoint, and plenty of solitude, all of which make it well worth your time and attention.

DIRECTIONS Drive Interstate 84 east to Cascade Locks, take Exit 44, and almost immediately veer right to loop around and cross the Columbia River on the Bridge of the Gods (a $1 toll applies, as of 2007). Turn right on State Highway 14, go 6.1 miles, and then turn left (north) on the signed road to Carson. After 0.9 mile you go straight at a junction in the middle of Carson, and then proceed 7.9 miles to a junction. Turn left (west) on Hemlock Road, following signs to Wind River Work Center, and go 1.3 miles to a junction marked with a small sign saying Canopy Crane Research Facility just before a bridge over Trout Creek. Turn right on Forest Road 43, drive 1.4 miles, and then park at the unsigned but obvious crossing of the Pacific Crest Trail where a concrete trail bridge crosses Trout Creek on your left.

Walk across the bridge and immediately come to an excellent campsite complete with bench, metal fire pit, and tent pad. The trail then curves to the right and heads upstream through a stately, moss-draped forest of tall western hemlocks, western red cedars, and Douglas firs. After an easy 0.3 mile in the flatlands near Trout Creek, you make a bridged crossing of a small but lovely tributary stream and soon begin climbing more noticeably. As always with the Pacific Crest Trail the route is well graded, so the uphill is gentle and not too tiring.

A pair of long switchbacks takes you to a junction atop a minor ridgetop at 1.3 miles. The 50-yard dead-end trail to the right leads to an excellent rocky viewpoint above the canyon of loudly cascading Trout Creek. Farther away you can see the Wind River Valley, Bunker Hill (Trip 23), and countless forested ridges and canyons. This viewpoint makes an excellent destination if you want a shorter hike.

To do the longer loop, go left at the ridgetop junction and continue up the PCT. The trail remains in dense forest, ascending long lazy switchbacks with few highlights other than a partial view to the east of Mt. Adams at 2.7 miles. Finally at 4 miles you come to long-abandoned Forest Road 41, which now serves as a wide trail.

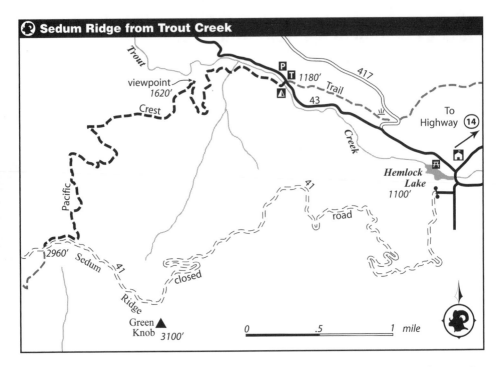

Sedum Ridge from Trout Creek

viewpoint
1620'

Trout

Crest

Pacific

2960' Sedum 41

Ridge

Green ▲
Knob 3100'

closed

41

road

1180'

Trail

43

417

Creek

*Hemlock
Lake*
1100'

To
Highway **14**

0   .5   1 *mile*

For the nearest viewpoint, go right (west) on the road/trail. In about 2 miles you come to the junction with the old spur road to the vistas atop Mowich Butte (see Trip 17 for details). To make the loop, however, turn left on the road/trail and gradually descend through lovely but viewless forest in long twists and turns for 5.2 miles to a gate and a cluster of Forest Service buildings. Walk past the buildings to the main paved road, turn left, cross a bridge over Trout Creek, and then almost immediately turn left again on Road 43. From here, it is a 1.4-mile road walk back to your car.

Pacific Crest Trail bridge over Trout Creek

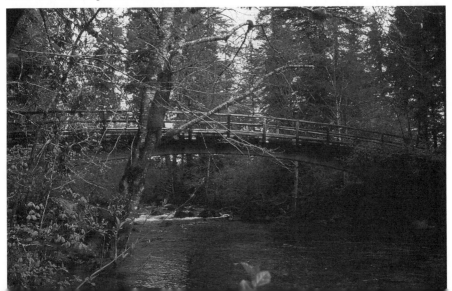

TRIP 22 Whistle Punk Loop

Distance	2.2 miles with side trip to canopy research site, Loop
Elevation Gain	50 feet
Hiking Time	1 hour
Optional Map	Use trailhead brochure
Usually Open	March to December
Best Time	Any
Trail Use	Good for kids, dogs OK, wheelchair accessible
Agency	Mount Adams Ranger District, Gifford Pinchot National Forest
Difficulty	Easy
Note	Good in cloudy weather

HIGHLIGHTS Here is your chance to learn all about Choker Setters, Whistle Punks, and Donkey Punchers—and, no, these aren't members of the latest rock band. All of these colorful terms, and many more, are explained on signs along this fascinating trail that highlights the logging history of the Pacific Northwest. Although this relatively new trail winds through an attractive second-growth forest and visits a wildlife-rich wetland, the real attraction is the area's history. So don your best Paul Bunyan–style plaid shirt and explore this trail with the proper frame of mind.

DIRECTIONS Drive Interstate 84 east to Cascade Locks, take Exit 44, and almost immediately veer right to loop around and cross the Columbia River on the Bridge of the Gods (a $1 toll applies, as of 2007). Turn right on State Highway 14, go 6.1 miles, and then turn left (north) on the signed road to Carson. After 0.9 mile you go straight at a junction in the middle of Carson, and then proceed 7.9 miles to a junction. Turn left (west) on Hemlock Road, following signs to Wind River Work Center, and go 1.3 miles to a junction marked with a small sign saying CANOPY CRANE RESEARCH FACILITY just before a bridge over Trout Creek. Turn right on Forest Road 43, drive 0.6 mile, and then turn right onto gravel Road 417. Drive 0.4 mile to the trailhead on the right.

The wide, gravel, wheelchair-accessible trail starts in an open meadow, but almost immediately enters a second-growth forest composed mostly of western hemlocks. After 80 yards you come to a junction and the start of the loop.

To follow the proscribed nature trail itinerary, bear right and soon pass through a seasonally flooded area where deciduous trees crowd out the conifers. Soon after reentering a coniferous forest, a series of interpretive signs explain the interesting logging history of this region. Keep an eye out for bits of rusted logging equipment scattered around the forest.

At about 0.3 mile you bear right at a junction with a shorter loop trail option and then continue to the north end of the loop where a wooden platform provides an overlook of a marsh. Wildlife here includes red-winged blackbirds, wood ducks, and roughskin newts. From here, the trail crosses a boardwalk over a corner of the wetland and then comes to a junction with a narrow road. A 0.7-mile round-trip side trip to the right up this road takes you to a fascinating research facility where scientists use a huge crane to access the tree canopy. From this perch they are able to study the numerous

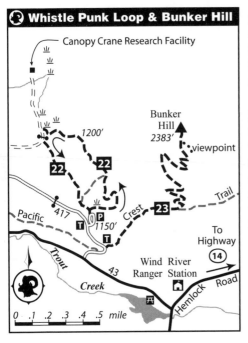

Whistle Punk Loop & Bunker Hill

plants and animals that call this lofty environment home. The research facility is not always open to the public and is often not is use, but it is well worth checking out when access is allowed.

The main loop trail turns left at the junction with the Canopy Research Road and then goes 50 yards to a gate at the edge of a large meadow. Once through the gate you bear left at a junction (the road goes right), soon walk through another gate, and reenter forest. Another 0.4 mile takes you past a junction with the shorter loop option trail and back to your car.

TRIP 23 Bunker Hill

Distance	3.8 miles, Out-and-back
Elevation Gain	1200 feet
Hiking Time	2 hours
Optional Map	Green Trails *Wind River*
Usually Open	Mid-March to November
Best Time	Any
Trail Use	Good for kids, dogs OK
Agency	Wind River Ranger District, Gifford Pinchot National Forest
Difficulty	Moderate

HIGHLIGHTS Although it bears no resemblance to the Revolutionary War battlefield in Massachusetts, Washington State's Bunker Hill is a fun place to visit. Historical interest may be lacking, but there is plenty of scenic interest with a pretty forest and a fine viewpoint that provides an unusual perspective of the Wind River Valley.

DIRECTIONS Drive Interstate 84 east to Cascade Locks, take Exit 44, and almost immediately veer right to loop around and cross the Columbia River on the Bridge of the Gods (a $1 toll applies, as of 2007). Turn right on State Highway 14, go 6.1 miles, and then turn left (north) on the signed road to Carson. After 0.9 mile you go straight at a junction in the middle of Carson, and then proceed 7.9 miles to a junction. Turn left (west) on Hemlock Road, following signs to Wind River Work Center, and go 1.3 miles to a junction marked with a small sign saying CANOPY CRANE RESEARCH FACILITY just before a bridge over Trout Creek.

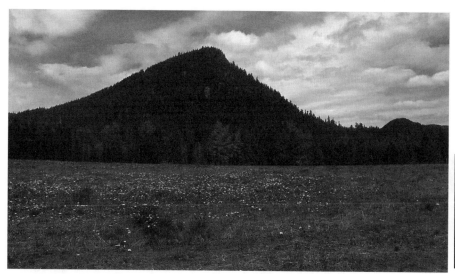

Bunker Hill from the south

Turn right on Forest Road 43, drive 0.6 mile, and then turn right onto gravel Road 417. After 0.25 mile you pass the signed crossing of the Pacific Crest Trail. Since there is almost no room to park here, drive another 0.15 mile to the trailhead for the Whistle Punk Trail and leave your car there.

Walk back along the road to the Pacific Crest Trail, and turn left (northbound) on that famous path. The trail initially passes along the edge of a large open area, which provides a stellar view of hulking Bunker Hill to the northeast. Heading directly toward that enticing goal, the nearly level trail soon enters forest and then begins a gradual climb to a fork at 0.4 mile.

You bear left (uphill) and settle in for a steady but not-too-difficult climb. Maintaining a fairly consistent moderately steep grade, the trail ascends a total of 11 irregularly spaced switchbacks on its way to the top. The entire way is in relatively open forest but features no views. In fact the views remain disappointing—nonexistent, to be more precise—once you reach the top, where trees get in the way. The only interesting features here are the concrete foundations of a long-gone lookout tower. To find the view, bushwhack 120 yards south along the narrow summit ridge to a moss-covered rock outcropping. From here you'll enjoy a fine view of the Wind River Valley, Oregon's Mount Defiance, and even a snippet of the Columbia River.

Chapter 3
Portland & the Willamette Valley

Since the overwhelming majority of the people in the Portland/Vancouver region reside in the fertile lowlands between the Coast Range and the Cascade Mountains, it is not surprising that most of the land here is plowed under, paved over, subdivided, or otherwise altered from its natural state. In other cities this would mean that hikers would be forced to look farther afield to find somewhere with wild trails to explore. Happily, that is not the case in the Portland/Vancouver region. In fact some of the finest trails in the area are either right in the city or just on its doorstep. And for pedestrians looking to keep in shape during those long wet months of winter, almost all of the trails at these lower elevations are open year-round.

Most of the available hiking is in a large network of city, state, county, and regional parks. But these aren't your typical city parks with picnic tables, ball fields, and playgrounds. No, these are truly *wild* preserves with dense forests, acres of wildflowers, lovely waterfalls, sparkling creeks, and plenty of wildlife. In addition to the parks, several local wildlife refuges feature hiking trails that are open to human visitors during seasons when the wildlife won't be disturbed.

Both Oregon and Washington have excellent trails in these heavily populated lowlands. On the north side of

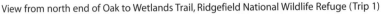
View from north end of Oak to Wetlands Trail, Ridgefield National Wildlife Refuge (Trip 1)

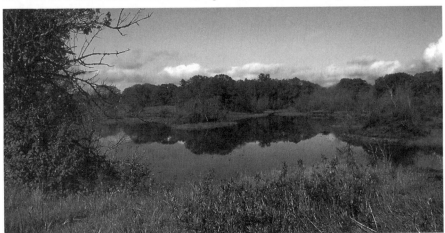

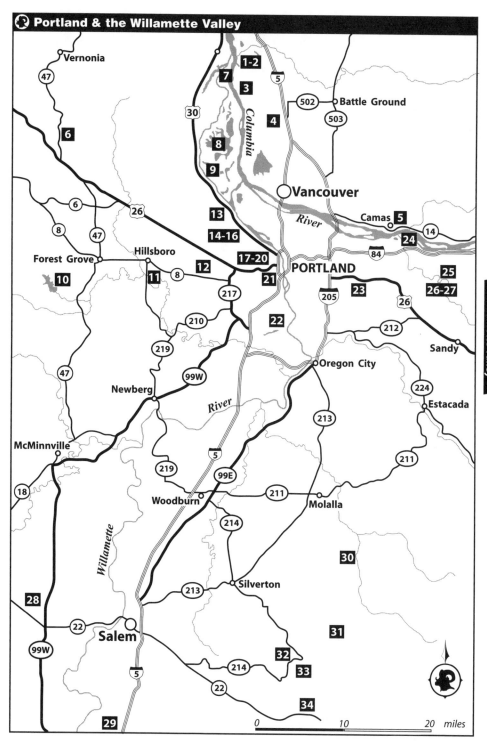

Vernonia

47

Battle Ground

502

503

6

30

Columbia

7

1-2

3

5

4

8

9

Vancouver

River

Camas 5

13

14-16

14

24

84

Hillsboro

17-20

PORTLAND

26

Forest Grove

6

8

47

12

21

25

26-27

10

11

8

217

23

26

205

22

210

212

Sandy

219

99W

Oregon City

Newberg

River

224

213

Estacada

McMinnville

5

211

18

219

99E

211

Woodburn

Molalla

214

30

213

Silverton

31

28

22

32

Salem

33

99W

5

214

34

22

29

0   10   20 miles

Portland & the
Willamette Valley

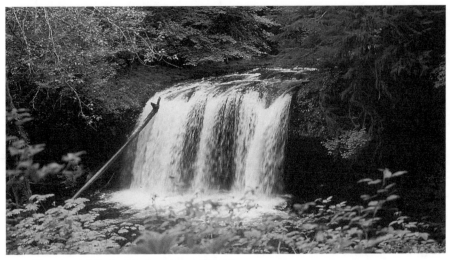

Upper Butte Creek Falls, Santiam State Forest (Trip 31)

the Columbia River the explorer will find plenty of good hiking in Ridgefield National Wildlife Refuge, one of the premier wildlife-viewing areas in the Portland region. And while fast-growing Vancouver offers very little for the hiker, the much smaller mill town of Camas proudly boasts Lacamas Creek Park, an outdoor treasure with scenery to rival any of the area's more famous (and distant) locations.

Just down the Columbia River from Portland sits Sauvie Island, a popular outdoor playground for local residents. The entire northern half of this large, nearly flat island is a state wildlife refuge filled with lakes, marshes, cottonwood forests, and fields that are home to waterfowl, bald eagles, sandhill cranes, and a host of other birds. There are trails here as well, and although visitors must purchase a day-use pass to park here, the rewards are well worth the price.

Scattered around the farmlands and small towns of the Willamette Valley south, west, and east of Portland are several parks and wildlife refuges featuring fine hiking trails. At Jackson Bottom, Ankeny Refuge, and Baskett Slough Ref-

uge wildlife sightings are virtually guaranteed, while Oxbow Regional Park and other sites along the Sandy River feature great scenery along a beautiful salmon stream amid old-growth forests. But top honors must go to Silver Falls State Park, where a dozen of the region's most spectacular waterfalls are bunched together in a wild forested canyon with scenery that will take your breath away.

Finally, even within the city limits are some outstanding hiking opportunities on surprisingly wild paths. Powell Butte Nature Park features stunning views while Tryon Creek State Park has excellent wildflower displays in a remarkably wild urban canyon. But for sheer urban hiking delight nothing in the region (in fact, nothing in the country) compares to Forest Park. At over 5000 acres, this is the largest forested city park in the U.S., and it truly is "wilderness"—the only human-made "improvements" are trails. The place is wild enough, in fact, that elk and even the occasional black bear live in the park. With many miles of interconnected trails and extremely easy access just blocks from downtown Portland, Forest Park is an urban hiker's dream.

TRIP 1 Ridgefield Refuge: Oak to Wetlands Trail

Distance	2.1 miles, Loop
Elevation Gain	150 feet
Hiking Time	1 hour
Optional Map	Use trailhead handout.
Usually Open	All year
Best Times	Winter for wildlife, late April for flowers
Trail Use	Good for kids, no dogs
Agency	Ridgefield National Wildlife Refuge
Difficulty	Easy
Note	Good in cloudy weather

HIGHLIGHTS This fine wildlife trail hits the most diverse and scenic terrain in Ridgefield National Wildlife Refuge, a generally overlooked local resource. Its easy circuit travels through habitat of a rich array of wildlife, including large concentrations of waterfowl in fall and winter. A visit in late April will delight you with colorful wildflowers. In winter and spring, the trail is often very muddy, so wear boots. Pets are not allowed in the refuge.

DIRECTIONS Take Exit 14 off Interstate 5 north of Vancouver, and drive west on State Highway 501 for 3 miles to the community of Ridgefield. At the west end of town, turn right at a T-junction with Main Street. After 1.1 miles, turn left on a well-signed gravel road that, in 200 yards, arrives at a large parking area at the trailhead.

A paved trail drops from the parking lot to an information kiosk where you can pick up a map and interpretive brochure for the nature trail. From here the trail climbs over an elaborately large, arcing bridge that spans three sets of railroad tracks. Immediately on the other side of the bridge, turn right at a junction and follow the Oak to Wetlands Trail through country that is entirely true to its name. Initially, the path wanders through grassy areas punctuated by large specimens of Oregon white oak, tangles of blackberries, and a wide variety of birds. Look for rufous-sided towhees, various sparrows, black-capped chickadees, ring-necked pheasants, and the ubiquitous American robin.

Soon the path passes a recreated Native American Cathlapotle plankhouse (visitors are welcome on weekend afternoons in spring and summer) and then drops to a viewing area for Duck Lake and its surrounding marshes, where the abundant avian life changes to such species as mallards, red-winged blackbirds, and marsh wrens. Unfortunately, another form of flying wildlife, mosquitoes, also make their home here. Other animals to look for are painted turtles and nutrias, which look like large muskrats, as they sun themselves on the opposite bank of the lake.

Stand of oak trees along the Oak to Wetlands Trail

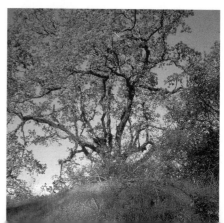

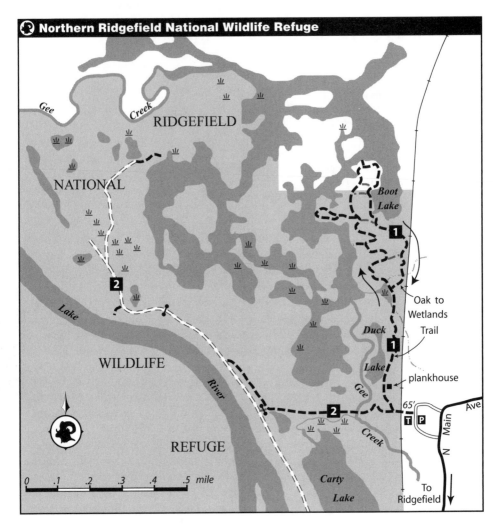

Northern Ridgefield National Wildlife Refuge

Past Duck Lake the trail returns to the oaks, crosses a small creek on a bridge, and shortly thereafter arrives at a fork. Both directions are part of the loop, but for now bear left and hike through a swath of blackberry brambles, whose rapidly growing vines have sharp thorns that rip through both skin and clothing, so keep your distance. Soon after entering a forest of Douglas fir, you veer left at another trail junction and continue to a 150-foot side trail to Site 9 on the nature trail, on a little bluff overlooking part of the marsh. The main trail goes through

lush forests with an understory of sword ferns and spring wildflowers like wood violet, twinflower, Oregon grape, and star-flowered smilacina.

Just as you emerge from the trees, you arrive at a junction with a trail that leads to a very worthwhile side trip visiting the most attractive terrain on this hike. To explore this area, go left at the junction. Some 10 feet later you will arrive at another junction with a smaller side loop to Site 11 on the nature trail. This side route leads to a nice overlook of the marsh, where you may see a great blue heron or double-crested cormorant. In late April, this overlook supports an abundance of wildflowers, especially yellow buttercups and pink onions.

To see the trip's best scenery, return from Site 11 and turn north on a trail that soon comes to a detour route that avoids the private property you are about to enter. The detour is mandatory from October 1 to the end of February, when the private property is closed to the public. In spring and summer, continue straight and hike up to Site 12, an open knoll with fine views of lakes, marshes, and woodlands. Carpeted with wildflow-

ers in late April, especially blue camas and pink onion, the knoll is indeed a choice lunch spot.

To return to your car, first complete the side loop that goes up and down along the shores of tranquil Boot Lake, and then turn left at the junction with the main loop and wander through lush, dense woods of Douglas fir, bigleaf maple, western red cedar, and Oregon white oak. You may hear trains going by on the nearby railroad tracks, but otherwise this is a pleasant, woodsy walk that takes you back to the junction with the return trail near Duck Lake.

TRIP 2 Ridgefield Refuge: Gee Creek Exploration

Distance	3.7 miles, Out-and-back
Elevation Gain	100 feet
Hiking Time	2 hours
Optional Map	None
Usually Open	All year (sometimes flooded in winter)
Best Times	Winter for wildlife, late April for flowers
Trail Use	Good for kids, no dogs
Agency	Ridgefield National Wildlife Refuge
Difficulty	Moderate
Note	Good in cloudy weather

HIGHLIGHTS If you didn't get enough exercise on the Oak to Wetlands Trail (Trip 1) or you're simply looking for a change of pace from established paths, try this excellent route. The trail here isn't officially maintained for hikers, but this entire portion of the refuge is open to the public. By exploring away from established routes, you can enjoy more solitude in a scenic setting. This area was originally set aside for the benefit of the many wildlife species that live here. To protect that wildlife, pets are strictly prohibited from the trail.

DIRECTIONS Take Exit 14 off Interstate 5 north of Vancouver, and drive west on State Highway 501 for 3 miles to the community of Ridgefield. At the west end of town, turn right at a T-junction with Main Street. After 1.1 miles, turn left on a well-signed gravel road that in 200 yards arrives at a large parking area at the trailhead.

A paved trail drops from the parking lot to an information kiosk and then climbs over a large, arcing bridge that spans three sets of railroad tracks. Immediately on the other side of the bridge,

the Oak to Wetlands Trail goes off to the right, but to explore the Gee Creek area you turn left.

The trail goes past some restrooms and then drops to a plank bridge over sluggish Gee Creek. From the bridge the path goes along a marsh at the north end of Carty Lake, where you are likely to see several species of water birds. In winter, look for ducks like mallard, pintail, and wigeon, as well as tundra swan and the ubiquitous great blue heron. In the adjoining marsh grasses and willow hedgerows are song sparrows and red-winged blackbirds. Much of this section will be muddy, and in some years it may even be flooded at this time of year, so rubber boots are best.

Where the trail comes to a gate, you turn right and parallel a brushy fence line. Follow this fence for several hundred yards to where you merge with a refuge maintenance road coming in from the left. Follow this rarely used road as it travels beside a thick hedgerow of blackberries, willows, and large cottonwood trees. The road goes through a usually open gate, cuts to the left through the trees, and emerges at an open area. From here, a 50-yard side trail on the left goes to an overlook of Lake River, a backwater slough of the Columbia River, where you may see double-crested cormorants, red-tailed hawks, and northern harriers.

This overlook is an acceptable turn-around point, but a much better one is still ahead. About 0.1 mile past the side trail, the rapidly diminishing road splits. The route to the left heads through more wet fields and hedgerows before petering out altogether amid grasses and scattered oak trees. The more interesting and attractive option from the road split goes to the right and travels through a strip of trees to reach a larger meadow with a nice view of snow-capped Mt. St. Helens.

Continue hiking northeast on the overgrown road to a fence, which you climb over on a metal ladder, and then ascend a little to a small, grassy, oak-covered knoll. The trail disappears here, but take the time to explore the many nearby oak-covered hills. Your efforts will be well rewarded with photogenic trees, spring wildflowers, and fine views of a large lake to the south. Birds you may see on this lake include great egrets, hooded mergansers, tundra swans, and various species of ducks. Bring a blanket, binoculars, and a sack lunch to sit in the grass under the shade of the oak trees and watch the wildlife in style. Once you've had your fill, return the way you came.

Gee Creek

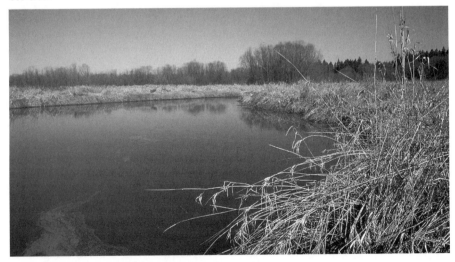

TRIP 3 Ridgefield Refuge: Kiwa Trail Loop

Distance	1.5 miles, Loop
Elevation Gain	Negligible
Hiking Time	1 to 2 hours
Optional Map	Use trailhead handout.
Usually Open	May 1 to September 30
Best Time	May
Trail Use	Good for kids, no dogs, wheelchair accessible
Agency	Ridgefield National Wildlife Refuge
Difficulty	Easy
Note	Good in cloudy weather

HIGHLIGHTS Wildlife is the star attraction of this nearly level hike. Birds in particular seem to be everywhere—standing in the marshes, flitting in the trees, floating on the lakes, swimming in the sloughs, and hunting among the meadow grasses. Experienced birders can easily identify 40 or 50 species in a single morning. The likely candidates include ducks, geese, herons, bitterns, rails, coots, sparrows, warblers, waxwings, eagles, hawks ... the list goes on and on. Mornings are especially productive, and spring brings the greatest variety (if not the greatest number) of birds. The trail is open from 8:30 AM to dusk from May 1 to September 30. Pets are not allowed in the refuge.

DIRECTIONS Drive Interstate 5 north from Vancouver, take Exit 14, and drive 2.6 miles west on State Highway 501 to the middle of Ridgefield. Turn left (south) on South 9th Avenue, which soon becomes Hillhurst Road, go 0.6 mile, and then turn right (west) on a gravel road at a large brown sign for Ridgefield National Wildlife Refuge. Drive 0.6 mile, cross a long wooden bridge, and soon come to a junction and a station where you must pay a day-use fee ($3 per vehicle, as of 2007). Turn right at the junction onto a one-way loop road and slowly proceed 1.5 miles to the signed trailhead parking lot.

The wide, gravel, wheelchair-accessible path goes north from a large trailhead signboard, crosses a bridge over sluggish Bower Slough, and soon comes to a junction at the start of the loop. For a counterclockwise tour turn right and enter a deciduous woodland alive with the sounds of birds. Warblers are especially common, but you may also see and hear towhees, vireos, sparrows, and flycatchers. This unusually diverse feathered assortment is the result of a unique mix of habitats. Woodlands, hedgerows, wet meadows, dry meadows, sloughs, marshes, and open water are all bunched together here, and the trail samples each of these zones.

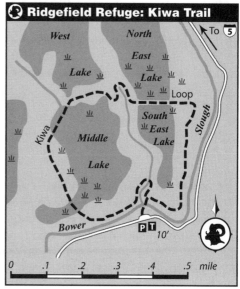

Ridgefield Refuge: Kiwa Trail

The first part of the hike travels through a pretty woodland environment between Bower Slough and South East Lake (really more of a marsh). At 0.5 mile, the trail turns left and passes a large wet meadow, where marsh birds are often seen. Look for American bitterns, marsh wrens, red-winged and yellow-headed blackbirds, and Virginia rails, among many others. On the nearby open water of South East Lake, ducks such as cinnamon teals, northern shovelers, mallards, and gadwalls are usually present.

You take a bridge over the end of a small slough, pass a hedgerow, and walk through more meadows. When the trail turns south it crosses a long boardwalk over the waters of marshy Middle Lake where geese, ducks, and pied-billed grebes are often seen. You then go through a drier meadow before crossing another boardwalk at the southwest end of Middle Lake. After turning east, the trail goes through the woods beside Bower Slough

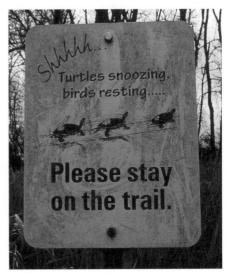

A sign along the Kiwa Trail

where turtles can sometimes be seen sunning themselves on logs. Finally, you cross a bridge over a small slough and return to the junction at the start of the loop. Turn right and retrace your steps to the parking lot.

TRIP 4 Whipple Creek Park Loop

Distance	2.7 miles or more, Loop
Elevation Gain	200 feet
Hiking Time	1½ hours
Optional Map	USGS *Ridgefield* (trails not shown)
Usually Open	All year
Best Time	April
Trail Use	Dogs OK, horseback riding
Agency	Clark County Parks
Difficulty	Easy
Note	Good in cloudy weather

HIGHLIGHTS Whipple Creek Park is a 375-acre county-owned wild area that has none of the ballfields, campgrounds, or other amenities usually associated with county parks. The only "improvements" in the park's heavily forested terrain are trails and even these have no signage to keep visitors from going astray. The park makes for fine exploring and even though the scenery does not rival that found at some of our area's mountain lakes or high viewpoints, the forest here is pretty and very peaceful. Despite this park's proximity

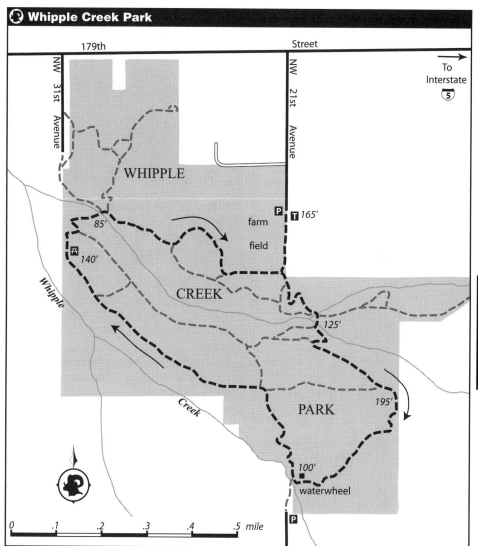

to an interstate, there are no highway sounds to disturb your walk, and serenity reigns supreme. Combine this with the area's easy access from Vancouver and Whipple Creek Park deserves more attention from the hiking community than it currently receives (close to none).

The park is adjacent to a riding stable and is very popular with equestrians. As a result, the trails can get quite muddy, especially in winter. Try to visit after a dry spell.

DIRECTIONS Drive Interstate 5 north from Vancouver and take Exit 9 for 179th Street. Turn left (west), go 1.6 miles, and then turn south on single-lane paved NW 21st Avenue, which is marked only with a DEAD END sign. Proceed 0.4 mile to the road's end and park in a large gravel lot.

There are dozens of possible hikes here, depending on which of the numerous trails you decide to explore. The loop described here sticks to the outer perimeter of the preserve, which makes it the longest option available. It is also one of the nicest because it visits some of the prettiest sections of forest, passes through a small meadow ideal for picnicking, and takes you past a historic waterwheel.

Hike 150 yards south on a wide and obvious dirt path to a junction at the southeast corner of a farm field. The path to the right, which travels the edge between the farm field and the park's forest, is the return route of the recommended loop.

You bear left and immediately enter a tangled forest of second-growth Douglas firs with some western red cedars, bigleaf maples, and Oregon white oaks mixed in. Just 50 yards after your first junction is the next one, and the start of dozens more, none of which are signed. Carefully follow the description here and the accompanying map to ensure that you remain on course. You keep left at the junction and make a brief but steep descent into a ravine where there are several more junctions and a bridged crossing of a tiny creek.

The recommended loop goes straight at two quick junctions on either side of the bridge and soon takes you over another creek and to another fork, where you veer left. This path quickly climbs out of the ravine to yet another junction, where you turn left again. The forest in this area is particularly lush and attractive, with plenty of wildlife, ranging in size from large black-tailed deer to tiny winter wrens. Ignoring yet another side path coming in from the right, you loop around the east side of the park, briefly passing a fenced pastureland, but mostly staying in attractive woodlands. In April,

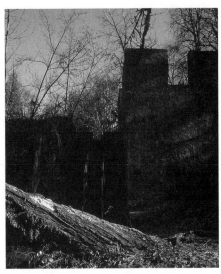

Old waterwheel near the park's southern end

forest wildflowers make their appearance, especially the cheerful white blossoms of trillium.

The up-and-down route eventually leads to the southern end of the park and the remains of an old waterwheel, which was nicely restored by a local church group in 1997. Nearby is a junction with a spur trail coming in from the south. Keep right, wind uphill for 0.2 mile, and then keep left at the next two junctions, which come in rapid succession. These turns keep you on the outer loop trail, which here is highlighted by views of marshy Whipple Creek below you on the left. You also pass two magnificent old bigleaf maple trees, the limbs and trunks festooned with moss and licorice ferns. Just after the second of these trees you keep left at a junction and soon pass through a small brushy meadow filled with grasses and bracken ferns. A picnic table at the northwest corner of this meadow makes an ideal lunch spot.

A brief downhill from the meadow leads to another junction, where you veer left (downhill) and walk 120 yards to a crossing of a small creek and, what else, another junction. Go right this time, and right again just 30 yards later where a narrow trail branches uphill to the left. You climb a bit, leaving the creek, and come to yet another junction. Turn left, walk 0.15 mile, go left again, and very

quickly reach the southwest corner of the farm field you passed at the start of the trip. Walk along the southern edge of the field to the junction at its corner and then make a final left turn to complete your hike.

TRIP 5 Lacamas Creek Park Loop

Distance	3.4 miles, Semiloop
Elevation Gain	400 feet
Hiking Time	2 hours
Optional Map	Use trailhead signboards.
Usually Open	All year
Best Time	Late April to early May
Trail Use	Good for kids, dogs OK, fishing
Agency	Clark Parks & Recreation Department
Difficulty	Easy
Note	Good in cloudy weather

HIGHLIGHTS Camas is a small, unassuming mill town on the Washington side of the Columbia River that most outdoor lovers drive right past on their way to better-known attractions in the Columbia River Gorge. But the 6000 or so residents of this town have a secret that outsiders have yet to discover. Lacamas Creek Park, a 325-acre preserve, is one of the wildest and most attractive city parks in the country. Hidden in this park are unusually varied and attractive woods, beautiful waterfalls, a tranquil lake, lots of birds, and some of the best low-elevation wildflowers in the Portland area. This loop hike visits all of the park's numerous highlights and is one of my favorite easy hikes in the Portland/Vancouver area. It perfectly showcases the subtle charms of our region.

DIRECTIONS From Vancouver, drive east on State Highway 14 about 6 miles past the junction with Interstate 205 and take Exit 12 to Camas. Drive the exit road for 1.4 miles and then turn right at a four-way flashing stoplight. After three blocks, turn left on N.E. 3rd Avenue and 0.8 mile later, just before you cross Lacamas Creek, turn left on an unsigned lane that looks like a private driveway. About 50 yards down this road is a small trailhead parking lot. Be sure not to block a small, private gravel driveway when you park.

Walk north past a house and go around the park's entry gate to a trailhead signboard. The wide gravel path wanders north, staying above the rushing waters of Lacamas Creek and traveling through bigleaf-maple woods that in April and May come alive with the sounds of songbirds. Under the maples are common shrubs like holly, salmon-

berry, and thimbleberry, while the forest floor features the blossoms of false Solomon's seal, wild strawberry, bleeding heart, and fairybells.

After 0.25 mile you go straight at a junction with a side trail that goes off to the left and climbs to a residential area. The main trail rolls up and down through a forest where the bigleaf maples are

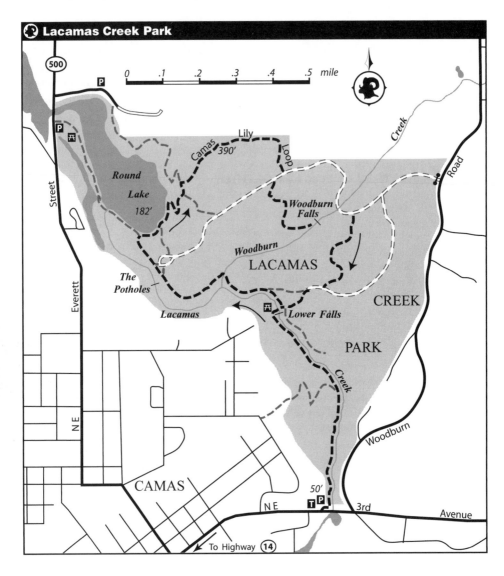

joined by stately Douglas fir and western hemlock. The forest floor is crowded with at least four different types of ferns: lady fern, maidenhair fern, bracken fern, and sword fern. A little more than 0.3 mile from the last junction, the trail comes to a pair of picnic tables and then crosses Lacamas Creek on a sturdy metal bridge just upstream from Lower Falls, an impressive sliding cascade.

On the east side of the bridge is an unsigned four-way junction. To the right,

a winding, unofficial trail goes downstream along the east bank of Lacamas Creek providing some decent views of Lower Falls. To begin the loop, you turn left and walk upstream beside the beautifully cascading creek to a wooden bridge across smaller Woodburn Creek. Above this bridge you go through a grove of lovely western red cedar before climbing a little to an open rocky meadow. In late April this meadow is filled with perky blue camas. Take the time to sit in this scenic meadow and look down on a short but impressive waterfall on Lacamas Creek called the Potholes.

Just a few feet past the meadow, you reach the end of a gravel service road and skirt around the left side of the road's turnaround loop. The path goes north for about 100 yards, past several unmarked side trails, to a junction with a wide path beside tranquil Round Lake. Turning left here takes you to a busy, manicured playground and picnic area typical of most city parks. For a wilder experience, turn right, and you will soon reach a junction at the southeast corner of the lake. You turn left here and make two short switchbacks up a hillside covered with vine maple and Douglas fir, to a junction near the top of the hill.

Turn left at the junction and after 100 yards turn right on the Camas Lily Loop. Although most trails in this park are open to mountain bikers, the Camas Lily Loop goes through a designated natural area that is open only to foot travel. The path climbs steeply but briefly to an open meadow surrounded by Oregon white oak and white avalanche lilies. In the meadow itself is an abundance of blue camas. This is probably the best place in the Portland area to enjoy this lovely flower, which in the centuries before pavement and plowed fields was very common in the natural meadows of the Willamette Valley.

There are many side trails exploring the meadow, all of which are worthwhile, but for the loop you stay left at all questionable junctions. The main path skirts the outside edge of several meadows and then descends through evergreen woods to a junction with a closed gravel access road. For a fine short side trip here, go right about 100 yards, turn left, and walk downhill on a 0.2-mile side trail that dead-ends at the base of joyful Woodburn Falls, which cascades over a mossy rock ledge.

To complete the loop, return to the closed gravel road and walk east. The road loops down to the right to cross small Woodburn Creek on a wide bridge before ascending briefly to a junction. You turn right and walk a narrow gravel route through strikingly attractive mixed woods. In the spring, you might hear the eerie, high-pitched cries of ospreys, which live in this area. Here they find good nest sites in the tall snags, and plenty of fish to eat from Lacamas Creek, Round Lake, and the nearby Columbia River. The trail drops to a poorly marked junction with a wider gravel path, where you turn right and almost immediately return to the bridge just above Lower Falls. Cross the bridge and return the way you came.

Woodburn Falls

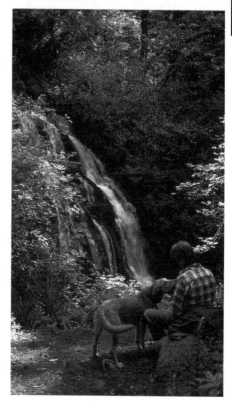

TRIP 6 Stub Stewart State Park: Linear Trail

Distance	4.3 miles, Out-and-back
Elevation Gain	300 feet
Hiking Time	2 hours
Optional Map	USGS *Buxton*
Usually Open	All year
Best Time	Any
Trail Use	Good for kids, dogs OK, wheelchair accessible, mountain biking, horseback riding
Agency	Stub Stewart State Park
Difficulty	Easy
Note	Good in cloudy weather

HIGHLIGHTS The Banks-Vernonia State Linear Trail is easily both Oregon's longest and its narrowest state park. The 21-mile route follows the grade of an abandoned logging railroad and is quite popular with hikers, equestrians, and mountain bikers. Although attractive, the rural landscape of pastures, woodlots, and farm fields is not "wild," so most of the trail has been excluded from this hiking guide. The section north from the Buxton Trailhead, however, travels through heavily forested terrain, where the sights and sounds of cars and farm machinery are left behind. Most of this area is now one of Oregon's newest state parks.

With its opening in late spring of 2007, 1654-acre Stub Stewart State Park is Oregon's first new full-service park in decades and will eventually include car campgrounds, picnic areas, and many miles of trails. As of this writing, the construction, especially of trails, was still underway. In years to come, hikers can expect plenty of interesting new paths to explore, but for now the 4 miles of the Linear Trail that passes through the new park is the best option for pedestrians.

DIRECTIONS Drive U.S. Highway 26 west from Portland to its junction with State Highway 47 near milepost 45. Turn right (north) on Highway 47, drive 0.3 mile, and then turn right on Fisher Road. Proceed 0.5 mile to a T-junction and turn left on Bacona Road. Go another 0.6 mile, and then turn right into the large Buxton Trailhead parking lot.

Before hiking the recommended trail, take a few minutes to check out the Buxton railroad trestle just 100 yards south of the trailhead. This impressive monument to early railroad engineering towers 100 feet over the meadow-lined banks of Mendenhall Creek and really should not be missed. Although the top of the trestle is closed to hikers, the structure can easily be viewed from the trail below and explored at either end.

Once you've checked out the trestle, walk the paved path going northwest from the trailhead, pass a tiny pond, and soon come to the turnoff of the access road to the parking lot. The northbound Linear Trail starts on the west side of Bacona Road behind a prominent gate just to the left (south) of a private driveway. For its entire distance, the trail is about 12 feet wide and has a gravel surface. Since it used to be a railroad grade, the trail is very gentle with a barely noticeable uphill grade and no sharp turns.

For its first 200 yards the trail is within sight of roads and farms, but as the route gradually curves to the right (north) these sights are replaced by the more natural

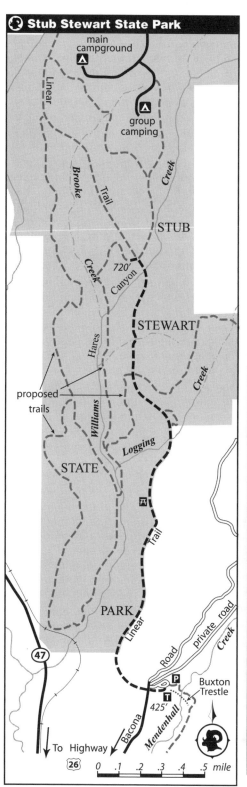

Stub Stewart State Park

appearance of a dense second-growth forest of mostly Douglas firs. As you head north the trail crosses numerous small ravines, where the conifers give way to a thick tangle of red alders and other deciduous trees. Several openings along the way provide nice views of the Coast Range to the west. Closer at hand, on the hillside immediately above the trail, you pass several areas that were replanted after clear-cutting and/or forest fires.

At 1 mile is a horse-hitching post and a remote picnic area with two tables. From here the trail continues north, soon crossing a deep alder-choked ravine resonating with the cheerful sounds of Logging Creek far below. Just 110 yards later a new foot trail, marked only with an old yellow railroad crossing sign, branches off to the

Old Buxton railroad trestle

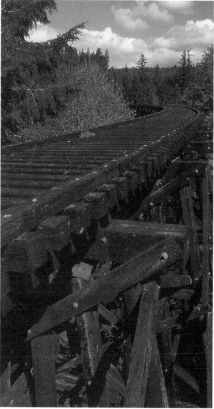

right and goes steeply uphill. This is the first of several new paths you will see in the park. Though hikers should ignore this one, which simply loops back to the main trail in about 200 yards, other trails provide more interesting diversions. One such route is an on-again-off-again foot trail that closely parallels the Linear Trail on the left (west side). It provides the same woodsy scenery but takes you away from the occasional piles of equestrian "leftovers" found on the main trail.

At 1.7 miles is a four-way junction. Go straight on the Linear Trail and soon cross yet another ravine. Interpretive signs describe how this ravine was once spanned by a wooden railroad trestle (now long gone). About 0.3 mile later you cross Williams Creek, which flows through heavily forested Hares Canyon, Stub Stewart State Park's dominate geographic feature.

Just past the road fill spanning Hares Canyon, and 2.1 miles from the trailhead, is another four-way junction. To the right a trail (still closed as of early 2007) is scheduled to go uphill to the park's group camping area atop a view-filled knoll. The trail to the left goes 100 yards to an overlook just above the rotting remains of another railroad trestle. This is the logical turnaround point, because north of here the Linear Trail soon reaches the more developed parts of the park and is less of a wilderness experience.

TRIP 7 Warrior Rock

Distance	6.8 miles, Out-and-back
Elevation Gain	Negligible
Hiking Time	3 to 4 hours
Optional Map	None needed
Usually Open	All year
Best Time	All year
Trail Use	Good for kids, dogs OK (on leash only)
Agency	Sauvie Island Wildlife Area
Difficulty	Moderate

HIGHLIGHTS At the northern tip of Sauvie Island is a quiet sandy beach that is ideally suited for watching ocean-going ships sail past while enjoying views of the city of St. Helens just across the water. In season, the hike provides opportunities either to observe wildlife (winter) or to pick delicious blackberries (summer). If you bring the family pet, keep in mind that all dogs must be on leash.

DIRECTIONS Drive U.S. Highway 30 northwest from downtown Portland about 10 miles to a traffic light where you turn right and immediately cross a bridge onto Sauvie Island. Once across the bridge, the road curves north and in 0.2 mile reaches Sam's Grocery, where you can purchase a day-use parking pass ($3.50 per vehicle as of 2007). Now that you can legally park on the island, continue north on Sauvie Island Road 1.8 miles, and then turn right on Reeder Road. Stick with this road for 4.2 miles through a few minor intersections to a stop sign. Go straight, still on Reeder Road, and follow it for 6.3 miles until the road becomes gravel. Then follow it another 2.3 miles until it ends at a gravel turnaround.

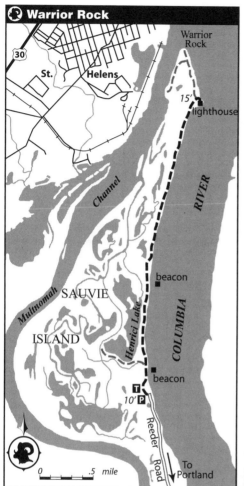

of the route is lined with huge cottonwood trees and a tangle of blackberry brambles. In mid- to late August, the abundant berries of these thorny plants afford an irresistible temptation to turn your tongue and fingers purple, so allow plenty of time for picking and eating.

At several points along the way unsigned side roads and trails go off to the left, visiting various lakes and small ponds. At all junctions stick to the main road, which always stays straight or bends to the right. In the spring, the mud along the road is a good place to look for the tracks of deer and raccoons.

After nearly 3 miles, the narrowing road fades away as it enters a small grassy meadow and comes to a fork. A couple of hundred yards to the right is a tiny lighthouse (closed to the public) and a secluded beach, the ideal spot for watching freighters go by. If you go left at the fork, you follow a foot trail beside a beach on the north shore of the island. After 0.5 mile you'll find some pilings where there is a nice view of the historic town of St. Helens to the west.

Warrior Rock Lighthouse

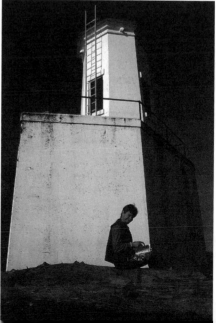

You go through a fence stile on the west side of the parking lot and then follow an overgrown jeep track that loops north through a pasture where you'll have to step carefully to avoid smelly cow pies. In addition to cows, this grassy field often accommodates a flock of geese in winter. If you see the birds suddenly scatter for no apparent reason, be sure to check the skies for one possible cause: bald eagles, several of which spend the winter here.

At the north end of the field, go over or around another gate and pick up the rough refuge-maintenance road that you will follow for the rest of the hike. Much

TRIP 8 Oak Island Loop

Distance	2.4 miles, Semiloop
Elevation Gain	Negligible
Hiking Time	2 hours
Optional Map	None needed
Usually Open	April 16 to September 30
Best Time	Any time it's open
Trail Use	Good for kids, dogs OK (on leash only)
Agency	Sauvie Island Wildlife Area
Difficulty	Easy
Note	Good in cloudy weather

HIGHLIGHTS Oak Island is technically a peninsula because the shallow, murky waters of Sturgeon Lake surround only three sides. But why worry about technicalities when you can enjoy such a splendid spot? This easy nature trail is probably the nicest hike on Sauvie Island because of its diversity of habitats, good views, and abundant wildlife. You can even learn something by picking up the trailhead handout, which explains the natural and the Native American history at various marked stops along the way. Dogs must be on a leash.

DIRECTIONS Drive U.S. Highway 30 northwest from downtown Portland about 10 miles to a traffic light, where you turn right and immediately cross a bridge onto Sauvie Island. Once across the bridge, the road curves north and in 0.2 mile reaches Sam's Grocery, where you can purchase a day-use parking pass ($3.50 per vehicle as of 2007). Now that you can legally park on the island, continue north on Sauvie Island Road for 1.8 miles and then turn right on Reeder Road. Drive this route 1.1 miles and then veer left onto N.W. Oak Island Road. Follow this road 3.1 miles to the end of pavement at a gate that is closed at 10 PM, to enforce the refuge's day-use only policy. Go straight through the gate and drive 1.0 mile farther, following signs for a nature trail, to the parking lot beside a second gate and signboard at the road's end.

A fter walking around this gate you will immediately come to a fork in the road. Bear left onto a lesser-used jeep route signed with a small yellow hiker symbol. This route goes north through oak woodlands, past lots of blackberry brambles, and into some open areas where a few blue camases bloom in late April and May. As you hike, you may enjoy the sight of cute little cottontail rabbits or fast-running California quail scurrying away into the brush. Also making their home here are black-tailed deer, northern flickers, song sparrows, various warblers, mourning doves, and other wildlife.

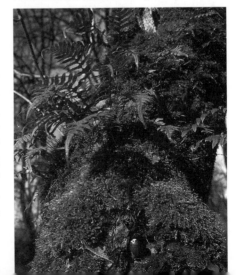

Ferns and moss on a tree trunk, Sauvie Island

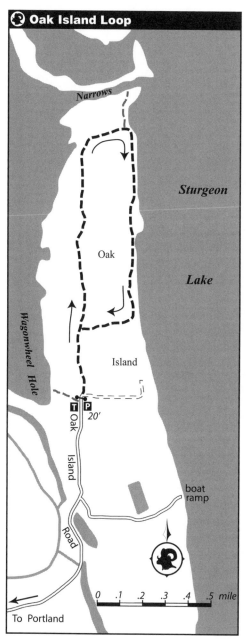

Oak Island Loop

Narrows

Sturgeon

Oak

Lake

Island

Wagonwheel Hole

T P
20'

Oak
Island
Road

boat
ramp

0   .1   .2   .3   .4   .5 mile

To Portland

At a junction after about 0.2 mile, the trail forks to form the loop. For a clockwise loop, go straight and hike beside a large cultivated field on the left and a wild oak woodland on the right. After going north for about 0.8 mile, the trail goes through a small stand of cottonwoods, where colorful northern orioles nest, and then turns right. The route now heads east for a short distance to the shores of Sturgeon Lake. To the northeast, snowy Mt. St. Helens looms like a conical, flat-topped cloud. In the shallow waters of the lake, large carp rise to the surface and make quite a ruckus with their splashing.

The trail turns south at the lake and follows its shore for about 0.8 mile to a small, rocky beach. Here the trail veers to the right at a yellow hiker sign and closes the loop with an easy stroll through oak woodlands to the junction north of the parking lot.

If you still have a bit of energy, it is worth your time to take an unmarked trail that goes 0.1 mile to the west from the parking lot across a grassy area to Wagonwheel Hole, a shallow lake with nice views of the wooded hills to the west. Animal tracks are common in the mud near the water.

TRIP 9 Virginia Lake Loop

Distance	2.2 miles, Loop
Elevation Gain	Negligible
Hiking Time	1½ hours
Optional Map	None needed
Usually Open	April 16 to September 30
Best Time	Any time it's open
Trail Use	Good for kids, dogs OK (on leash only), fishing
Agency	Sauvie Island Wildlife Area
Difficulty	Easy
Note	Good in cloudy weather

HIGHLIGHTS This very easy loop goes around a marshy, wildlife-rich lake and visits Multnomah Channel, where anglers can try their luck in the Columbia River backwater. Like all trails on Sauvie Island, this is a good choice for hikers with children, as the trail sports lots of wildlife and doesn't gain any significant amount of elevation. In August, both kids and parents will enjoy eating the delicious blackberries that ripen there. Dogs must be on a leash.

DIRECTIONS Drive U.S. Highway 30 northwest from downtown Portland about 10 miles to a traffic light, where you turn right and immediately cross a bridge onto Sauvie Island. Once across the bridge, the road curves north and in 0.2 mile reaches Sam's Grocery, where you can purchase a day-use parking pass ($3.50 per vehicle as of 2007). Now that you can legally park on the island, continue north on Sauvie Island Road for 1.8 miles to a junction where you go straight. After 0.6 mile you turn left into a small gravel parking lot for the Wapato Greenway Access.

You hop over a gate across a maintenance road and hike west 100 yards on a jeep route beside a hedgerow. At an unsigned junction a hiking trail veers to the left, while the jeep road goes right. For a clockwise loop, follow the trail to the left, which goes along the edge of a grassy field beside a brushy area of blackberry brambles and cherry trees. As you hike, listen and watch for song sparrows, western meadowlarks, American robins, rufous-sided towhees, yellowthroats, and a variety of other songbirds. After 0.1 mile you hit a junction with a wide gravel track and turn left.

This trail stays in the shade of tall black cottonwoods as it loops around the edge of a large marsh called Virginia Lake. Along the way you pass a wildlife-viewing blind, a little before crossing over the end of the marsh. Then you wander through a cottonwood forest to the next unsigned junction, where a 150-yard dead-end trail goes off to the left to Hadley's Landing, a fishing pier and boat dock on Multnomah Channel.

If you go right at the loop trail junction, you travel north through a shady strip of cottonwoods and brush with Multnomah Channel on the left and Virginia Lake on the right. Although poison oak is rare here, there are more than enough thorny blackberry vines and stinging nettles to discourage off-trail exploration. In the spring, this stretch of trail is especially nice early in the morning when all the birds are singing.

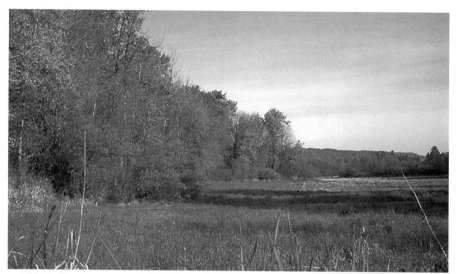

Virginia Lake

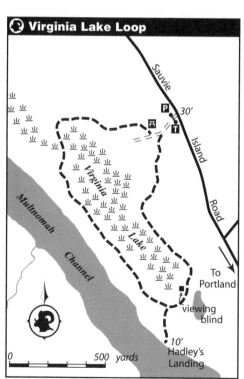

After about 1 mile, the trail curves right and crosses the end of the Virginia Lake marsh on a short boardwalk. Now you climb very briefly and then turn south on slightly higher ground past farms, grassy fields, and scattered oaks and Douglas firs. If you brought binoculars, you will have the chance to search the marsh for great blue herons, cinnamon teals, red-winged blackbirds, mallards, and other water-loving birds that make the marsh home. After about 0.6 mile, you come to a junction beside a covered picnic shelter, where you turn left and close out the loop with a short stroll back to your car.

TRIP **10** Henry Hagg Lake Loop

Distance	13.1 miles, Loop
Elevation Gain	250 feet
Hiking Time	6½ hours
Optional Map	Unnecessary
Usually Open	All year
Best Time	Early to mid-April
Trail Use	Dogs OK, mountain biking, fishing
Agency	Bureau of Reclamation
Difficulty	Difficult

HIGHLIGHTS The trail around Henry Hagg Lake, an artificial reservoir built in 1975, comes as something of a surprise to wilderness lovers. You'd never expect to find such a pleasantly wild footpath around a reservoir, especially one with a good paved highway circling it. But the trail builders did such an admirable job of routing this path that hikers can enjoy something close to a wilderness experience, despite nearby distractions.

If you visit in the first part of April, when the developed recreation sites surrounding the lake are not yet open, the wilderness feeling is greatly enhanced. Fortunately, early April is also a particularly scenic time to take this hike because of the abundance of forest wildflowers and the budding leaves on the trees. You will have to carry all of your own water at this time of year, however, because the piped water sources at the picnic areas will not yet be available. The path is closed to horses but is open to mountain bikes and, in fact, the circuit is a wonderful trip for bicyclists.

DIRECTIONS Drive State Highway 47 south from Forest Grove almost 4 miles and turn right (west) on the well-signed road to Scoggins Valley Park and Henry Hagg Lake. Continue for 4 miles to the large earthen dam that creates the reservoir. An elaborately large fee booth collects a day-use charge from late April through September ($5 per vehicle as of 2007). There are at least a dozen places you could start this loop trip, but if you visit before the recreation sites are open, you'll have to park at one of the lots beside the main road or, as recommended here, at the gravel parking lot below the dam just south of the entrance booth.

From the lower lot you follow a narrow gravel road up a grassy slope to the top of the dam. For a counterclockwise loop, cross the road atop the dam and follow a fence line about 0.2 mile to a paved road that is gated and closed in the off-season. As at all places where the trail touches a road, the trailhead is marked by a rust-colored post.

To pick up the trail, walk down toward the lake and look for the path leaving the parking area about 100 yards north. The surprisingly quiet trail goes up and down as it zigzags in and out of

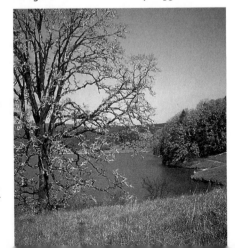

Along the north shore of Henry Hagg Lake

forested side canyons with picturesque bridges over trickling creeks. The forests are surprisingly open, and feature pretty April-blooming wildflowers like wood violet, trillium, and slender toothwort. The murky, greenish waters of the lake are almost always visible through the trees, and you will often hear waves lapping up against the shore. As you hike this circuit you will pass dozens of short spur trails (far too many to list in this text) that take off to the right leading to the road, but in all cases the proper route for continuing to circle the lake is unmistakable. Somewhat less frequent but more worthwhile are the many short routes leading down to the lake. Almost all these paths end at choice picnic spots.

After 1.3 miles, you cross a paved boat-ramp parking area. The trail resumes at the west end of the lot as an all-accessible paved trail. You walk past a couple scenic picnic sites, then path becomes dirt again, and you make a long detour through pleasant forests around a large arm of the reservoir. In these woods listen for the surprisingly loud song of winter wrens and, in the spring, the drumming of ruffed grouse. You can see an inviting and attractive grassy hillside on the opposite shore of the lake. The trail continues to the end of the lake arm, where you cross a small creek over a culvert and then briefly touch the road at a trailhead.

The path now passes several sturdy picnic tables before emerging on the grassy hillside you saw from the opposite

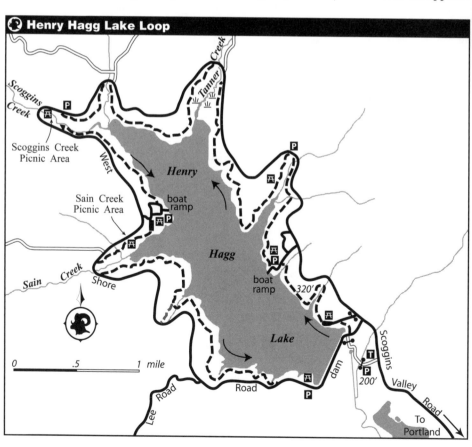

Henry Hagg Lake Loop

Scoggins Creek

Scoggins Creek Picnic Area

Tanner Creek

West

Henry

Sain Creek Picnic Area

boat ramp

Sain Creek

Shore

Hagg

boat ramp

320'

Lake

0   .5   1 mile

Lee Road

Road

Road

dam

200'

Scoggins

Valley Road

To Portland

shore, a fine place to lazily lie in the grass and enjoy a tranquil view. From this grassy area you return to a second-growth forest of western red cedar, Douglas fir, red alder, grand fir, and bigleaf maple, as the up-and-down trail alternates between woods and grassy overlooks framed by oak trees. After passing through more woods, the path travels just below the road, along the edge of a marshy area, before climbing briefly to the road shoulder.

The route then follows the road shoulder for about 250 yards to cross a bridge over Tanner Creek, where you return to a true trail. This path travels through more scenic grassy areas and marshes alive with red-winged blackbirds. You must negotiate several muddy spots as you round two small arms of the lake, before coming to a large gravel parking area. Follow the road for 0.4 mile past the attractive Scoggins Creek Picnic Area and then go over a road bridge that spans clear, rushing Scoggins Creek.

Not far from this creek, you turn left onto a footpath and then make several steep little ups and downs near the lake in a pleasant mix of woods, artificial rocky areas, and grassy slopes. You then come to a large boat ramp and picnic area, which are very busy in the summer months. You cross two large parking lots before returning to the trail. Another 0.3 mile of hiking takes you to the more intimate Sain Creek Picnic Area, after which you round yet another arm of the reservoir and follow the road again to cross Sain Creek itself.

The final segment of the path is more of the same—skirting arms of the lake, passing through woods alive with flowers like calipso orchid and wood violet, and crossing grassy areas. You often approach but never quite reach the road. The footpath ends about 0.2 mile before you reach the south end of the dam. From here you follow the road past a large gravel parking area and then over the dam and back down to your car.

TRIP **11** Jackson Bottom Wetlands Loop

Distance	1.8 miles, Semiloop
Elevation Gain	100 feet
Hiking Time	1 hour
Optional Map	Trailhead handout
Usually Open	All year
Best Time	November to April (for wildlife)
Trail Use	Good for kids, no dogs
Agency	Jackson Bottom Wetlands Preserve
Difficulty	Easy
Note	Good in cloudy weather

HIGHLIGHTS As science increases human understanding of natural ecosystems, our appreciation of what used to be considered wasteland has changed. For example, what used to be worthless jungles are now seen as invaluable rain forests, the loss of which is now widely considered a global crisis. On a domestic level, there once were swamps, which had to be drained and put to more "productive" uses. Now they are wetlands with recognized value as wildlife habitats, flood-control areas, and natural filters for water pollutants. Like tropical rain forests, the loss of wetlands is now seen as a matter of grave concern.

Jackson Bottom is a precious remnant of the Willamette Valley's once extensive wetlands. With all but a few such areas long since filled and converted into shopping malls or agricultural land, wildlife is increasingly dependent on the tiny wetlands that remain. A visit to this 650-acre preserve gives hikers a chance to see a great blue heron colony, rafts of waterfowl, and aquatic mammals such as muskrats, beavers, and river otters. Pets are not allowed on the trails in this wildlife preserve.

DIRECTIONS Begin by driving to downtown Hillsboro, about 15 miles west of Portland. Turn south on State Highway 219 (South First Avenue), and 1.4 miles later turn left into the large paved parking lot for the Clean Water Services Wetland Education Center.

From the southwest corner of the parking area, the trail drops on wooden steps into dense riverside vegetation and turns downstream. For tangible proof of the abundance of wildlife in Jackson Bottom, take some time to look beside the slow-moving water in search of tracks in the mud. In the spring, warblers fill the air with their distinctive songs, and in winter the sounds of honking geese give hikers a thrill.

The dirt path (sometimes muddy in winter) follows the river to a junction with a trail that is covered with wood chips to reduce the mud problems. You turn right at this junction and travel between the

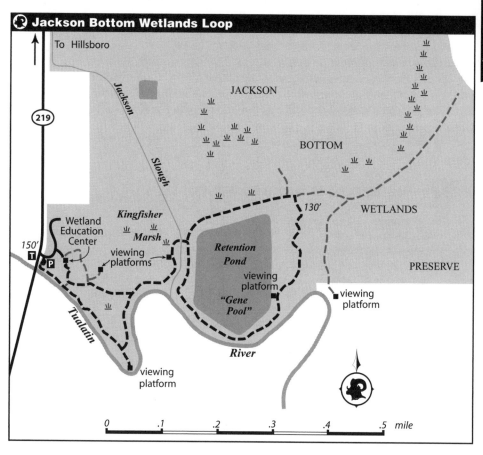

Jackson Bottom Wetlands Loop

To Hillsboro

Jackson

JACKSON

219

Slough

BOTTOM

WETLANDS

130'

Wetland
Education
Center

Kingfisher

Marsh

150'

viewing
platforms

*Retention
Pond*

PRESERVE

viewing
platform

*"Gene
Pool"*

viewing
platform

Tualatin

River

viewing
platform

0   .1   .2   .3   .4   .5   mile

dense riparian vegetation on your right and grassy Kingfisher Marsh on your left. Numerous interpretive signs, all drawn and written by local elementary-school children, add to the enjoyment of this hike, as do the many benches where you can rest and listen to the birds. Hundreds of bird houses erected by local wildlife enthusiasts are clearly appreciated by our feathered friends, who happily make use of these nesting sites.

The level path comes to a dead end at a viewing platform at a curve in the Tualatin River. To return to the loop trail, retrace your steps about 100 feet, and then turn north on a trail that soon reconnects with the woodchip-covered route you left earlier. The trail now travels north beside small Jackson Slough and soon comes to a viewing shelter that overlooks Kingfisher Marsh to the west and a large retention pond (sometimes called the "Gene Pool") to the east. You will cheer for the swallows that zip past your head here in search of insects, as there seems to be no shortage of blood-sucking mosquitoes.

The trail crosses a bridge over Jackson Slough, where you may hear the raucous call of marsh wrens. It then splits to loop around the retention pond. Turn right and walk through the tall grasses back to the trees beside the Tualatin River, and then curve left and pass between the river and the retention pond through an area of overgrown shrubbery. After leaving the trees, you come to another viewing shelter and then zigzag through grassy areas to a junction with a maintenance road at the northeast corner of the pond. For a longer hike you can turn right here and explore trails leading to more wetlands and viewing platforms to the east and southeast, but for the recommended loop turn left and walk the sometimes muddy road back to the junction at the bridge over Jackson Slough.

For variety on the return trip, you can skip the riverside path and take the trail in the grasses north of the river. This path passes a spur to yet another viewing platform, shortly before ending amid the maze of paved trails near the Wetland Education Center and parking area.

TRIP 12 Tualatin Hills Nature Park Loop

Distance	2.1 miles, Loop
Elevation Gain	50 feet
Hiking Time	1½ hours
Optional Map	Use trailhead handout.
Usually Open	All year
Best Time	All year
Trail Use	Good for kids, no dogs
Agency	Tualatin Hills Park & Recreation District
Difficulty	Easy
Note	Good in cloudy weather

HIGHLIGHTS The Tualatin Hills Nature Park does not provide a wilderness experience. At just 220 acres, this little suburban oasis is too small to truly escape the sights and sounds of the outside world. In addition, the park is so popular you are almost constantly in the company of other park users pushing baby carriages, jogging, or quietly enjoying the trails. But the park itself and its landscapes are still quite wild, and in at least one way they are even more natural than many locations farther from the city. In the park, efforts have been made to remove nonnative plants like English ivy, so the mosaic of species here consists primarily of native vegetation. There is also a wide assortment of wildlife to enjoy, including muskrats, beavers, roughskin newts, and dozens of species of birds. Bring a pair of binoculars and several nature guides to fully enjoy this hike.

DIRECTIONS The best access is from the Interpretive Center in the southeast corner of the preserve. To reach it, take Murray Boulevard either 0.3 mile north from State Highway 8 (the Tualatin Valley Highway) or 2.1 miles south from the Murray Road exit off U.S. Highway 26. In either case, you reach a traffic light and turn west on Millikan Way. Take this route 0.7 mile past a traffic light, and turn right at the well-signed turnoff into the parking lot.

The trailhead on the north side of the Interpretive Center is marked by a large signboard, where you can gather general information about the park and pick up a trail map. The paved trail goes for about 200 feet to a junction that, like

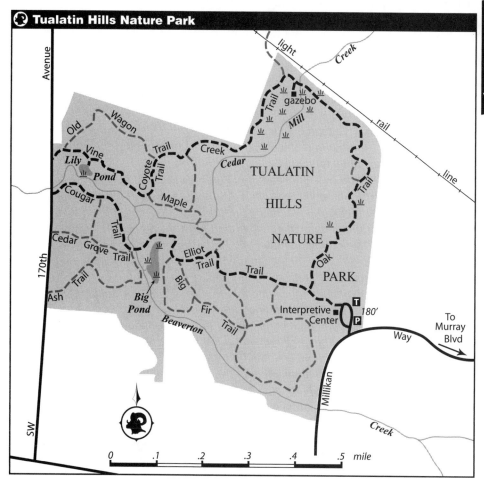

Tualatin Hills Nature Park

all the junctions in the park, is marked by a small post identifying the trails and distances. There are many good options from this point. For the recommended loop, turn right on the paved Oak Trail and wander this circuitous path through lovely second-growth forests.

The trees are a mix of Douglas fir, red alder, Oregon white oak, western red cedar, Pacific yew, and grand fir. Not far into the hike you come to some out-of-place ponderosa pines, a very unusual species for the west side of the Cascades. In early April the park features a variety of woodland wildflowers, as well as numerous migrating and resident birds, most prominently black-capped chickadees, winter wrens, and rufous-sided towhees. Many benches and interpretive signs along the trail offer good opportunities to stop and to enjoy both flowers and birds.

The remarkably level, paved route uses boardwalks to cross marshes and wet areas. The most extensive network of these boardwalks takes you over Cedar Mill Creek, where a spur from the main trail leads to a romantic little gazebo overlooking the marsh. In this area you will probably hear the trains of Portland's light-rail transit system zipping past, but fortunately these intrusions are brief and the trains remarkably quiet compared to typical trains.

Just after the end of the last boardwalk is a junction. To do the full loop, leave the paved trail here and turn left onto Creek Trail, a woodchip-covered path that is often muddy and may be closed in winter. This trail follows the edge of a marshy area where thick-stalked rushes line the path. The calls of red-winged blackbirds draw your attention away from the warehouse complex just outside the preserve, on your right.

You soon turn away from the warehouse area and reenter wilder woods, just before coming to a junction with the Old Wagon Trail. Turn right on this woodchip-and-gravel-covered path and less than 0.1 mile later turn left on Coyote Trail, which goes a short distance to a junction with the paved Vine Maple Trail.

At this junction you have the option of returning to the Interpretive Center by turning left, but for more exercise and a longer loop, turn right. This pleasant route goes 0.2 mile to where the pavement ends at a short spur to Lily Pond. After taking this side trip, you follow the main route, which goes straight and soon reaches busy S.W. 170th Avenue. You turn left, following the road shoulder. At the south end of the bridge over Beaverton Creek, look for the Cougar Trail back into the park. In winter, avoid this path because it is usually flooded.

As an alternate route you can continue on the highway shoulder for another 0.1 mile and then take the much drier Cedar Grove Trail to rejoin the loop. In drier conditions, follow the Cougar Trail as it goes through muddy areas beside the creek to a junction, where you go straight

Sword fern in Tualatin Hills Nature Park

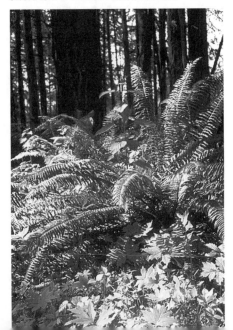

and continue near the creek to a four-way junction next to a bridge. A 100-yard walk up the trail that goes straight here takes you to a good view of Big Pond, where you are likely to see ducks, geese, great blue herons, belted kingfishers, and other water-loving birds.

Back at the bridge, you cross the creek and then skirt the marsh of Big Pond to a junction with the Elliot Trail. From here you can follow either the woodsy Big Fir Trail to the right, or follow the Elliot Trail directly back to the paved Vine Maple Trail. In either case, once you reach the Vine Maple Trail, turn right and join the legions of joggers and baby strollers heading back to the Interpretive Center and trailhead.

TRIP 13 Far North Forest Park

Distance	5.1 miles, Point-to-point
Elevation Gain	300 feet
Hiking Time	2½ hours
Optional Map	None needed
Usually Open	All year
Best Times	April and early November
Trail Use	Dogs OK
Agency	Portland Parks Bureau
Difficulty	Moderate
Note	Good in cloudy weather

HIGHLIGHTS Starting in Washington Park near the Oregon Zoo, the Wildwood Trail has been gradually extended over the years so that it now travels almost 30 miles through the wilderness parks in the hills of northwest Portland. The entire route is a joy, and any section makes an excellent option for Portlanders seeking exercise and the quiet contemplation of nature. The last section to be completed was the 5.1 miles through the far northern part of Forest Park.

This hike is pleasant in any season, but the trail is most enjoyable in April, when the forest flowers are in bloom, or in November, when the bigleaf maples put on a fine fall-color display. In theory, the route is open only to pedestrians, although in practice you will see lots of mountain biking tracks.

DIRECTIONS To reach the N.W. Germantown Road trailhead, follow U.S. Highway 30 (N.W. St. Helens Road) through northwest Portland to the St. Johns Bridge. Just north of the bridge, turn sharply left at a traffic light and follow the bridge-access road 0.1 mile to the junction with N.W. Germantown Road. Here you turn right and drive 1.5 miles to the small trailhead parking area on the left. Unless you are just being dropped off, don't start this hike from its north end at N.W. Newberry Road, since there is no parking or identifiable trailhead.

The northbound Wildwood Trail starts from a log-lined parking pullout about 100 yards downhill from the signed parking area. The remarkably level route immediately begins the pattern it will retain throughout its length—zigzagging into little gullies and around small ridges on a quiet forested hillside. Light-blue

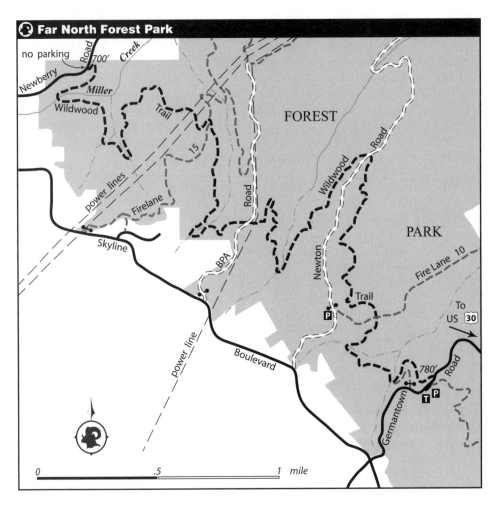

diamonds painted on tree trunks mark the route but really are unnecessary as the route is always evident.

The woodsy scenery rarely changes, but it is not monotonous—unless you don't like lush forests, delicate ferns, stately trees, and forest wildlife.

Remarkably, even though you never leave Portland's city limits, you rarely hear the sounds of traffic or anything else unnatural. The forest alternates between areas dominated by evergreens like western red cedar, Douglas fir, and western hemlock and those places dominated by deciduous trees, especially bigleaf maple and red alder.

Ferns are abundant throughout and always lovely. The most common variety is sword fern. Bracken fern predominates in areas that get a bit more sun, and maidenhair fern on the wetter slopes. Delicate licorice fern hang from the trunk of almost every tree. Other forest-floor species include native Oregon grape and thimbleberry, and nonnative blackberry and English ivy, which grow out of control and are slowly taking over everything.

Since this description applies to every mile of this hike, all that remains is a listing of the other landmarks and junctions. Major junctions are marked with signs showing a map and distances to the nearest .01 mile (as if it really mattered whether a trail is 5.12 or 5.13 miles long).

After 0.8 mile, you cross Firelane 10, one of several former roads now used as trails. In another mile, more woodsy zigs and zags take you to abandoned N.W. Newton Road. Another mile, mostly a gentle uphill, brings you to a power line and the BPA Road. One more gentle mile, and you cross Firelane 15 and a second set of power lines. You finish off with a mile of attractive forest walking and a quick trip into the headwaters of Miller Creek. Done as a one-way car shuttle, this trail makes a very easy dayhike.

TRIP 14 Northern Forest Park Loop

Distance	4.5 miles (with many other options), Loop
Elevation Gain	300 feet
Hiking Time	2 to 3 hours
Optional Map	None needed
Usually Open	All year
Best Times	April and early November
Trail Use	Good for kids, dogs OK
Agency	Portland Parks Bureau
Difficulty	Moderate
Note	Good in cloudy weather

HIGHLIGHTS The length and difficulty of this fun, woodsy loop can be tailored to meet the preferences of just about any hiker. From a short outing of just 2.4 miles to long loops of 16 miles or more, the topography of Forest Park allows plenty of options. The Wildwood Trail and N.W. Leif Erikson Drive, which form the outgoing and returning legs of the loop, run parallel to one another, and there are numerous connecting routes, so there is always an option for crossing over and shortening or lengthening this hike. Like other trails in Forest Park, this loop keeps to deep woods. The forest is always shady and enjoyable, with lots of lush greenery in spring and early summer. In early November, the less popular northern parts of Forest Park are more attractive than the southern regions because more of the trees are deciduous and the fall colors are on display.

DIRECTIONS To reach the N.W. Germantown Road Trailhead, follow U.S. Highway 30 (N.W. St. Helens Road) through northwest Portland to the St. Johns Bridge. Just north of the bridge, turn sharply left at a traffic light and follow the bridge-access road 0.1 mile to the junction with N.W. Germantown Road. Turn right here and drive 1.5 miles to the small trailhead parking area on the left.

A s it does elsewhere in Forest Park, the Wildwood Trail here contours across steep, forested hillsides, extending to the ends of minor ridges and down the little gullies and canyons of seasonal trickling creeks. Small woodland wildflowers brighten the forest floor in the spring, especially white trillium and yellow wood violet in April. Taller shrubs include Oregon grape and salmonberry, with an abundance of sword fern scattered throughout.

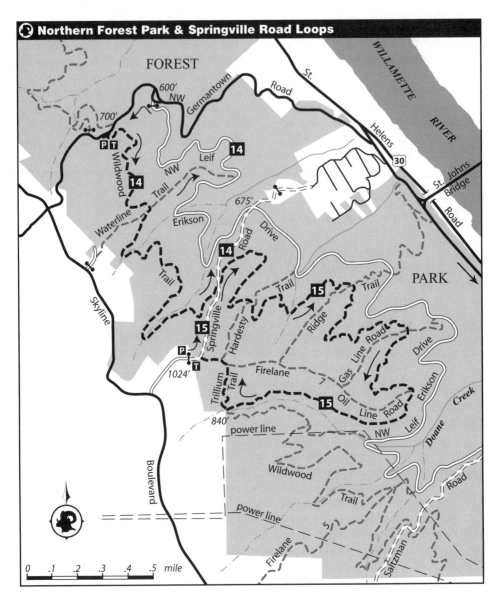

How far you go depends entirely on how much exercise you want and the time available. There are many points where your route intersects trails or old roads and you can cut it short by descending about 150 feet to go back on N.W. Leif Erikson Drive. The first of these comes after just 0.6 mile, at the intersection with the Waterline Trail. After this the Wildwood Trail continues into deep little canyons lush with maidenhair fern and tiny creeks spanned by quaint little bridges. About 1.5 miles farther on comes the recommended place to turn left, on Springville Road, a closed dirt-and-gravel route. A quick look at the map reveals dozens more alternatives in the miles to come on the Wildwood Trail.

Gradually descend 0.3 mile on Springville Road to a junction with Leif Erikson

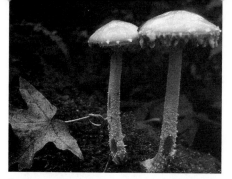
A species of Stropharia mushroom in Forest Park

Drive, where you turn left. The road here is relatively free of joggers and bicyclists, so the gentle walk along this overgrown old route is quiet and pleasant. It is about 1.8 miles along N.W. Leif Erikson Drive back to N.W. Germantown Road, where you turn left and walk uphill 0.3 mile back to the Wildwood Trailhead.

TRIP 15 Springville Road Loop

Distance	5.1 miles, Loop
Elevation Gain	400 feet
Hiking Time	3 hours
Optional Map	USGS *Linnton*
Usually Open	All year
Best Time	March to May
Trail Use	Good for kids, dogs OK
Agency	Portland Parks Bureau
Difficulty	Moderate
Note	Good in cloudy weather

HIGHLIGHTS This loop explores a relatively remote section of Forest Park and is arguably the most outstanding hike in this urban preserve. The forest setting is soothing and beautiful, the wildflowers are abundant in spring, and wildlife is unusually common. Add to this the almost complete solitude in a forest setting less than 15 minutes from downtown Portland, and you have a real winner.

DIRECTIONS Drive Skyline Boulevard either 0.9 mile south from its junction with Germantown Road or 3.9 miles north of the Cornell Road intersection. Turn east on gravel Springville Road, and proceed 0.2 mile to the road turnaround and small trailhead parking area.

Walk around the gate at the southeast end of the parking area, and go 30 yards to a junction with Firelane 7 and the start of the loop. Bear left (downhill) on Springville Road, which has been closed to traffic for so long it is now more of a wide trail. The route descends at a moderate grade through a strikingly attractive and open forest of red alders, bigleaf maples, western hemlocks, and western red cedars that hosts a lovely array of the usual wildflowers from late March through May. Look for red-flowering currant, serviceberry, trillium, false

Solomon's seal, and wood violets, among others. At 0.4 mile is a junction with the Wildwood Trail.

Veer right on the southbound Wildwood Trail and settle in for a long and exceptionally attractive hike. As is typical of this pedestrian-only trail, there are only very minor ups and downs along the way as you spend most of your time contouring into small gullies and out to forested ridgelines. The forest here is unusually open, especially in early spring before the deciduous trees have leafed out, allowing for some partially obstructed views as you hike. Probably the most noteworthy feature of this walk, however, is the solitude. Since this part of the park is far from major trailheads, it gets a lot fewer visitors. In fact, on weekdays you stand a good chance of having the route all to yourself. Wildlife also appreciates the quiet, giving you a reasonable chance of seeing such forest denizens as black-tailed deer, gray fox, and pileated woodpecker, all of which usually avoid the more crowded areas in the preserve.

Remain on the Wildwood Trail for 4.3 very easy and enjoyable miles passing junctions with, consecutively, Hardesty Trail, Ridge Trail, Firelane 7/Gas Line Road, and Oil Line Road. Turning right at any of these junctions will provide a shorter loop option than the full recommended itinerary. Eventually the Wildwood Trail makes a particularly long inward "zig" on its zigzagging course and comes to a wooden bridge over a usually flowing little creek. Immediately before this bridge is an unsigned junction. Turn

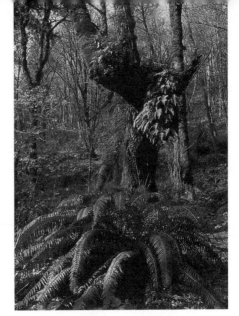

Along Wildwood Trail

right on an obvious but unofficial boot path, known locally as the Trillium Trail, and follow this route for 0.25 mile as it steeply climbs through open woods to a junction with Firelane 7. Turn left, soon pass a signed junction with Hardesty Trail, and then climb a bit more back to a reunion with Springville Road and your car.

TRIP 16 Central Forest Park Loop

Distance	8.2 miles, Loop
Elevation Gain	500 feet
Hiking Time	4 hours
Optional Map	None needed
Usually Open	All year
Best Time	Late March to mid-April
Trail Use	Good for kids, dogs OK
Agency	Portland Parks Bureau
Difficulty	Moderate
Note	Good in cloudy weather

HIGHLIGHTS This loop hike, through the central part of the preserve, is one of the wildest options in Forest Park. Other hikes require the use of the biker-and-jogger thoroughfare of N.W. Leif Erikson Drive on your return. On this outing, however, almost all of the route keeps to hiker-only trails by linking the Maple Trail with a typically attractive section of the Wildwood Trail, which makes for a beautiful and quiet circuit through the hills.

DIRECTIONS Drive on U.S. Highway 30 from northwest Portland toward St. Helens. Just past milepost 5, turn left on N.W. Saltzman Road and drive 0.9 mile to a gate. Be sure not to block the gate when you park.

You begin with an easy uphill walk of 0.4 mile on N.W. Saltzman Road to a junction with the Maple Trail, where the loop begins. For a clockwise loop, turn left and follow the narrow footpath as it ascends through a forest of western hemlock, Douglas fir, and—true to the trail's name—bigleaf maple, which put on a nice show of bright yellow leaves in early November. Down on the forest floor is the characteristic assortment of sword fern, Oregon grape, and the invasive English ivy, along with a smattering of forest wildflowers, such as trillium, wood violet, and vanilla leaf, which peak in early April.

You cross a jeep track beneath a set of power lines and then wind very gradually uphill as the trail explores these heavily forested ridges and creek canyons. The trickling creeks are spanned by quaint little wooden footbridges. Since you're not heading to an end point at some lake, viewpoint, or waterfall, take the opportunity to clear your mind of the hiker's disease of destinationitis. Enjoy the glories of the hike itself, especially the subtle charms and intimate beauty of this quiet forest. It won't be long before you realize that the white blossom of a trillium, the mosses and licorice ferns hanging onto the limbs of a maple tree, or the

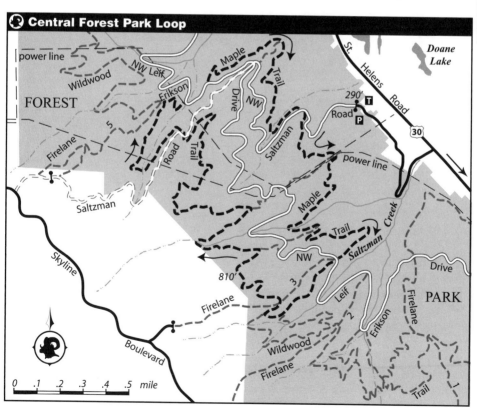

Central Forest Park Loop

deep-green fronds of a sword fern afford as much beauty as more "spectacular" mountain lakes or vistas.

Stay on the Maple Trail, keeping left at one possibly unsigned junction, all the way to N.W. Leif Erikson Drive. Since it is far from the nearest trailhead, this part of the closed road sees fewer joggers and only a handful of bicyclists. Your route crosses the road, staying to the left with the Maple Trail rather than the parallel old fire road on the right. You then climb a little to a junction with the Wildwood Trail.

To do the recommended loop, turn right on the Wildwood Trail and amble along this famous path as it contours across the forested slopes of the park. As usual, the Wildwood Trail rarely gains or loses any noticeable elevation, featuring only brief ups and downs for the next 3.2 miles. You'll cross several creeklets, a small clearing beneath a power line, and three old jeep roads, but the basic forest scenery remains unchanged throughout, and the proper course is always well marked. At one of the many small ridges along the way, you reach the end of Fire-lane 5, a closed jeep road going up to the left. Turn right onto a possibly unsigned but obvious foot trail that loses about 150 feet in 0.3 mile before arriving back at N.W. Leif Erikson Drive. You turn right on this closed road, and a little less than 0.2 mile later, you turn left at a small grassy area, returning to the Maple Trail. This path goes 1.2 miles through more of the same kind of uneventful but pleasant forest scenery back to the junction with N.W. Saltzman Road.

TRIP **17** Southern Forest Park Loop

Distance	8.6 miles, Loop
Elevation Gain	700 feet
Hiking Time	4 hours
Optional Map	None needed
Usually Open	All year
Best Time	Late March to mid-April
Trail Use	Dogs OK
Agency	Portland Parks Bureau
Difficulty	Moderate
Note	Good in cloudy weather

HIGHLIGHTS Even if Forest Park lacks any really spectacular scenery, you can't beat it for convenience. With a less than five-minute drive you can go from the hectic world of downtown traffic and skyscrapers to the quiet woods of this massive park. Outdoor-loving office workers come here for a short hike or a jog during their lunch break, while others take advantage of the long evenings of early summer to go for a hike after work.

This route in the southern part of the park is especially convenient since it has the shortest street access to the big city. Interestingly, most visitors aren't hikers at all; N.W. Leif Erikson Drive is closed to cars but hosts a cross-section of Portland's fitness fanatics, joggers, bicyclists, and inline skaters, all taking advantage of this scenic, traffic-free opportunity to pursue their chosen form of exercise. But don't be dissuaded from a visit just because part of the loop is heavily traveled by nonhikers. The upper segment of the

Southern Forest Park Loop

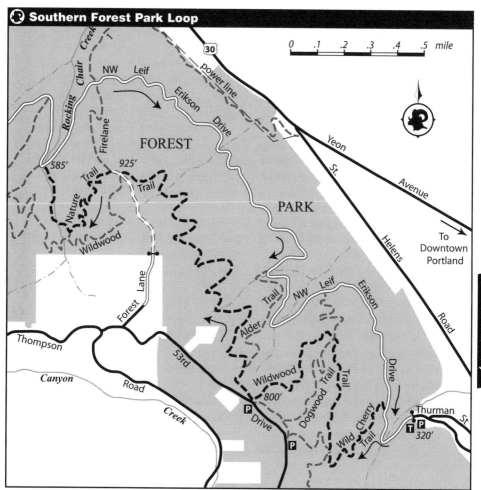

0   .1   .2   .3   .4   .5   mile

route, along the Wildwood Trail, is for pedestrians only and therefore much less crowded than other parts of the park.

DIRECTIONS From Interstate 405 in downtown Portland, take Exit 3 for U.S. Highway 30 toward the town of St. Helens. From this off-ramp you immediately exit onto N.W. Vaughn Street, which you follow for 0.3 mile to the traffic light at N.W. 26th Street. Turn left, and then two blocks later turn right onto N.W. Thurman Street. Follow this road uphill over a tall bridge and through a quiet neighborhood for 1.2 miles, and then keep going straight where the road switchbacks to the left. In about 100 yards you'll reach a small parking area and a gate across the start of N.W. Leif Erikson Drive.

Begin your hike by going around the gate and gradually climbing the wide surface of the partly paved, partly gravel road. After 0.3 mile you part with the stream of joggers and bicyclists in favor of the hiker-only Wild Cherry Trail, which goes off to the left. This pleasant path climbs moderately steeply on a sometimes muddy tread to a signed junction with the Wildwood Trail. Turn right and follow this practically level path as it wanders along the heavily forested hillsides of Forest Park. The route is very easy, and since there are no viewpoints or other highlights causing you to linger, the miles go by quickly.

The forest here is predominantly Douglas fir, with some western red cedar, Pacific yew, and bigleaf maple for a little variety. The forest floor affords plenty of variety, but it is dominated by the usual sword fern and Oregon grape. Just 0.6 mile beyond the Wild Cherry Trail you come to a four-way junction with the Dogwood Trail. For a very short loop, you can turn right here, and drop to N.W. Leif Erikson Drive to return to your car. For more exercise and forest scenery, however, go straight and continue the level hike on the Wildwood Trail. The path comes within spitting distance of a trailhead on N.W. 53rd Drive and then takes you to a junction with the Alder Trail, another option for a shortened loop.

For the full recommended trip, veer left, sticking with the Wildwood Trail a little below the ridge crest on your left, for another uneventful but soothing 1.8 miles. Along the way you pass through several nearly pure stands of bigleaf maple, which are particularly fetching with the new green leaves of spring or the old yellow leaves of early November. Eventually, the nearly level, wandering Wildwood Trail comes to a junction with Firelane 1, a closed dirt road. The Wildwood Trail crosses this road, but a better option is to turn right and follow the fire lane downhill for a little over 100 yards and then bear left onto the Nature Trail.

This trail switchbacks downhill for 0.4 mile before arriving at a small open spot, the site of now dismantled Rocking Chair Shelter. Beyond this point the Nature Trail continues a short distance to a junction where you turn right (downhill) and descend along small but attractive Rocking Chair Creek, past an old dam site to a junction with N.W. Leif Erikson Drive. To complete the loop, turn right and follow this attractive winding road as it goes past a couple of decent viewpoints of the city. It gets steadily more crowded with other visitors. In the 3.4 miles from Rocking Chair Creek, you pass junctions with Firelane 1, Alder Trail, Dogwood Trail, and finally Wild Cherry Trail, all the way back to the starting point.

Mushrooms in Forest Park

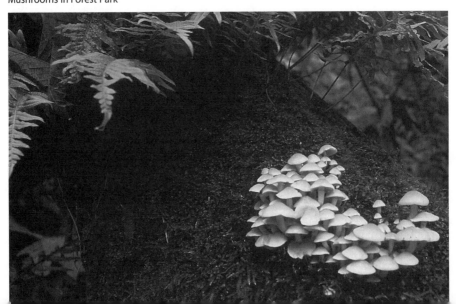

TRIP 18 Balch Creek & Wildwood Trail Loop

Distance	4.8 miles, Loop
Elevation Gain	700 feet
Hiking Time	2 to 2½ hours
Optional Map	None needed
Usually Open	All year
Best Time	Late March to mid-April
Trail Use	Good for kids, dogs OK
Agency	Portland Parks Bureau
Difficulty	Moderate
Note	Good in cloudy weather

HIGHLIGHTS This easy loop provides a perfect sampling of the charms of Forest Park. You start by hiking up a first-rate urban stream canyon, follow a particularly attractive segment of the Wildwood Trail across heavily wooded slopes, and finish with a short walk through a quiet city neighborhood. Probably no other major city in North America can match this type of wild variety within its city limits.

While this path is open and enjoyable in any season, it is most attractive from late March to mid-April, when the forest floor comes alive with wildflowers. Most abundant are Oregon grape, trillium, twinflower, and wood violet—which, despite that old rhyme about violets being blue, are mostly yellow in this area. Wear boots or shoes that you don't mind getting muddy, as the path is usually a sloppy mess in winter and spring.

DIRECTIONS From Interstate 405 in downtown Portland, take Exit 3 for U.S. Highway 30 toward the town of St. Helens. From this off-ramp you immediately exit onto N.W. Vaughn Street, which you follow for 0.3 mile to the traffic light at N.W. 26th Street. Turn left and then right in less than a block onto N.W. Upshur Street. Follow this road for 0.5 mile to its end at a small parking lot and turnaround, directly beneath a tall suspension bridge on N.W. Thurman Street.

The paved trail starts by going through a small picnic area under the imposing bridge. This bridge is a favorite roosting and nesting site for pigeons, so you will probably be serenaded with their soft cooing sounds as you hike. You pass a catch basin where the waters of Balch Creek, flowing toward you, disappear beneath the pavement and then continue along the lovely wild creek above. In the 19th century, this stream was used as a water source for the city, and even though it flows entirely within the city limits, it remains clean enough today to provide habitat for native cutthroat trout.

The trail crosses the creek on a bridge, shortly after which the pavement ends and the scenery changes suddenly from city to wilderness. Though you are only a few hundred yards from the street grid, homes, and apartments of the big city, that all seems worlds away as the forested canyon effectively shields you from the human-made sights and sounds. Just a few steps into your hike and you are already enjoying the sounds of birds and a bubbling creek, happily enclosed in a wilderness.

After the first crossing of Balch Creek, the wide path parallels the stream, which tumbles over rocks and small waterfalls under an overhanging canopy of salmonberry and western red cedar. The cliffs and tree trunks near the stream are

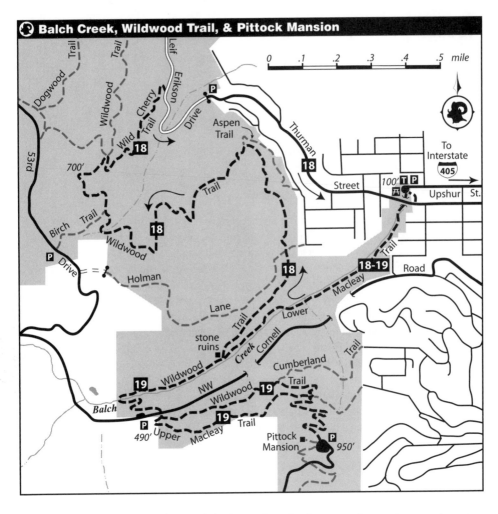

covered with mosses and ferns, while the forest floor is carpeted with sword fern, Oregon grape, and trillium.

You recross the creek on a bridge just below a particularly fetching little falls and then pass a huge old Douglas fir as you make your way upstream. Not long after this, the path arrives at some old stone ruins beside a junction with the Wildwood Trail.

To do the recommended loop, turn sharply right just in front of the ruins and gradually climb the Wildwood Trail on a mostly open hillside. One of the most common plants here is English ivy. This plant looks attractive as it spreads out on the forest floor and climbs the trees trunks, but it is actually an unwelcome introduced species that crowds out native vegetation. Park officials and volunteers wage a never-ending battle to rid the park of this menace.

You intersect closed Holman Lane just above a small meadow, and go straight on the hiker-only Wildwood Trail. This path quickly demonstrates its characteristic pattern, rarely gaining or losing much elevation, opting instead to zig into small forested gullies and zag out to equally heavily wooded ridges. Here in south-

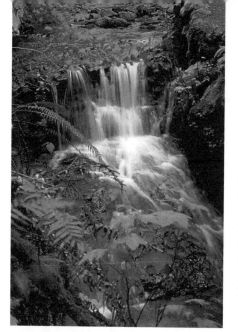
Falls on Balch Creek

switchbacks and then make a straight-forward ascent of a sword-fern-covered slope. After this you level off and resume the pattern of zigzag level hiking. There is an abundance of birds in these woods, so bring binoculars to enjoy black-capped chickadees, rufous-sided towhees, dark-eyed juncos, hairy woodpeckers, American robins, winter wrens, and others.

Go straight at a junction with the Birch Trail and, about 0.3 mile later, meet the Wild Cherry Trail. To close the loop, turn sharply right and lazily descend a woodsy hillside to N.W. Leif Erikson Drive, which is closed to vehicles but teeming with joggers and bicyclists. You turn right on this road and soon arrive at a gate and small parking area.

To finish off the loop, follow the sidewalk beside N.W. Thurman Street as it goes gently downhill through a quiet neighborhood with lovely homes and colorful gardens. After about 0.7 mile, you cross Balch Creek Canyon on a tall bridge, at the far end of which are a staircase and a trail dropping to the parking area and your car.

ern Forest Park the trees are nearly all conifers, mostly Douglas firs, with a few western hemlocks and Pacific yews.

You keep left at an intersection with the Aspen Trail, after which the Wildwood Trail makes one of its few noticeable climbs. In the next 0.5 mile you gain approximately 300 feet in four short

Portland & the Willamette Valley

TRIP 19 Balch Creek to Pittock Mansion

Distance	4.4 miles, Out-and-back
Elevation Gain	1000 feet
Hiking Time	2½ hours
Optional Map	None needed
Usually Open	All year
Best Time	Late March to mid-April
Trail Use	Good for kids, dogs OK
Agency	Portland Parks Bureau
Difficulty	Moderate

HIGHLIGHTS Historic Pittock Mansion, with its carefully manicured lawns, exquisite gardens, and popularity with car-bound visitors, hardly qualifies as a wilderness destination. But its setting on a scenic high point in Portland's woodsy West Hills, with views that extend to five volcanic peaks, hardly makes it seem like a typical spot for city sightseeing either.

It's well worth anyone's time to tour the beautiful old house and stroll through the grounds—whether you arrive by car or by trail, but it is the trail that qualifies this hike as sufficiently wild for inclusion in this book. Following almost the entire length of wild Balch Creek and then ascending a hillside of stately conifers, this trail retains its wilderness character for all but the last couple of hundred yards. So this trip gives you the best of both world's—God's wild forests on the way and a stunning human-made attraction at the end.

DIRECTIONS   From Interstate 405 in downtown Portland, take Exit 3 for U.S. Highway 30 toward the town of St. Helens. From this off-ramp you immediately exit onto N.W. Vaughn Street, which you follow for 0.3 mile to the traffic light at N.W. 26th Street. Turn left and then right in less than a block onto N.W. Upshur Street. Follow this road for 0.5 mile to its end at a small parking lot and turnaround, directly beneath a tall suspension bridge on N.W. Thurman Street.

Begin the adventure by ascending the gorgeous trail up the canyon of Balch Creek, as described in Trip 18. This trip diverges from that one after 0.9 mile, at the stone ruins where you meet the Wildwood Trail. This time, instead of turning right, you go straight on the path beside Balch Creek and for the next 0.4 mile remain close to the north bank of this creek as it tumbles through a scenic woodsy canyon. Every foot of the trail is a joy, as you travel through the lush creekside vegetation. You finally cross the

creek on a bridge and reluctantly leave the stream. Three switchbacks help you climb out of the canyon to a crossing of busy N.W. Cornell Road, the source of those traffic sounds you've been hearing for the last 0.2 mile.

The Wildwood Trail crosses N.W. Cornell Road at a grassy trailhead and reenters a lovely forest traveling a short distance to a junction with the Upper Macleay Trail. Either trail will get you to Pittock Mansion, and the best option is to combine the two paths into an enjoyable

Stone ruins along Balch Creek

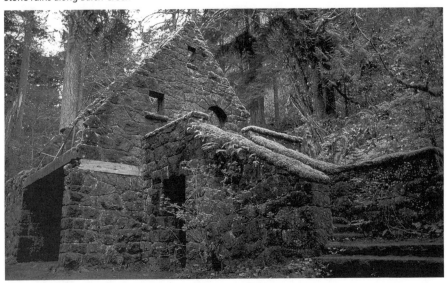

loop. For now, veer left on the Wildwood Trail and wander along at a nearly level grade on the hillside above N.W. Cornell Road. After about 0.5 mile, you bear right at a junction with Cumberland Trail and begin the 500-foot climb to Pittock Mansion. The sweat is offset by the joy of traveling through extremely attractive woods, with lots of beautiful old Douglas firs and lush greenery on the forest floor. About 0.1 mile from the last junction, you come to a four-way junction with the Upper Macleay Trail, the end of the semi-loop mentioned above. To finish your climb to Pittock Mansion, go straight and ascend five well-graded switchbacks before the uphill rather abruptly ends and you arrive at a large parking lot for visitors to Pittock Mansion. Be sure to allow some time to explore the gardens, enjoy the view, and, if it's open, tour the old mansion. Tours of this 16,000-square-foot brick palace, built between 1909 to 1914, run daily from 1 PM to 5 PM and require a small entry fee ($7 for adults as of 2007).

Continuing south from Pittock Mansion, the Wildwood Trail drops to cross very busy W. Burnside Road and then wanders through the human-made plantings of Hoyt Arboretum and the manicured lawns in Washington Park. Both of these locations are worth visiting, but they aren't wild enough to be included in this book.

TRIP 20 Audubon Sanctuary Loops

Distance	2.3 miles (both loops), Loops
Elevation Gain	400 feet
Hiking Time	1 to 2 hours
Optional Map	Trail brochure available from Nature Center
Usually Open	All year
Best Times	April and May
Trail Use	Good for kids, no dogs
Agency	Portland Audubon Society
Difficulty	Easy
Note	Good in cloudy weather

HIGHLIGHTS Although relatively small in size, the 160-acre Portland Audubon Wildlife Sanctuary is perhaps the nicest single sampling of Portland's West Hills. In addition to the usual attractive forests, you can enjoy Balch Creek, a lovely urban stream, and sit beside a quiet, lily-pad-filled pond. Concentrated throughout the preserve are lots of wildflowers and wildlife. The trails are open to the public year-round from dawn to dusk, but dogs are prohibited.

DIRECTIONS From northwest Portland, drive west on N.W. Lovejoy. This road bears to the right after crossing N.W. 25th, where it becomes N.W. Cornell Road. Continue on N.W. Cornell Road for 1.5 miles through two tunnels to the Audubon Sanctuary. There is a small parking lot in front of the bookstore, nature center, and wildlife rehabilitation buildings on the north side of the road. Additional parking is available in the gravel overflow lot on the south side of the road. If you are coming from the west, the Audubon Sanctuary is 1.5 miles east of the junction of N.W. Cornell Road and N.W. Skyline Boulevard.

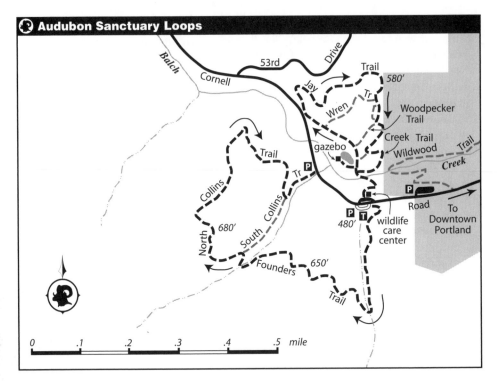

Audubon Sanctuary Loops

There are trails on both sides of N.W. Cornell Road, but if you have time for only a short stroll, stick with the trails to the north, as they are more interesting. A good gravel path begins from the east side of the parking lot, next to the wildlife care building, and drops quickly to a bridge over Balch Creek. This lovely urban stream drains a 2000-acre watershed, most of which is protected in either wild city parks or the Audubon Sanctuary itself, so the water remains reasonably clear, and even supports native cutthroat trout.

On the other side of the bridge is the first of many junctions with trails that split off in many directions, all of them marked by names on green signs. Not surprisingly in an Audubon Society sanctuary, the trail names tend to have an avian theme—Woodpecker, Wren, and Jay—in addition to the Creek Trail along Balch Creek.

For now, go left at two successive junctions to quickly arrive at a small, lily-pad-filled pond. A wooden gazebo here provides an ideal viewing platform to look at the many roughskin newts that laze about in the water. After enjoying the pond, you have a choice of trails. For a 0.9-mile circuit of the preserve, a loop follows the pleasant Jay Trail through the trees and near the surrounding fences, roads, and homes that ring the sanctuary grounds.

The dense native vegetation along this route features a canopy of western hemlock, western red cedar, bigleaf maple, and a wide variety of wildflowers. In April and May, you can expect to see trillium, candyflower, twisted stalk, wood violet, star-flowered smilacina, and false Solomon's seal, among many others. Also in these spring months you will be treated to an unusual abundance of songbirds. This area is a favorite of local birders in search of migrating warblers, grosbeaks, sparrows, and other feathered songsters. The loop ends at the junction near the bridged crossing of Balch Creek.

For a longer loop that provides more exercise and some fine forest scenery, try the Founders and Collins trails on the south side of Cornell Road. Cross the road and find the sign for the Founders Trail beside the Audubon maintenance building at the east end of a small parking area. The wide gravel trail makes one quick uphill switchback and then travels 150 yards to a flat area used for storage. The trail then narrows and goes lazily uphill beside a seasonal creek through a pretty forest of western red cedars and western hemlocks. You cross a bridge over the creek and then go generally west, zigzagging into and out of small gullies. The forest here is lush and beautiful with a notable lack of the invasive and nonnative English ivy, which so often plagues other parks in our area. The lack of ivy allows native plants such as trillium to grow in profusion, with their distinctive cheerful white blossoms brightening the forest from late March to mid-April. Also of interest are several tall snags covered with shelf fungus and licorice ferns. The mass of greenery and lack of traffic sounds make it easy to forget that you are still within the limits of a major U.S. city.

Shortly after descending to cross a seasonal creek at 0.6 mile, you come to a junction with the North and South Collins trails. Go left (uphill) on North Collins Trail and stick with this wind-

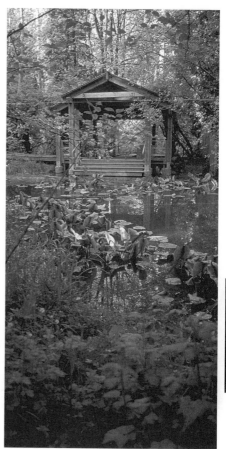

Pond and gazebo in the Portland Audubon Wildlife Sanctuary

ing route as it climbs through forest and then loops back down to a junction with South Collins Trail. Turn left and walk 150 yards to a small gravel parking area on Cornell Road. It is a short 0.1-mile walk along the road to your car, but there is no shoulder and traffic can be heavy, so be very careful.

TRIP 21 Marquam Nature Park Loop

Distance	1.3 to 8 miles, Loop
Elevation Gain	300 to 1500 feet
Hiking Time	1 to 4 hours
Optional Map	None needed
Usually Open	All year
Best Times	Late March to mid-April and early November
Trail Use	Good for kids, dogs OK
Agency	Portland Parks Bureau
Difficulty	Easy to Moderate
Note	Good in cloudy weather

HIGHLIGHTS For proof of the claim that Portland is a city that includes wilderness within its borders, you need look no further than Marquam Nature Park. Downtown office workers looking to withdraw temporarily from the rat race can literally walk to this unspoiled gem on their lunch hour for a healthy dose of the medicine that only wilderness provides. This little park protects an amazingly wild canyon of dense forests. It's hard to believe that it is only a few blocks away from the world of skyscrapers and traffic.

DIRECTIONS From downtown Portland, simply follow S.W. 6th Avenue south to the overpass at Interstate 405 and the traffic light just to the south. Stay on S.W. 6th Avenue, following signs to Oregon Health Sciences University (OHSU), and travel 0.3 mile to a traffic light where S.W. Terwilliger Boulevard goes left. Go straight on S.W. Sam Jackson Road, and

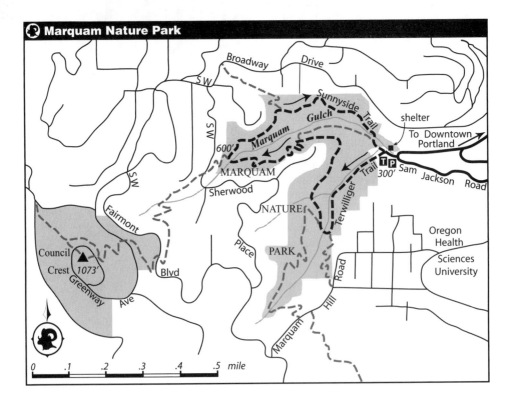

continue 0.2 mile to where the road makes a hairpin turn to the left. You turn to the right and immediately arrive at the tiny parking lot next to the Marquam Nature Park Shelter. All of this can be done as an easy half-hour walk from downtown or by taking the regular Tri-Met bus service to either OHSU or the S.W. Terwilliger Boulevard turnoff. If you are driving, note that there is a two-hour limit on parking.

A network of trails radiates from this trailhead, giving you a wide variety of destinations and choices. The easiest alternative, a loop in the lower forested canyons, is also the wildest. Longer trails head off for more distant locales and connect with trail systems in other parts of the West Hills. Immediately above the open-sided shelter, the wide gravel trail splits at the start of the loop. Either direction is fine, but for a clockwise loop turn left on the Terwilliger Trail and hop over a low chain across the path.

This gravelly old road is now just a wide trail that climbs fairly steeply up a densely wooded canyon. Wooden catch basins trap the water in the gully beside you, eliminating what once was a pretty little creek. The trail itself is often wetter than the gully leading to several muddy spots, so don't wear your dressiest shoes. After 0.3 mile you come to a junction where the old road continues straight on its way to S.W. Marquam Hill Road and S.W. Terwilliger Boulevard. For the short loop, turn sharply right on a narrow foot trail that traverses back along the forested hillside and, after just 50 yards, comes to another junction.

For the recommended loop, stay straight on the lower trail and soon hop over a tiny, splashing creek. After this, the trail very gradually gains elevation and then contours as it curves left into the next canyon. The forests in this remarkably wild canyon are a mix of Douglas fir, western hemlock, western red cedar, and bigleaf maple. Below these big trees are lots of shrubs, especially red elderberry, vine maple, and thimbleberry. English ivy is incredibly abundant, and while it looks attractive, the dense mat covering the forest floor has effectively crowded out most of the native plants and flowers.

When you come to the next junction you have a choice. The quickest way to return to your car is to veer right and drop directly back down to the shelter. For a longer trip, bear left and climb several gently graded switchbacks to the next junction. If you want a long hike with a good view as a payoff, turn left and follow this trail for 1 mile as it switchbacks uphill, crosses three neighborhood roads, and tops out on Council Crest, the highest point in the city of Portland. There are sweeping views here, which makes this spot well worth visiting, but it isn't really a wilderness destination, since it has paved road access, manicured lawns, and a radio tower.

To stay on the wilder lower loop, bear right at the junction, and hike on the Sunnyside Trail as it zigzags downhill and comes to a junction with a trail going left to S.W. Broadway Drive. You close the loop by going straight and losing elevation for another 0.3 mile. The last part of this descent is through a brushy area with blackberry brambles and a grassy meadow. The trail ends at a junction about 50 yards above the Marquam Nature Park Shelter.

TRIP 22 Tryon Creek State Park Loop

Distance	1 to 7 miles, Loop
Elevation Gain	100 to 400 feet
Hiking Time	30 minutes to 3 hours (depending on route)
Optional Map	Tryon Creek State Natural Area brochure
Usually Open	All year
Best Time	Early April
Trail Use	Good for kids, dogs OK
Agency	Tryon Creek State Natural Area
Difficulty	Easy
Note	Good in cloudy weather

HIGHLIGHTS Tryon Creek State Park is a tiny wilderness treasure. Although surrounded by busy roads and housing developments, the park's forested canyon effectively isolates the visitor in a cocoon of wilderness where the sounds of birds and babbling creeks overwhelm the distant hum of traffic and trains. The 645-acre park is a treat any time of year but is most enjoyable the first week of April when the preserve's signature flower, the white-blooming trillium, is on full display. This time of year is also when other flowers, such as skunk cabbage, salmonberry, and wood violet, are most prominent. In addition, the red alder trees have yet to grow their summer leaves, so the forest feels more open and inviting. Despite these ideal conditions, in midweek the trails are lonesome, most of the visitors being schoolchildren on field trips.

The park is laced with a confusing network of trails. Some paths are specifically designed for bicyclists, others for equestrians, and still others for hikers. It is very easy to take a wrong turn when faced with so many junctions and choices. Fortunately, the park is relatively small, so it's impossible to get too far off course. You can easily create your own itinerary amid the maze of footpaths. The route described here is only one suggestion.

DIRECTIONS From downtown Portland, go south on Interstate 5 and then take S.W. Terwilliger Boulevard Exit 297. Drive south on S.W. Terwilliger Boulevard 2.2 miles, through several traffic lights and junctions. Turn right into the main parking area for Tryon Creek State Park.

From the north end of the parking area follow the Maple Ridge Trail for a short distance to Jackson Shelter where it turns right. This gentle path wanders downhill amid a forest of western red cedar, western hemlock, Douglas fir, and red alder, with common understory species like Oregon grape, sword fern, and licorice fern keeping everything green. The path is covered with gravel, so mud is at a minimum, which does not hold true for most trails in the park.

You remain on the Maple Ridge Trail all the way down to High Bridge over Tryon Creek, which you cross, and then turn left onto the Middle Creek Trail. This creekside route goes downstream 0.2 mile—part of it across a boardwalk that provides dry access over a skunk-cabbage bog—to a junction. Turn right onto the Cedar Trail and make a short, brisk climb past some excellent trillium displays to the canyon rim. Listen carefully in this area for the calls of screech owls in the trees, especially in the early morning and

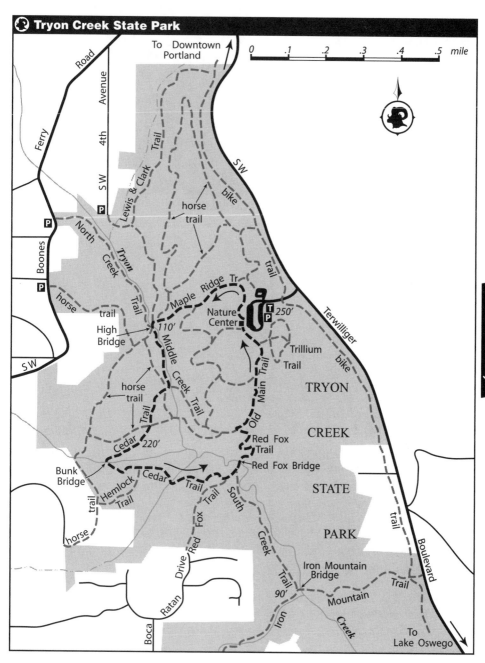

around dusk. You keep going straight at a four-way junction with the West Equestrian Loop, following signs for Red Fox Bridge, and then go up and down a little

to Bunk Bridge, which spans a trickling side creek.

From this bridge, walk a short distance further to a junction with the Hemlock

Trail, a short spur route that leads to S.W. Englewood Drive. You go straight for about 0.4 mile and then turn left at the intersection with the Red Fox Trail, where you turn left. This path descends to a junction with the South Creek Trail, where you go straight and then cross Red Fox Bridge. To return to your car, climb four short switchbacks to a junction with Old Main Trail, and turn right. The final section of your tour follows a nearly level route past the Nature Center and back to the parking lot.

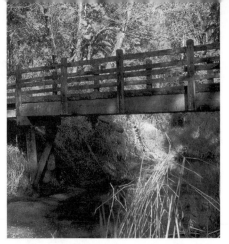

Iron Mountain Bridge at the junction of South Creek and Iron Mountain trails

TRIP 23 Powell Butte Loop

Distance	3.5 miles (with many other options), Loop
Elevation Gain	300 feet
Hiking Time	1 to 4 hours
Optional Map	Use trailhead brochure (still inadequate).
Usually Open	All year
Best Time	Late March to May
Trail Use	Good for kids, no dogs, partly wheelchair accessible
Agency	Portland Parks Bureau
Difficulty	Easy

HIGHLIGHTS Powell Butte Nature Park is a surprisingly wild 570-acre urban oasis that protects the slopes of an extinct volcano between Portland and Gresham. Most of the rolling peak is covered by a rare, low-elevation, grassy meadow, while the northern and western slopes host beautiful forests more typical of our region. You'll never realize it as you hike, but underneath the trail is a 50-million-gallon reservoir used by the Portland Water Bureau as the apex of its distribution system to more than 700,000 users in the Portland area. The park's 9 miles of official trails are a recreational haven for all types of outdoor lovers, in part because off-road vehicles are prohibited. Keep in mind that, except for the wild coyotes and foxes that you might see, all dogs are required to be on leash.

DIRECTIONS Follow S.E. Powell Boulevard (U.S. Highway 26) 3.4 miles east from its junction with Interstate 205 and then turn right (south) at the light for S.E. 162nd Avenue. This road goes up a hill and in just 0.5 mile dead-ends at a large gravel parking lot, just inside Powell Butte Nature Park.

A wild confusion of trails goes off in all directions from the parking lot and, for that matter, all over the mountain. Most of these are unsigned and are not part of the official trail inventory, but they are indistinguishable from the official paths. Although the park makes a point of stressing the need for visitors to stay on established trails, this becomes very difficult since there are no signs identifying trails that are not part of the established system. Do your best but you should expect to make at least a few wrong turns. Fortunately, it is impossible to get really lost, and since all the trails are equally attractive, you can't go wrong.

For a trip that includes all of the park's major environments, try taking a large circle on the trails around the perimeter. Start by following the paved wheelchair-accessible Mountain View Trail that leaves from the northwest end of the parking lot and goes southeast, climbing gradually for 0.6 mile, in one long switchback to the rolling meadows atop Powell Butte. As you ascend, you will pass several unsigned trails and cross a service road, but it's best to stick with the paved path. In the spring, expect to see lots of woolly bear caterpillars doing their best slinky-toy impersonations across the pavement in front of you. Be careful not to step on these colorful and cuddly native residents.

At the top of your climb, the paved route ends at a junction with a dirt trail. For the outer loop of the park, turn left and walk along the scenic ridgeline of Powell Butte, past a few inviting picnic tables in an old walnut orchard. Also here is a useful "mountain finder," where railroad ties in the ground point toward distant snow peaks and lesser nearby summits. Bear right at an unsigned junction just past the mountain finder and then cross a shallow depression to come to another unsigned junction.

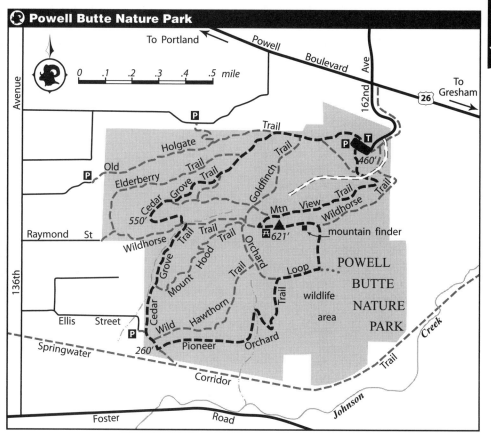

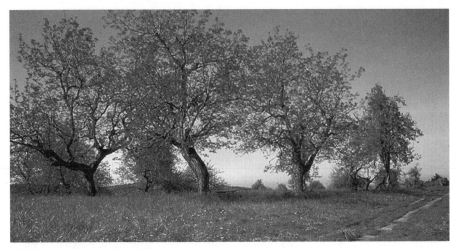

Old walnut orchard atop Powell Butte

For the recommended route, turn right here and walk beside a designated wildlife area on your left that is closed to public access. The wildlife seems to appreciate this concern, as you are likely to spot rabbits, sometimes deer, and lots of songbirds, especially various warblers, towhees, and sparrows, all taking advantage of the people-free environment.

At the next signed junction, turn left onto the Pioneer Orchard Trail, which drops below the meadowlands and enters some exceptionally attractive woods. Western red cedar, Douglas fir, and red alder are dominant here, while the forest floor hosts many woodland wildflowers, such as yellow violets, candyflower, fairy bells, and twisted stalk. From here, the path descends steadily to cross a gully with a seasonal trickle of water and then curves to the west and drops some more. You may see a house or two through the foliage or hear the distant sounds of traffic on Foster Road to the south, but in general the hike stays wonderfully wild.

Eventually you come to a junction at the southwest corner of the park, where you turn right and, just 10 yards later, bear left at a junction with the Wild Hawthorn horse trail. You are now on the Cedar Grove Trail. You ascend slowly through deep forest and then go straight through at a junction with a spur trail, which goes left to a trailhead on nearby S.E. Ellis Street. A little while later, you go straight again where the Mt. Hood Trail leads off to the right. Climb up the woodsy canyon of a seasonal creek, passing some enormous old Douglas firs and lots of western red cedars, with their distinctive sinewy bark. When you reach a confusing four-way junction with the Wildhorse Trail, you make a short jog to the left to cross the tiny creek and then turn right and resume travel on the Cedar Grove Trail.

After climbing a little, you top a low ridge and come to a series of very confusing unsigned junctions. The "proper" route is as much a matter of opinion as anything else, but generally try to avoid any major turns to the left and you will soon break out of the forest and enter the extensive meadows on Powell Butte. From here, simply follow any of several trails and old service roads that all tend to head generally northeast and converge on their way back to the parking lot and your car.

TRIP 24 Sandy River Delta

Distance	4.2 miles, Out-and-back
Elevation Gain	100 feet
Hiking Time	2 hours
Optional Map	None are adequate.
Usually Open	All year (may be flooded in winter)
Best Time	All year
Trail Use	Good for kids, dogs OK
Agency	Columbia Gorge National Scenic Area
Difficulty	Moderate
Note	Good in cloudy weather

HIGHLIGHTS North of Interstate 84, on the east side of the Sandy River, is an undeveloped area of U.S. Forest Service land that protects a flood-prone region of meadows, cottonwood bottomlands, and backwater sloughs. Although there are no signed trails, the entire region is open to hikers and it is laced with a network of unofficial trails and old roads. There isn't any real destination, but the walking is easy and enjoyable with diverse wildlife and nice views of the surrounding mountains in a surprisingly quiet and wild setting. The area is especially popular with dog lovers, who come here to exercise their pets in an unrestricted environment. The hike described here visits the area's most noteworthy feature, the confluence of the Columbia and Sandy rivers.

DIRECTIONS Leave Interstate 84 eastbound at Exit 18 for Lewis & Clark State Park. The exit road makes a cloverleaf loop and comes to a road junction, where you turn right, go under the freeway, and 0.2 mile later park at a gated road on the left. Be sure not to block access to this road when you park.

The road splits immediately on the other side of the gate. The road that continues straight runs too close to Interstate 84 to be enjoyable. You turn left and follow the northbound road atop an old dike, which goes through a black-cottonwood forest. Lining the route are lots of blackberries, which ripen in August, providing a delicious diversion for hikers. Although several unsigned side paths on the left drop to fishing spots on the Sandy River, the main road always goes straight, taking you to a meadow where you bear to the right off the dike.

As you travel north, the freeway sounds fade away and are gradually replaced by the songs of rufous-sided towhees, American robins, and song sparrows. The road passes numerous unsigned paths that invite further exploration, but the route of the main road is evident at all intersections, and it is your best choice for this hike. In winter, there is a lot of standing water on the road and even more on the side routes, so wear boots that keep your feet dry. In the mud surrounding these puddles, look for tracks of raccoon and deer.

The road crosses a sandy backwater slough of the Columbia River, goes through a gate, and passes under two sets of power lines in a large grassy area. To the east and southeast, you will see Mt. Hood and the distinctive profile of Larch Mountain, among other landmarks. Bring binoculars to get a closer look at the deer in this area that bound away at the sight of hikers. Also look for red-tailed hawks circling overhead in search of a meal.

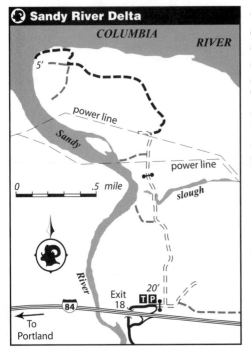

Sandy River Delta

COLUMBIA
RIVER

5'

power line

Sandy

power line

0   .5 mile

slough

River

Exit   20'
18   T P

To
Portland

track. Not far past the power lines, you come to a fence line that curves in front of the road. Turn right, go through the dilapidated fence, and climb to an old dike on the other side of a low grassy vale. To reach the Columbia River—the closest thing to an identifiable destination in this area—turn left on a trail that slowly curves to the west. After about 0.6 mile you'll reach a four-way junction. Turn right and in about 400 yards you should reach the sandy shore of the Columbia River beside a large sign warning river dredges of an underground pipeline. The two industrial towns across from you, in Washington, are Camas and Washougal.

To check out the confluence of the Sandy and Columbia rivers, walk west for about 0.2 mile along the beach to the meeting of the waters, a fine place to take a leisurely lunch while you watch the gulls and bald eagles usually found here. Return the way you came, or take the time to explore some of the many side routes if you are looking for more exercise.

Keep going straight where the road splits again beneath the second power line, and follow an overgrown grassy

TRIP 25 Oxbow Regional Park: North Side

Distance	1.8 miles, Out-and-back; 3.8 miles (including road walk), Loop
Elevation Gain	350 to 450 feet
Hiking Time	1 to 2 hours
Optional Map	USGS *Sandy, OR; Washougal, WA*
Usually Open	All year
Best Time	All year
Trail Use	Good for kids, no dogs
Agency	Oxbow Regional Pak
Difficulty	Moderate
Note	Good in cloudy weather

HIGHLIGHTS This attractive hike offers a much quieter alternative to the more popular routes in the developed south side of Oxbow Park (see Trip 26). Here the trails are unsigned and little traveled, but they are just as scenic and host a wider variety of wildlife. So even though finding this trail is a little tricky, it is well worth the effort. Pets are not allowed in Oxbow Park.

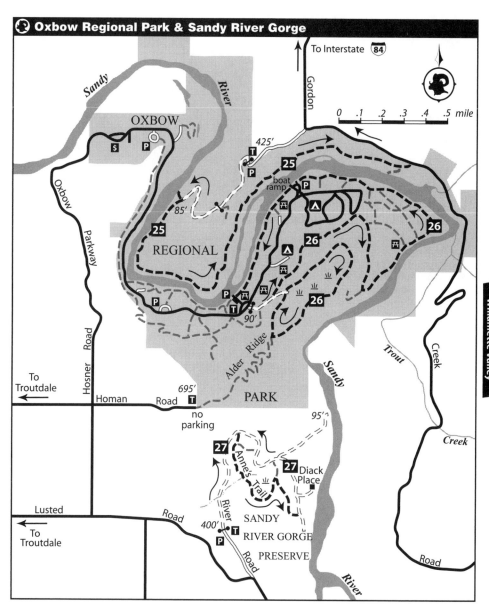

DIRECTIONS Drive Interstate 84 east from Portland, and take Exit 18 (immediately after the bridge over the Sandy River). Turn south on Jordan Road, which after 0.5 mile merges with the Historic Columbia River Highway. Stay on this road for 4.9 additional miles. Come to a fork and turn right on Hurlburt Road. Drive 2.1 miles to a four-way junction where you turn right on Gordon Creek Road. After 0.6 mile, where the road makes a sharp left turn and begins to go downhill, you turn right on a narrow gravel road marked only with a sign saying dead end. (Although it looks like a driveway, this is actually a public road.) Proceed on this road, keeping left at several driveways along the way, for 0.35 mile to a gate where the road enters Oxbow Regional Park. There is room here to park 3 or 4 cars.

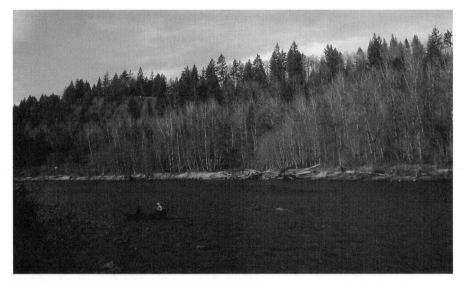

Sandy River from the northeast shore trail

Walk around the gate and down the dirt road as it passes through a relatively young and open forest of Douglas firs, western red cedars, and red alders. In winter, when the deciduous trees are bare, there are some nice views along the way of the scenic Sandy River Gorge. The closed road slowly descends across wooded hillsides and through level areas for 0.4 mile to a second gate. Here an unsigned foot trail drops to the left. Although initially promising, this trail is soon blocked by washouts and deadfall, so stick with the abandoned road as it descends in two wide turns to a river-level bench beside the rushing Sandy River.

Short spur trails lead to good fishing and picnic spots on the sandy beaches beside this well-named and beautiful stream. From the bank you can expect to see wildlife (ospreys in summer and great blue herons and river otters all year), cars on the road on the other side of the river, and boaters drifting by (their occupants casting for steelhead in the winter and looking for rafting fun in the summer). If you want a short trip, turn around here.

For a more complete experience of this wilder part of Oxbow Park, continue walking upstream, now on a narrow foot trail. The trail climbs briefly and then returns to river level on a wide, sandy bench populated by deer, raccoons, foxes, pileated woodpeckers, and other interesting wildlife. The vegetation is dominated by deciduous trees, especially black cottonwoods and bigleaf maples, but the understory is a mix of various thorny bushes, so off-trail travel is not recommended. There are no particular highlights along the way, but the hiking is very enjoyable and the solitude is nearly complete. The trail goes gradually uphill following the hillside a bit above the river before eventually ending at an unsigned and unofficial trailhead on Gordon Creek Road. The road shoulder here has room for a few cars to park, but signs direct that parking is prohibited between May 1 and October 1. To return to your car, walk 0.6 mile uphill along Gordon Creek Road to the gravel road turnoff, turn left, and then walk along this road to your car. Gordon Creek Road is narrow and has almost no shoulder—be very careful of traffic.

TRIP 26 Oxbow Regional Park: South Side Loop

see map on p.159

Distance	2.0 to 5.5 miles, Loop
Elevation Gain	100 to 500 feet
Hiking Time	1 to 4 hours
Optional Map	None are adequate.
Usually Open	All year
Best Time	All year, especially late September
Trail Use	Good for kids, no dogs
Agency	Oxbow Regional Park
Difficulty	Moderate
Note	Good in cloudy weather

HIGHLIGHTS Oxbow Regional Park is a justifiably popular preserve that provides the perfect mix of natural and artificial attractions. In addition to manicured campsites and picnic areas, complete with all the amenities, there are wild forests, quiet ridges, lots of wildlife, and dozens of tranquil riverside locations perfect for relaxing. An intricate network of trails gives you access to the entire park, with every foot of every path providing very pleasant scenery. In late September and early October, the river comes alive with spawning salmon, making this one of the best and most popular places to observe these magnificent fish struggling to complete their life cycle. Pets are not allowed in the park.

DIRECTIONS Leave Interstate 84 at Exit 17 in Troutdale. The exit road parallels the freeway for about 0.5 mile to a junction with S.W. 257th Drive. Turn right on this road, signed MOUNT HOOD COMMUNITY COLLEGE, and drive 2.8 miles. Then turn left onto N.E. Division Street. Follow Division (which becomes S.E. Oxbow Road) for 4.4 miles through a couple of intersections. Bear left at a fork to stay on the main road. In 0.7 mile you arrive at a four-way junction where the main road turns 90 degrees to the right. You turn left, following signs to Oxbow Regional Park, and drive 1.5 miles on Hosner Road (also known as Oxbow Parkway) to the park entrance station, where you must obtain a day-use pass. After paying the entry fee ($4 per car as of 2007), drive the park road past several pullouts and picnic areas. There are numerous places to start hiking, but the recommended one is at Group Area A, at a large gravel pullout on the left.

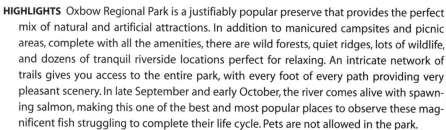

From Group Area A, you begin hiking by crossing the park access road and picking up a gravel service road that climbs Alder Ridge. In about 200 yards you come to a junction with a trail that goes off to the left. The park's main loop route follows this trail, but for a highly recommended and enjoyable side trip, stay on the service road. This road continues climbing through areas of lush, wet vegetation, with maidenhair ferns and horsetails especially abundant. In about 0.2 mile, a trail crosses the route,

just before the road tops a ridge. Before taking this trail, continue on the road for another 50 yards to see a large, scenic meadow, rimmed by tall flowers like foxglove and cow parsnip.

To make the pleasant loop in the trees around this meadow, retrace the 50 yards back to the trail junction and turn either way. This horse trail wanders through open red-alder and bigleaf-maple forests, along an almost perfectly level course. The trails on Alder Ridge are the quietest in the park, providing a welcome change

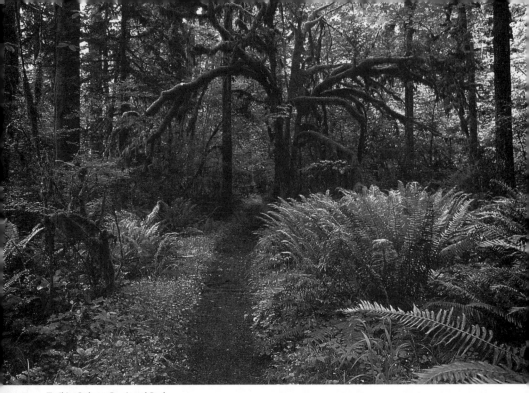

Trail in Oxbow Regional Park

from the popular routes closer to the river and road. But beware of the overhanging stinging nettles, which grow abundantly along the trail. Avoid touching this plant because contact with exposed skin causes a temporary but very painful stinging sensation. The deer don't seem to mind, however, as they frequently use this path, and in muddy areas you are likely to see deer tracks, and perhaps some of the hoofed creatures themselves. On the far side of the meadow, you pass several nice clifftop viewpoints some 300 feet above the rushing Sandy River. If you feel the need for some extra exercise, take a side trip off the loop on a trail that climbs a heavily wooded ridge to the southwest. This path climbs a dozen short switchbacks in coniferous woods to a trailhead at the end of a residential road. (Don't try to start your hike here as there is no legal parking.)

After completing the loop around the meadow, walk back down the gravel service road to the trail junction mentioned earlier, and turn right (downhill) on a narrow trail that descends to the valley floor. This route takes you to a tiny opening and a wooden fence near the campground and then through a lovely woodland, with dense thickets of sword fern under a canopy of old-growth Douglas fir and bigleaf maple. You pass a couple of junctions with unmarked side trails and then come to a fork in the trail with a signpost simply labeled "J". Bear right here, looping gradually around the end of Alder Ridge, and eventually reach a junction with the riverside trail beside the Sandy River.

The trail to the right dead-ends, so turn left and follow the river downstream. Several side trails lead down to the water, and you'll want to check out as many as time allows because the scenery and wildlife viewing are excellent. Birdwatchers will delight in watching the swallows zip over the water in search of insects and the fast-flying merganser ducks zooming upstream, just above the surface of the water. You might also want to join the human anglers trying their luck in the river, but be prepared to share the action with such natural anglers as river otter, great blue heron, osprey, and an occasional bald eagle. Using much less sophisticated methods, these creatures seem to fare just as well as those of us using expensive poles and tackle. Another tempting activity, especially on hot summer days, is to take a dip in the water. Stick to wading in the shallows, however, as the river is dangerously swift and the water is very cold, so swimming isn't recommended.

The trail passes a rustic picnic shelter and then slowly curves around the looping bend in the river that gave Oxbow Regional Park its name. Along the way, you may be confused by several side trails to the left and by a few places where flooding has washed out the main trail, requiring detours. Stay on the main loop trail at all junctions, and the route will eventually lead you to a boat ramp. You cross the parking lot here and then climb a little to follow the loop trail on a bench above the river. On your left, you will be very close to the well-kept picnic areas and horseshoe pits of the park, but despite these unnatural intrusions, the trail retains a remarkably wild character, especially on weekdays. On these quiet days, you may see rabbits hopping away from you into the brush or, in spring and early summer, you may even be visited by a spotted fawn tentatively coming out of the woods to have a look. About 0.3 mile from the boat ramp, you reach Group Area A and your car.

Portland & the Willamette Valley

TRIP 27 Sandy River Gorge Loop

Distance	2.6 miles, Semiloop
Elevation Gain	500 feet
Hiking Time	2 hours
Optional Map	None are adequate.
Usually Open	All year
Best Time	All year
Trail Use	Good for kids, no dogs
Agency	The Nature Conservancy
Difficulty	Moderate
Note	Good in cloudy weather

see map on p.159

HIGHLIGHTS Immediately upstream from popular Oxbow Regional Park is a much quieter area owned by The Nature Conservancy, a private nonprofit group that works to protect biodiversity. The Sandy River Gorge Preserve is a 436-acre parcel of land set in a 700-foot-deep gorge with fine examples of old-growth Douglas fir and western red cedar. The Nature Conservancy manages the land for its educational and scientific attributes, and to this end they prohibit visitors from camping or building campfires. You also are not allowed to travel by motorcycle, bicycle, or horse, and dogs are prohibited. Groups of 10 or more people need a special use permit, which you can obtain by contacting The Nature Conservancy at (503) 230-1221.

The Diack brothers owned part of this property and worked hard for its preservation. Their noteworthy accomplishments in conservation included tireless and successful efforts to get the Sandy River officially protected in both the Oregon and the federal scenic rivers systems. In addition to their conservation work, these two doctors were important community leaders. Dr. Arch Diack, a surgeon, invented the heart defibrillator, while his brother, Sam, is the father of the Oregon Museum of Science and Industry (OMSI).

DIRECTIONS Leave Interstate 84 at Exit 17 in Troutdale. The exit road parallels the freeway for about 0.5 mile to a junction with S.W. 257th Drive. Turn right on this road, signed MOUNT HOOD COMMUNITY COLLEGE, drive 2.8 miles, and then turn left onto N.E. Division Street. Follow Division (which becomes S.E. Oxbow Road) for 4.4 miles through a couple of intersections, bear right on Altman Road, and go 0.4 mile to a four-way junction. Here you turn left onto Lusted Road and follow this rural route 1.7 miles to the bottom of a steep downhill section. Immediately at the bottom of this downhill, turn left on unsigned River Road, in front of some farm buildings. Follow this gravel road 0.3 mile to a gate. Be sure not to block this gate when you park.

The hike begins when you go around the gate and immediately come to a large sign on your left. Here you will learn about the area's natural history, as well as the history of its preservation. Unfortunately, the trail map shown on this sign is incomplete and inaccurate, so don't rely on it.

River Road descends across private property, passes below and to the left of a farmhouse, and then enters wilder, forested terrain. The woods are composed mostly of lovely western red cedar and moss-draped bigleaf maple, mixed with some western hemlock, Douglas fir, and Pacific yew. The most abundant under-

Sandy River Gorge Preserve

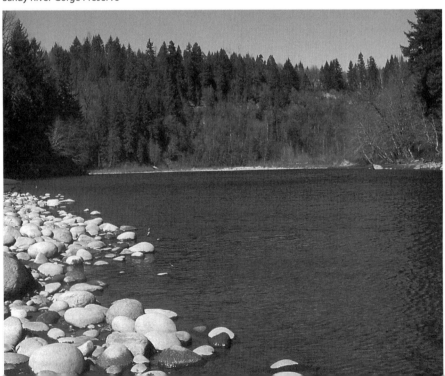

story species are sword fern, holly, and blackberry. As you descend, salmonberry becomes more common, and the impressive old-growth trees get larger, with some specimens up to 500 years old. Shortly after the road completes a sweeping turn to the right, you arrive at a junction with the rather faint Anne's Trail.

To do the loop, turn right on Anne's Trail, and 150 yards later bear right at an unmarked junction. Despite being a little muddy and overgrown, this route is enjoyable to hike, as it drops to a seasonal creek and then works around an open meadow frequented by a small band of elk. The sunny borders of the meadow are crowded with 3-foot-tall bracken ferns, which are liberally fertilized with piles of elk droppings. Watch your step.

Just past the meadow, the trail comes to a small grassy opening and a junction.

Anne's Trail goes left and soon returns to River Road. To explore more forest, turn right and follow a good trail that winds around in the trees to meet a small road. Turn left here to reach a junction with River Road. About 200 yards to the right are the buildings of the Diack Place.

To reach an even better riverside location, go left on River Road 0.2 mile to a road junction. Then go right on a jeep road 0.3 mile to a nice lunch spot on the rocky banks of the river. Nicely rounded by countless years of moving water, the rocks here make comfortable seats. There is also a good view downstream to the yellowish sandstone bluffs in Oxbow Regional Park. To return to your car, go back to River Road and follow it past two junctions with Anne's Trail and then up the woodsy hillside to the trailhead.

TRIP 28 Mount Baldy & Baskett Slough Loop

Distance	1.5 to 4.2 miles, Semiloop
Elevation Gain	300 feet
Hiking Time	1 to 2 hours
Optional Map	None needed
Usually Open	All year for Mt. Baldy Loop, May 1 to September 30 for rest of hike
Best Time	May
Trail Use	Good for kids, no dogs
Agency	Baskett Slough National Wildlife Refuge
Difficulty	Easy

HIGHLIGHTS In the mid-1960s, concern about the declining numbers of the dusky Canada goose led to the establishment of three national wildlife refuges in the Willamette Valley, the winter home of the goose. Thanks in part to these preserves, the goose's numbers have stabilized and even grown.

Hikers have also benefited from the refuges, which give them a chance to see what the Willamette Valley looked like before the land was largely transformed into farms. Baskett Slough, the most northerly of these refuges, has much to offer the outdoor lover. Here you will discover rolling hills covered with grasses and Oregon white oak trees, extensive lowland marshes, and lots of wildlife in addition to the geese. A handful of trails provide access to some of the best parts of the 2492-acre refuge. To protect its wildlife, the refuge prohibits dogs from the trail.

DIRECTIONS Take U.S. Highway 99W south from Tigard, and stay on this highway for 30 miles through Newberg to a junction with State Highway 18 south of McMinnville. Turn south, staying on Highway 99W toward Corvallis, and drive for 17 miles to a junction just shy of milepost 56. Turn right on gravel Coville Road, drive 1.5 miles, and then turn into the signed trailhead parking lot on the right.

You begin by climbing a grassy old road up a pleasant hillside covered with native vegetation including grasses, scattered Oregon white oak, blackberry, serviceberry, wild rose, and black hawthorn. In May, flowers like buttercup and a few camas add color to the scene. Thickets of head-high poison oak proliferate in almost every open area, so rule out any thoughts you might have of going off-trail.

After 0.2 mile, you come to an unsigned fork where you bear left and ascend to a ridgeline junction in a grassy saddle. You turn left here and wander up to the nearby summit of Mt. Baldy, with its oval-shaped wooden viewing platform. From here you'll enjoy a fine view of the distant Coast Range and the surrounding farmlands, as well as the wildlife-rich, shallow marshes nearby to the south.

As this is a wildlife refuge, there are, of course, lots of animals. You will probably hear the honking of geese on the marshes or flying overhead. Red-tailed hawks and American kestrels patrol the skies, while four-legged predators like coyotes and bobcats prowl the hillsides in search of a meal. Deer bound away from hikers, and many species of songbird nest in the oaks and shrubs.

From the viewing platform, return to the grassy saddle and bear left on an unsigned but obvious footpath, which departs from the open meadow and meanders through a surprisingly dense deciduous forest of Oregon white oak, bigleaf maple, and Oregon ash. Growing in the dappled sunshine of the forest floor are sword ferns, prairie star flowers,

and an abundance of poison oak. Oak woodlands like this have become rare ecosystems in the Willamette Valley, so this hidden treasure is a treat.

The trail's circuitous route across the slopes of Baskett Butte ends at a T-junction. To keep the trip short, you can turn right here and return to your car in just 0.5 mile. If you are visiting between October 1 and April 30, you will have to take this route because the rest of the refuge is closed to protect the wintering waterfowl. If you are visiting in late spring or summer, however, you can turn left and explore more of the refuge's diversity.

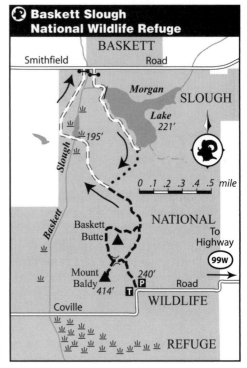

Baskett Slough National Wildlife Refuge

BASKETT Road

Smithfield

Morgan

SLOUGH

Lake 221'

195'

Slough

0 .1 .2 .3 .4 .5 mile

Baskett

NATIONAL

Baskett Butte

To Highway

99W

Mount Baldy 414'

240'

Coville

Road

WILDLIFE

REFUGE

For the longer trip, follow the path as it goes through a grassy swale and then curves to the left descending an oak-studded hillside to a lower area of fields and marshes. At the bottom of the hill, you meet the end of a quiet gravel service road and follow it as it goes north and west through several fields and past cattail marshes, to a dike across sluggish Baskett Slough.

In the marshy lakes on either side of the road, you will probably see and hear red-winged blackbirds, raspy-voiced marsh wrens, swooping northern harriers, and flocks of western sandpipers, who zip past in search of mudflats where they can feed. Killdeer nest in the drier open fields, and the adults are known to lead you away from their eggs and young by feigning a broken wing. From the marsh, the road continues north along a fence line on the border of the refuge, all the way to a gate at Smithfield Road.

Years ago, it was possible to return to Baskett Butte by way of a service road and a mowed trail that led past Morgan Lake. The trail portion of this route is no longer signed or maintained, but you can still follow its course. To do so, walk east on Smithfield Road to just past a large barn on the left, and then turn back into the refuge on the closed service road.

This road curves over to Morgan Lake and then crosses the dam forming the lake, where you will probably see geese and ducks on the water or spot a nutria sunning itself on the shore. To close out the loop, follow the overgrown road around the west side of Morgan Lake to a hedgerow near the lake's seasonal inlet creek. From here you wander southwest across a grassy field about 0.5 mile, back to the end of the quiet gravel service road below Baskett Butte.

TRIP 29 Ankeny National Wildlife Refuge: Rail Trail Loop

Distance	1.4 miles, Loop
Elevation Gain	Negligible
Hiking Time	1 to 2 hours
Optional Map	USGS *Sidney* (trails not shown)
Usually Open	April 1 to September 30
Best Time	Any time it's open
Trail Use	Good for kids, no dogs, wheelchair accessible
Agency	Ankeny National Wildlife Refuge
Difficulty	Easy
Note	Good in cloudy weather

HIGHLIGHTS Like Baskett Slough, its sister refuge to the northwest, Ankeny National Wildlife Refuge was set aside primarily to protect the wintering grounds of dusky Canada geese, but the preserve is also home to a wide variety of other birds, as well as numerous mammals, reptiles, and amphibians. A hike along the nearly level Rail Trail takes visitors through some of the refuge's best and most diverse wildlife habitat. To protect the wildlife, dogs are not allowed on the trail.

DIRECTIONS Drive Interstate 5, about 52 miles south of Portland (or 9 miles south of Salem), to Exit 243 for Ankeny Hill Road. Go right (west), drive 0.2 mile to a junction, and then go straight on Wintel Road. Continue 1 mile to another junction, go straight again, proceed 1.2 miles, and then turn left at a sign for Rail Trail. Drive 0.15 mile on this dead-end gravel road to the trailhead.

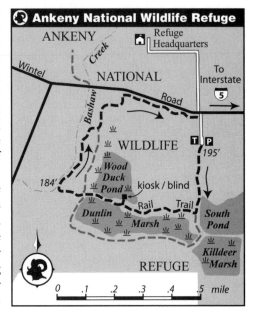

In a flatland dominated by grassy fields that are bordered by hedgerows, the wide, wheelchair-accessible trail goes south 0.2 mile to a junction. The mown-grass trail that goes straight visits South Pond and Killdeer Marsh, turns west to travel the edge of Dunlin Marsh, and then rejoins the recommended loop. This trail provides hikers with a little more exercise but misses the most interesting part of the hike.

The better choice is to turn right at the junction on a boardwalk trail that travels over a unique flooded-forest ecosystem. Here towering deciduous trees rise above a soggy marshland that simultaneously provides habitat for both tree-nesting songbirds, such as warblers, and water birds including coots, various ducks, bitterns, and rails. In spring, especially in the morning, the sound of birds singing seems to come from every direction. This is also ideal habitat for wood ducks, a spectacularly plumaged duck that nests in tree cavities.

At 0.35 mile a short spur trail branches off to the right and leads to an enclosed observation blind overlooking, appropriately enough, Wood Duck Pond. Look here, not only for the pond's namesake species, but also geese, various ducks, great blue herons, and red-winged blackbirds. The main trail continues on the winding boardwalk through more marshes and flooded forest, where visitors might see a yellowthroat (a small warbler) or a sora (a dark and secretive little rail). At 0.45 mile the boardwalk ends at a junction with a mowed trail atop a low dike. To the left is the alternate trail that looped around Dunlin Marsh. To the right is the shortest way back to your car. The best choice, however, is to angle about 5 feet to the left and then descend on a narrow, unmarked trail.

This circuitous trail winds through a relatively dry Oregon white oak woodland with lots of April-blooming wildflowers such as fringecup, buttercup, and camas. The forest also provides habitat for snakes, especially garter snakes, which often slither rapidly away from hiker's boots to avoid being stepped on. The trail has two muddy spots—insignificant obstacles and an excellent place to look for animal tracks. Common prints here include those of deer, raccoon, fox, and skunk. After 0.25 mile, you return to the mowed trail atop the dike. Turn left and

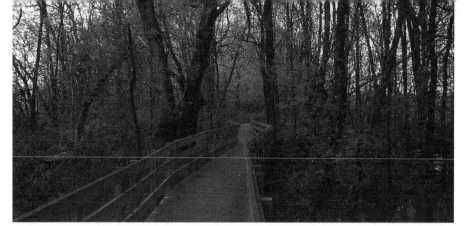

Boardwalk at Wood Duck Pond, Ankeny National Wildlife Refuge

walk past a seasonally wet meadow where long-billed marsh wrens seem to be singing constantly. The trail turns sharply right (east) just before reaching Wintel Road and then follows a hedgerow for 0.25 mile to a junction with the trailhead access road. Turn right and walk along the road back to your car.

TRIP 30 Lower Molalla River Trails Loop

Distance	3.3 miles, Loop
Elevation Gain	650 feet
Hiking Time	1½ hours
Optional Map	USGS *Fernwood* (trails not shown)
Usually Open	April 16 to November 14
Best Time	Any time it's open
Trail Use	Dogs OK, mountain biking, horseback riding
Agency	BLM *Salem District*
Difficulty	Moderate
Note	Good in cloudy weather

HIGHLIGHTS Flowing out of the Cascade foothills northeast of Salem, the Molalla River is a lovely stream that offers a wealth of recreational opportunities. The Bureau of Land Management owns most of the land along the river and has developed several trailheads, fishing spots, and primitive campsites. Although the corridor of public land is narrow, the trail network is impressively large, with more than 25 miles of interwoven paths and old roads. Equestrians use these trails extensively, so expect to encounter orchards of aromatic "horse apples" and some mud.

DIRECTIONS Leave Interstate 205 at Exit 10 just north of Oregon City, and go 16.5 miles south on State Highway 213. Turn left (east) on Highway 211, proceed 2.1 miles, passing through the town of Molalla, and come to a junction. Turn right (south) on S. Mathias Road, go 0.3 mile, turn left on S. Feyrer Park Road, and drive 1.7 miles to a T-junction. Turn right on Dickey Prairie Road, and proceed 5.4 miles to a poorly signed junction. Turn right at a small brown sign for Molalla River Recreation Corridor, immediately cross a bridge, and drive 3.6 miles on this narrow but scenic paved road to the prominent Hardy Creek Trailhead on the right.

The well-used trail curves northwest following an abandoned road as it slowly ascends from a river-level bottomland filled with deciduous trees to a hillside covered with western red cedars and Douglas firs. After 0.3 mile you come to the first of many junctions.

Since this area has no particular destination, hiking here generally consists of rambling through attractive forests while selecting trails more or less at random. It really doesn't matter which way you decide to turn at any given intersection. The route described here is just one of countless options, combining parts of several trails and old roads into a loop. With enough time and ambition you could easily spend several days wandering all the trails here.

The Huckleberry Trail is the return route of the recommended loop and follows the closed road that curves back to the left (south). For now, though, take Looney's Trail, which goes slightly right, also on an old road. After walking 50 yards, you come to a fork. Looney's Trail follows the road that goes straight (north). For this trip, however, turn left (uphill) at the fork, hike 20 yards to a possibly unsigned but obvious junction with the Rim Trail, and turn left onto this narrow foot path.

The Rim Trail climbs steeply for 0.1 mile, curves to the left (south), and becomes much more gradual with occasional views to the east of the forested ridges on the other side of the Molalla River Canyon. At about 0.6 mile is an unsigned junction. The Rim Trail angles slightly to the right (uphill), but for the recommended loop you should angle slightly left (staying level), now on the Deer Skull Trail, which is not named for any immediately apparent skeletal remains. This trail travels up and down (mostly down) for 0.2 mile to a junc-

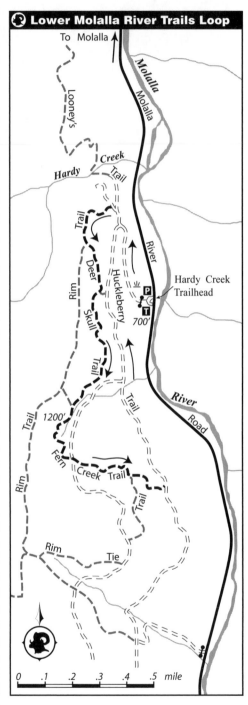

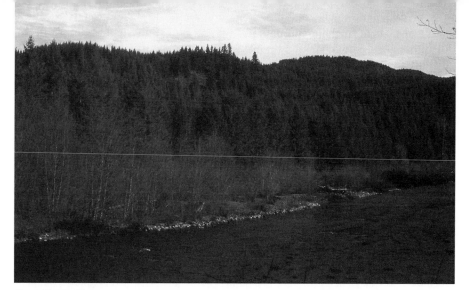
Along Molalla River

tion with a 40-yard spur trail down to the Huckleberry Trail. Go straight, still on the Deer Skull Trail, and follow this meandering path as it goes up and down through a young forest of 40- to 80-year-old Douglas firs. The trees in this area are scheduled for thinning, so don't be surprised to encounter logging activity along this section.

After 0.5 mile, the Deer Skull Trail reaches a T-junction. You turn left on the Fern Creek Trail, and stick with this sometimes dirt, sometimes gravel path as it curves left and down to a crossing of a side road from the Huckleberry Trail. After crossing the road, the Fern Creek Trail continues to show a strong preference for an indirect route, aimlessly wandering through the second-growth forest. Sounds along the way include the occasional unnatural roar from logging trucks on the Molalla River Road and the

loud rattling calls of pileated woodpeckers and the constantly cascading river in the canyon to the left (east).

About 0.3 mile from the road crossing the Fern Creek Trail comes to a junction with the Rim Tie Trail. As always, it really doesn't matter which way you elect to turn here. If you are eager to return, however, bear left (downhill) and rapidly descend for 0.15 mile to an unsigned junction with the Huckleberry Trail. Turn left and gradually descend this pleasant, woodsy route for about 0.3 mile to an unsigned junction with a road that goes left. Go straight, still on the Huckleberry Trail, and continue to the junction with the previously mentioned spur path to the Deer Skull Trail. Go straight and in 0.2 mile come to the junction with Looney's Trail and the close of the loop. Turn sharply right and retrace your steps 0.3 mile back to your car.

TRIP 31 Abiqua & Butte Creek Falls

Distance	2.0 miles (combined), Out-and-back
Elevation Gain	400 feet (combined)
Hiking Time	1½ to 2 hours (combined)
Optional Map	USGS *Elk Prairie* (trails not shown)
Usually Open	Mid-March to early December
Best Times	Mid-May and late October to early November
Trail Use	Dogs OK (but may be difficult for them in places)
Agency	Santiam State Forest
Difficulty	Moderate
Note	Good in cloudy weather

HIGHLIGHTS Hidden in the hills east of Silverton, Abiqua and Butte Creek falls are among the state's most spectacular waterfalls. Given their beauty, it is a shame that only a handful of Oregonians have ever heard of them. This lack of publicity is due entirely to the unmarked trail access rather than any deficiency in scenery. The same geologic conditions that created nearby Silver Falls State Park—basalt cliffs bisected by rushing streams—also created these natural wonders. And while the scenery isn't as concentrated as it is at Silver Creek Falls, the solitude more than compensates for the extra drive and effort.

DIRECTIONS For both destinations, begin by driving to the small community of Scotts Mills, reached by a well-signed road going east off State Highway 213 between Silverton and Molalla. From the southeast side of the bridge over Butte Creek, in the middle of town, turn south on Crooked Finger Road and climb this rural route 9.5 miles to the end of pavement. Exactly 1.5 miles past the end of the pavement is a junction with an unmarked gravel road on the right.

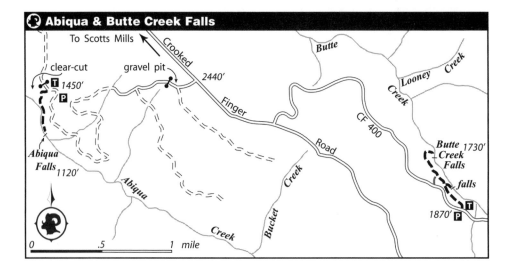

Abiqua Falls

To reach Abiqua Falls, turn right at the unmarked junction and drive 0.1 mile to a small gravel pit, where you go straight and pass through a gate. (This gate is usually open, but if not, you can just park here and walk, which adds 4.8 miles and 1000 feet of elevation to the round-trip hike.) Past the gate, you drive downhill, and go straight at another junction 0.3 mile beyond the gravel pit. About 2.1 miles from this last junction the sometimes rough road comes to a locked gate just inside a clear-cut. Park on the side of the road about 50 yards back from the gate.

To find the unsigned trail to the base of Abiqua Falls, leave the road about 100 yards before the gate and walk downhill on a small skid road. Follow it 100 yards and, just before entering a recently logged area, turn left on an obvious foot trail.

Tiny falls above Abiqua Falls

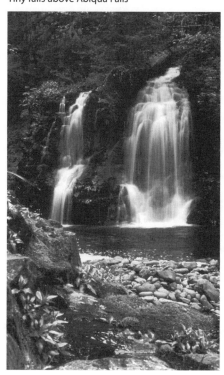

This steep route drops 0.2 mile to the banks of lovely Abiqua Creek, where you turn upstream.

From here the going is sometimes tricky, as you scramble over rocks and follow portions of a rough trail for 0.3 mile to the basalt amphitheater at the base of the falls. Birdwatchers will enjoy the sight of dippers zipping past and singing amidst the roar of the falling water, while photographers will delight in the excellent picture opportunities featuring foregrounds of the creek, mossy rocks, and overhanging trees. This is just the kind of lonesome spot that adventurous explorers love to discover.

With a bit of detective work, you can find a rough scramble trail that goes to the top of Abiqua Falls. The unsigned route leaves the access road at a small pullout about 0.3 mile before you reach the last gate. After about 150 yards the path splits. The steep trail to the right leads to a rather scary and dangerous overlook of Abiqua Falls, while the rugged and slippery path going straight leads to the top. Only confident and experienced hikers should contemplate taking either of these routes. Part of the hike to Abiqua Falls is on land owned by the Mount Angel Abbey. They have traditionally allowed hikers access to the falls but may close the area if problems with trash or accidents develop. Please be respectful and careful so hikers can continue to enjoy this area in the future.

Butte Creek Falls

From the turnoff for the road to Abiqua Falls, continue on Crooked Finger Road another 0.6 mile and then turn left on possibly unsigned Road CF 400. Drive exactly 1.9 miles and then pull into a small parking area on the left that is lined with large logs. The unsigned but well-beaten trail that leaves the parking

area has received some welcome maintenance in recent years, with gravel added
to the wet spots and boardwalks over the
dampest areas.

After just 0.2 mile, you come to a junction with a short spur trail that goes to
the right and leads to the 20-foot-high
upper falls, a broad spread of falling
water that is well worth a visit. From this
turnoff, the main trail passes a junction
with a spur trail back up to the road and
then continues downstream along the
canyon wall another 0.3 mile to a rocky
viewpoint of much more attractive Butte
Creek Falls. The mossy forest setting,
the 80-foot-high twisting cataract, and
the rocky gorge combine to make this
an ideal lunch spot. Don't forget your
camera and plenty of film, as the falls
demands to be captured from many different viewpoints.

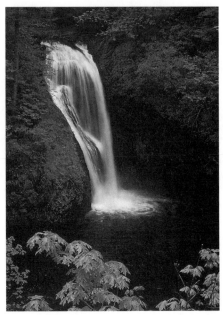

Butte Creek Falls

TRIP 32 Silver Falls State Park: Canyon Loop

Distance	7.8 miles, Loop
Elevation Gain	700 feet
Hiking Time	4 hours
Optional Map	Use park brochure.
Usually Open	All year (except during winter storms)
Best Time	All year
Trail Use	Good for kids, no dogs
Agency	Silver Falls State Park
Difficulty	Moderate
Note	Good in cloudy weather

HIGHLIGHTS Don't come to Silver Creek Falls in search of mountain views; the depths of this
forested canyon don't offer any. Don't come to Silver Creek Falls in search of flowers; it
has its share of forest wildflowers but no standout displays. And definitely don't come to
Silver Creek Falls in search of solitude; the place is overrun with your fellow *Homo sapiens*
practically every day of the year. But despite all that, absolutely do come to Silver Creek
Falls. With 10 spectacular falls tightly packed into a verdant canyon, including five that are
more than 100 feet tall, the park is a waterfall lover's paradise.

If this park were located in almost any other state, it would be a national park and
probably world famous. But in Oregon, which has an embarrassment of outdoor riches,
the park is well known only to residents of the Beaver State.

The hike is glorious in the spring when water flows are high and the sounds of falling water thunder out of the canyons. It is also a joy in summer when the shades of green are positively overwhelming. Fall is nice too, when bigleaf-maple leaves turn yellow and cover the trails in a crinkly bed of foliage. Even winter is spectacular, especially during a cold spell, when the falls become ice castles and occasional snowfalls make for stunning photographs. The best plan is to visit in all seasons, so you won't miss any of the park's faces and moods.

DIRECTIONS Drive south on Interstate 5 to Woodburn Exit 271, and turn east on Highway 214. Follow this road for 2 miles to a junction with Highway 99E, turn right (south), and then drive 1.5 miles to a junction with the continuation of Highway 214. Turn left (east) and proceed 28 miles, through the charming town of Silverton, to the North Falls parking lot and trailhead immediately before a bridge over North Fork Silver Creek.

You can start this hike at either of two trailheads. By far the more crowded one is South Falls, where a huge parking area also services a very popular picnic area. Much less crowded is the North Falls parking lot, on the north side of the bridge over North Fork Silver Creek. There is also a small parking lot at the trailhead above Winter Falls, but parking here is restricted to just two hours, which does not allow you enough time to complete the hike. Regardless of where you start, the park charges a day-use fee

($3 per vehicle as of 2007), and you must display a permit on your dashboard when parked in any of the lots. Permits are available either at the entrance station at South Falls or at the automatic pay station at North Falls.

If you start from the less crowded North Falls lot, you immediately drop to a footbridge over North Fork Silver Creek and come to a junction. For an excellent side trip, turn right here and loop under the highway bridge. Follow this route upstream for 0.2 mile to beautiful Upper

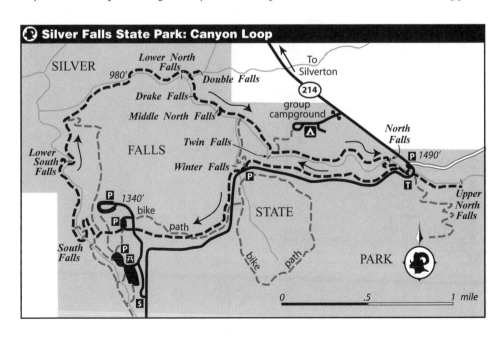

Silver Falls State Park: Canyon Loop

SILVER   Lower North Falls   To Silverton
980'   Double Falls
Drake Falls
group campground
Middle North Falls   North Falls
FALLS   Twin Falls   214
Lower South Falls   Winter Falls   P 1490'
1340'   STATE
bike
path
South Falls   PARK
Upper North Falls
bike   path
0   .5   1 mile

North Falls, which by itself would make this trip worthwhile, but is only a small sampling of the glories to come in this park.

Returning to the junction below the North Falls Trailhead, hike west and soon reach a second junction, which is the start of the loop. To save the best scenery for last, go left on the path toward South Falls, and traverse steep slopes covered with dense Douglas-fir and western-hemlock forests. On the rim of the canyon just above you is Highway 214, but the traffic sounds are never too intrusive. Most of the route is viewless, but at one point you come to a break in the trees and can look back up the canyon to towering North Falls.

Just short of 1 mile from the trailhead, you come to the small roadside parking lot for Winter Falls. If you want to visit this falls, turn right at the trail junction here, and then switchback downhill beside this

tall waterfall. If you want a short 2.9-mile loop, you can continue down the trail below Winter Falls to a bridge over Silver Creek, where you turn right and return to your car at North Falls.

For the complete loop, continue hiking on the trail paralleling the road, and you will soon come to a junction with a paved bike trail. You can follow either the hiker's trail or the bike route, as both wind through attractive forests for about 1.5 miles to the area around busy South Falls. There are several roads and trails in this area, some of them not well-signed, but you really can't get lost if you just keep going west.

From the north end of the main parking area, you pick up the paved trail that follows a fence line guarding the steep drop-off of the rim beside 177-foot-high South Falls. To pick up the loop trail, simply follow the crowds going north and drop down into the huge bowl holding

Middle North Falls

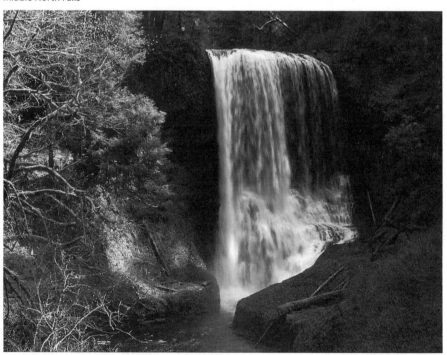

this classic falls. Snapping photographs all the way, you follow the paved trail as it takes you under the lip of a basalt cliff and into a huge, dry cavern behind the wall of water. This cavern, like the others you will find along the loop trail, was formed over millions of years as the falling water eroded the soft soils under a hard layer of basalt on the lip of the falls.

After this exciting walk, you come to a junction with a trail to the right, which goes over a bridge and returns most tourists to their cars at the South Falls parking lot. For the hiking loop, you go straight and leave the paved trail in favor of a quieter dirt path in the deep woods. The canyon is densely forested with Douglas fir, western hemlock, western red cedar, bigleaf maple, and lots of ferns. Trillium and other small wildflowers carpet the forest floor. The beautiful South Fork Silver Creek on your right is always a joy and provides many chances to observe cheerful dippers searching for food in the clear waters.

The next highlight is Lower South Falls, a 93-foot waterfall in another cliff-walled bowl. To reach this falls, the trail switchbacks several times and travels down a series of stairs, which may be dangerously icy in winter. At the bottom of the steps, the trail contours behind this impressive sheet of water and then climbs a little to a junction. Go straight and walk slightly downhill to a bridge over North Fork Silver Creek, which flows through a moss- and fern-lined slot canyon. The bridge here was washed out by floods in 1996, but the new one looks pretty sturdy.

The canyon walls become a little less steep but no less beautiful as the trail closely follows the cascading creek. At a bend in the stream, Lower North Falls makes a sloping 30-foot drop over a small cliff into a deep pool. Just past this falls is a junction with a 120-yard trail that goes up a side creek to tall and delicate Double Falls, an outstanding side trip.

The main trail travels above Drake Falls, which is difficult to see in a deep canyon on your right and then works its way up to the much more attractive Middle North Falls. A side trail contours around and curves behind this gorgeous falls in yet another eroded cavern.

A short distance past Middle North Falls is a junction with the trail up to Winter Falls. You go straight and continue up the lush canyon to Twin Falls, which anywhere else would draw rave reviews, but here seems rather prosaic. Just past this falls is a junction with a trail that goes up to the park's group camping area. Go straight, staying on the Canyon Trail, and cross increasingly steep slopes to the loud drop of awe-inspiring North Falls. This 136-foot-tall waterfall bursts out of a narrow chute on the lip of a basalt cliff and arcs down into the enormous bowl below. Photographers will love it. The trail goes through a cavern behind this fall and then switchbacks up the steep south side of the bowl, back up to the junction just a few hundred yards from your car.

TRIP 33 Silver Falls State Park: Perimeter Loop

Distance	10.3 miles, Loop
Elevation Gain	1750 feet
Hiking Time	5 hours
Optional Map	USGS *Drake Crossing, Elk Prairie, Lyons, Stout Mountain*
Usually Open	February to November
Best Time	Mid-March to May
Trail Use	Dogs OK
Agency	Silver Falls State Park
Difficulty	Difficult

HIGHLIGHTS This hike provides a quiet alternative to the extremely popular Canyon Trail in Silver Falls State Park (Trip 32). Although this route doesn't pass any waterfalls, its lovely moss-draped forests, babbling creeks, and solitude are rewards enough. Because the trail is not maintained as frequently as the Canyon Trail and it travels to higher elevations, the path is often closed in winter due to ice and blowdown.

DIRECTIONS Drive south on Interstate 5 to Woodburn Exit 271, and turn east on Highway 214. Follow this road for 2 miles to a junction with Highway 99E, turn right (south), and then drive 1.5 miles to a junction with the continuation of Highway 214. Turn left (east) and proceed 28 miles, through the charming town of Silverton, to the North Falls parking lot and trailhead immediately before a bridge over North Fork Silver Creek.

Walk south over the large hiker's bridge spanning North Fork Silver Creek and then loop down and to the right, following the paved trail that goes upstream toward Upper North Falls. Immediately after you pass under the road bridge over North Fork Silver Creek, you bear right (uphill) onto the Perimeter Trail.

The hiker-only trail switchbacks steadily uphill on a hillside covered with maples, Douglas firs, and western hemlocks with sword fern, deer fern, salal, and Oregon grape covering most of the forest floor. At several points along the climb the trail crosses tiny seasonal creeks on quaint wooden bridges. After 1 mile the trail levels off and then continues west to a junction with an old fire road at 1.6 miles.

You turn left and wander through a relatively open second-growth forest, at one point passing through a brushy meadow that is almost completely covered with bracken ferns. The hiking here is easy due to a mostly level grade with only a few minor uphills. After crossing an unnamed but reliable creek, the trail makes four short uphill switchbacks and then at 3.1 miles comes to a four-way junction with the Rockett Ridge Trail.

Go straight, still on the Perimeter Trail, and go sharply downhill through a forest with an unusually thick understory of salal. You cross another small creek, make a series of minor ups and downs, and then go steadily downhill in short switchbacks and long traverses to a crossing of another tiny creek. Just 0.1 mile later the trail comes to South Fork Silver Creek. You go upstream beside this lovely creek for 0.1 mile to a wooden bridge just 200 yards from the park boundary, a fact attested to by the sight of clear-cuts on the unprotected land to the east.

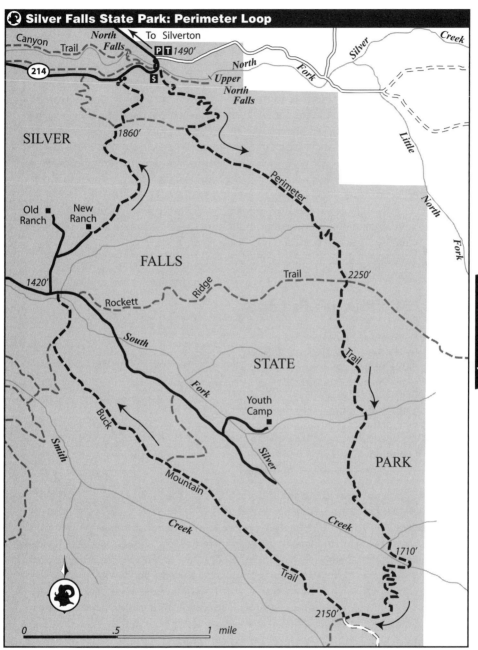

Silver Falls State Park: Perimeter Loop

You now ascend 10 well-graded switchbacks, make a few gradual turns on gentler uphill terrain, and come to four-way junction. To the left a fire road leads to the park boundary. You turn right on a route that until recently was a continuation of the fire road but is now the wide Buck Mountain Trail. About 1.2 miles along this gently descending ridgetop trail is a junction with another abandoned fire road that goes sharply right and downhill. You go slightly left, still on the Buck Mountain Trail, and continue going downhill. At 8 miles is the next junction, where you turn right on a long-abandoned gravel road. This route soon takes you to a bridged crossing of South Fork Silver Creek and a gate just before you meet a paved road. Turn left on this road, walk 100 yards, and then turn right (uphill) on the paved road providing access to "The Ranches."

After 0.2 mile this road forks in a large meadow. Bear right on the road to New Ranch, and walk 0.2 mile to road's end at the spacious and modern conference building. The trail resumes as an old fire road that starts behind the building near the dumpster. This route climbs moderately steeply for 0.6 mile to a forested ridgetop where there is an unsigned but obvious junction. You go right, walk 50 yards, and then veer left at another unsigned junction. This rather steep route (yet another long-abandoned fire road) winds 0.5 mile down to a gate where it meets Highway 214. Turn right and walk the narrow road shoulder for 0.2 mile back to your car at the North Falls parking lot.

TRIP 34 Shellburg Falls Loop

Distance	6.7 miles, Semiloop
Elevation Gain	1200 feet
Hiking Time	3 to 4 hours
Optional Map	USGS *Lyons*
Usually Open	All year
Best Time	April to June
Trail Use	Good for kids, Dogs OK
Agency	Santiam State Forest
Difficulty	Moderate
Note	Good in cloudy weather

HIGHLIGHTS Secreted away in the foothills of the Cascade Mountains, awe-inspiring Shellburg Falls is a delightful destination. Few hikers have made this discovery, however, because until fairly recently there were no developed facilities at the falls. A few years ago, however, the Santiam State Forest built a fine network of trails here and a small campground. Unfortunately, reaching these facilities remains problematic, since the most reasonable access road crosses private land and is closed to the public. Although it is possible to approach the area on a back road part of the year, the best way to reach the falls is to simply walk in along the closed lower road. This is perfectly legal, and a trailhead parking lot is available just below the closed gate. Regardless of how you get there, the destination is definitely worth it, since few falls in our area surpass the beauty found here.

DIRECTIONS Drive Interstate 5 south to Salem, take Exit 253, and then go 22 miles east on State Highway 22 to a junction in the small town of Mehama. Turn left (north) on Fern Ridge Road, drive 1.3 miles, and come to an unsigned junction with a gated gravel road going sharply right. Park in the gravel day-use lot immediately north of this junction. From May 20 to October 31 it is possible to reach Shellburg Falls from the north via remote gravel logging roads. Finding these sometimes rough roads is difficult, however, and really only worthwhile if you plan to car camp at the falls.

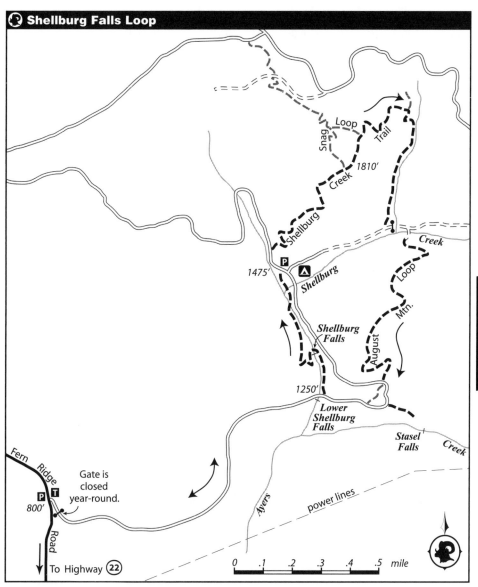

Shellburg Falls Loop

Snag Loop Trail

1810'

Shellburg Creek

1475'

Shellburg

Creek

Loop

Shellburg Falls

August Mtn.

1250'

Lower Shellburg Falls

Stasel Falls

Creek

Fern Ridge

Gate is closed year-round.

800'

Road

Ayers

power lines

To Highway 22

0 .1 .2 .3 .4 .5 mile

Walk around the gate and go gradually uphill on a narrow gravel road through an attractive rural landscape of small woodlots and pastureland. After about 1 mile the road enters forest, and then at 1.5 miles it reaches a bridge over Shellburg Creek. Just below the bridge you can hear (but not see) crashing Lower Shellburg Falls. The signed trail begins immediately on the east side of the bridge.

Walk up a stairway beside the stream, and then follow a gravel path that climbs moderately steeply in lush forest. Sword fern, salal, towering western hemlocks, moss-laden bigleaf maples, and a wide assortment of other greenery assault your senses in this junglelike environment.

After 0.15 mile you encounter the tall drop of 100-foot Shellburg Falls, an impressive column of water that drops over a basalt cliff.

The trail goes through a large cavern behind Shellburg Falls and then climbs stairways and a few short switchbacks to reach the creek above the falls. The trail follows the lovely stream for about 0.1 mile, crosses the flow on a bridge, and then crosses another bridge just 150 yards later before reaching the upper trailhead parking lot at 2.1 miles.

You can turn right here and walk the road back to your car, but to explore a longer loop through quiet forest, turn left on the road, walk 0.1 mile, and then veer right at a small brown sign for Shellburg Creek Trail. This often muddy path ascends 0.5 mile through a dense second-growth Douglas-fir forest to a junction with the Snag Loop Trail. You go straight, still ascending, and 0.1 mile later reunite with the upper end of the Snag Loop. Go straight again and climb a bit more to the top of a rise before beginning a long downhill. At 3.9 miles you go sharply right (downhill) at an unsigned junction, and then skirt a clear-cut and descend beside a small creek. A pleasant gradual descent of 0.3 mile through moss-draped woods leads to the end of a gravel road. You turn left on a section of closed road, cross a creek, and then turn right on another closed road that goes over Shellburg Creek. Almost immediately after this crossing you go left on August Mountain Loop Trail. This wooded route climbs over a low ridge and then winds down to a junction with the gravel access road.

Before exiting the area, it's worth your time to visit one more waterfall. To find it, go left and descend the gravel road for 0.1 mile to where it curves sharply to the right. Look here for an unsigned route (an old road) that goes left 0.15 mile to a viewpoint of towering Stasel Falls. The falls is on private land, so you cannot explore its base, but the viewpoint on public land is well worth a visit. To finish the trip, return to the gravel access road, walk downhill for 0.3 mile back to the lower trailhead, and retrace your steps to your car.

Shellburg Falls

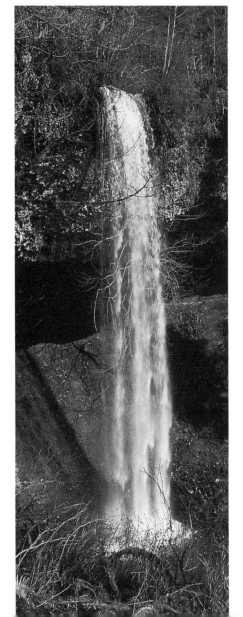

Chapter 4

Western Columbia River Gorge

The western Columbia River Gorge is a land of extremes. Here incredibly lush vegetation carpets amazingly steep slopes, dark cliffs tower thousands of feet above gentle river flats, and neck-craning views extend up and down one of North America's largest rivers as it cuts the only sea-level gap through one of the continent's longest and most important mountain ranges. A remarkable assortment of wildflowers and wildlife crowd this narrow strip, attracted by the fact that several life zones are literally stacked atop one another in this incredibly vertical landscape. And with all of that, I have yet to mention this region's most famous natural attraction, its waterfalls.

With its incredibly steep terrain and a generous portion of the Pacific Northwest's famous precipitation, it is not surprising that the western Columbia River Gorge boasts more waterfalls than almost anywhere else in North America. Dropping 620 feet, Multnomah Falls has no equal in Oregon and few in the country. And since this falls is conveniently located right beside Interstate 84, it is not surprising that some 2.5 million people visit this natural wonder every year, making Multnomah Falls Oregon's most popular

View east from Cape Horn Trail (Trip 1)

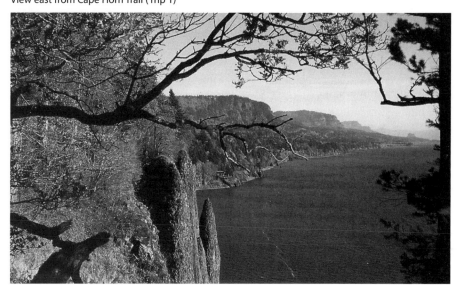

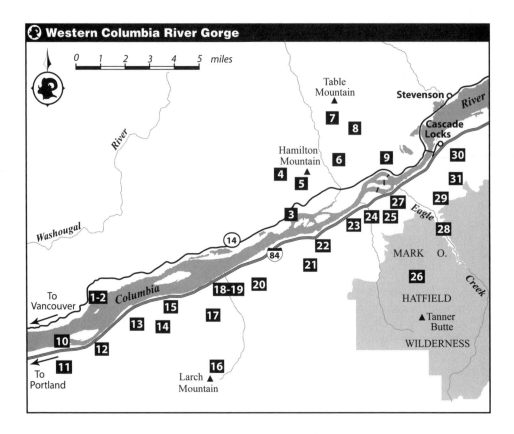

natural attraction by far. But the western Gorge hides literally hundreds of other waterfalls, and (hikers take note) most of these are only accessible by trail.

Most of the land in the Gorge, especially on the Oregon side, is publicly owned, either in a string of state parks, or as part of the Mount Hood National Forest. Even better, that public land is laced with hundreds of miles of excellent hiking trails, giving the dedicated pedestrian options for every season and enough to keep themselves busy for several years.

Getting here is ridiculously easy with Interstate 84 and the historic Columbia River Scenic Highway on the Oregon side and State Highway 14 on the Washington side giving Portland/Vancouver residents quick access to choice locations. And while both sides are worth seeing, the general rule of thumb is that Oregon has more waterfalls and trails, while Washington features better viewpoints and a southern exposure that ensures warmer weather and a longer hiking season than Oregon.

TRIP 1 Cape Horn

Distance	3.3 miles to Cape Horn Falls, Out-and-back
Elevation Gain	850 feet
Hiking Time	2 hours
Optional Map	USGS *Bridal Veil* (trail not shown)
Usually Open	All year
Best Time	Mid-March to May
Trail Use	Dogs OK (but trail is potentially dangerous for them in places)
Agency	Columbia River Gorge National Scenic Area
Difficulty	Moderate

HIGHLIGHTS Cape Horn is a cluster of dramatic cliffs that tower above the Washington side of the Columbia River east of Washougal. In recent years the U.S. Forest Service has purchased much of the land in this area, giving hikers access to several superb destinations that were previously off limits. So far, however, the only trails here are unofficial, so the routes are unsigned and are not shown on most maps. As a result, you'll need a little local knowledge (or this guidebook) to locate the starting points. Once found, however, the trails are easy to follow and among the most scenic in the entire Gorge. The area's most rewarding trail is this exciting path to several viewpoints and a lovely waterfall near the base of Cape Horn's cliffs.

DIRECTIONS Drive 21 miles east of Vancouver on State Highway 14, and park in an unsigned gravel pullout on the right (south) side of the road at milepost 24.6. If you come to the signed overlook at Cape Horn, you have gone about 0.4 mile too far.

The unsigned but obvious trail starts from the east end of the gravel pullout, winding south and slightly downhill through a relatively open forest of mixed deciduous and coniferous trees. After about 0.2 mile you go straight where an unmarked trail goes left and soon come to a second junction. The main trail goes right, but first you should go straight on a short, downhill, dead-end trail that leads to a wonderful viewpoint. (When the tread is wet, the clay soils along this trail

View west from Cape Horn Trail

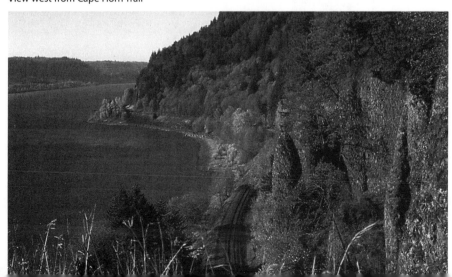

Western Columbia
River Gorge

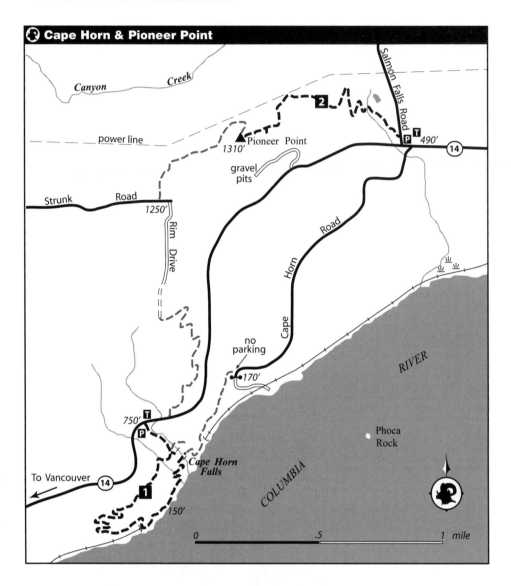

⊙ Cape Horn & Pioneer Point

Canyon *Creek*

power line

Strunk Road
1250'

Rim Drive

Salmon Falls Road

2

▲Pioneer Point
1310'

gravel
pits

P **T** 490'
14

Cape Horn Road

no
parking

•170'

750' **T**
P

RIVER

Phoca
Rock

To Vancouver **14**

1

Cape Horn
Falls

150'

COLUMBIA

0   .5   1 mile

can be very slippery.) In addition to providing great river vistas, this viewpoint is right above a falls on a small creek.

Back on the well graded and volunteer-maintained main trail you wander west through forest for 0.3 mile, coming ever closer to a steep drop-off, then switchback down a moss- and fern-covered talus slope to the first of several outstanding viewpoints atop a wall of rocky cliffs about 100 feet above the river.

The first viewpoint is right above where the railroad tracks go into a tunnel. More impressive than the railroad, however, is the view. The scene is breathtaking, with sheer drop-offs at your feet and views across the river to the high promontory of Oregon's Angels Rest and its rounded, forested companion, Devils Rest. As the main trail goes farther east along these cliffs, short side paths lead to more viewpoints where you can look east to nearby

Phoca Rock, poking its head out of the middle of the river, and distant Beacon Rock towering above the Washington shoreline about 9 miles away. You can also see portions of distant Dog and Augspurger mountains. Any of these rocky viewpoints makes a great lunch spot, although acrophobics may get a bit nervous, especially when it is windy, which is almost always.

At about 1.3 miles you leave the clifftop viewpoints and steeply climb a series of short, rocky switchbacks to the next big highlight of the trip. Spread out over an overhanging rock formation in a high shower of water, Cape Horn Falls (sometimes called "Salmon Falls") is an impressive sight. The falls is most spectacular in early spring when the small creek has plenty of water. By late summer the flow diminishes to a trickle. The trail drops a little in a rocky gully and then goes behind the falls, where you should expect to get wet. Cape Horn Falls is a good turnaround point.

You can extend the hike by going east, crossing a series of moss-covered talus slopes and steep, rocky gullies on an up-and-down trail that finishes off with a pleasant forest walk to Cape Horn Road. There is no legal parking here, so do not start your hike at this point.

A popular loop variation of this trip, which involves a fair amount of road walking, is to walk 2 miles up Cape Horn Road to Highway 14, turn left (west), and walk 0.1 mile to the Pioneer Point trailhead at the junction with Salmon Falls Road. From there hikers take the Pioneer Point Trail (Trip 2), and follow unmarked trails and roads back to the starting point. See Trip 2 and the accompanying map for details on this 7.2-mile loop.

TRIP 2 Pioneer Point

Distance	2.8 miles, Out-and-back
Elevation Gain	850 feet
Hiking Time	2 hours
Optional Map	USGS *Bridal Veil* (trail not shown)
Usually Open	All year
Best Time	April to June
Trail Use	Dogs OK
Agency	Columbia River Gorge National Scenic Area
Difficulty	Moderate

HIGHLIGHTS Although an unofficial and unsigned path, the Pioneer Point Trail is easy to follow and is an excellent option in the Cape Horn area. The trailhead is easy to reach, the hike is generally well-graded and not too difficult, and the forest is varied and attractive. Best of all, the destination provides a first-rate view of the entire western Columbia River Gorge. Like all trails in this area, this route was built and is maintained by volunteers. Please assist their efforts by doing some minor trail maintenance while you hike.

DIRECTIONS Drive 22 miles east of Vancouver on State Highway 14 to the junction with Salmon Falls Road near milepost 26. Park in the unsigned gravel pullout at the northeast corner of this junction. If you do not have a car, you can reach this trailhead by taking the Skamania County bus, which, conveniently enough, stops right at the Salmon Falls Road junction.

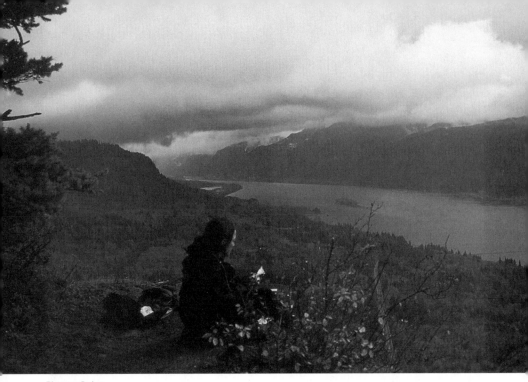

Pioneer Point

The unsigned trail begins at a low berm on the west side of Salmon Falls Road about 30 yards north of the Highway 14 junction. The trail gradually ascends through a mostly deciduous forest of bigleaf maples and red alders mixed with some western red cedars and Douglas firs. Traffic noise from Highway 14 dominates for the first 0.5 mile, but this is eventually replaced by the sounds of wind in the trees and singing birds. After crossing a trickling creek, the trail climbs six gently graded switchbacks and then connects with an old logging track that is now so overgrown it is hard to recognize as a road.

Your route follows the "road" for about 75 yards and then goes right on a narrow trail that steadily climbs a heavily forested hillside. Eventually you make a short, relatively steep climb just before the trail eases off near the top of the ridge. At 1.1 miles the trail briefly skirts a small, sloping meadow, reenters forest, and soon reaches the first of two stunning overlooks near the top of Pioneer Point. The second overlook, which is reached by a short spur trail, has outstanding views south to Oregon and east up the Columbia River. For another excellent viewpoint, continue 200 yards west to a grassy viewpoint at the top of a tall cliff about 400 feet above a gravel pit. There is plenty of room here to sit, eat lunch, and enjoy the view.

It is possible to continue this hike to the west and southwest along good but unmarked trails and old roads, generally keeping left at all intersections in an arc that takes you around fenced private land. This route eventually leads to paved Strunk Road, where you turn left (east), walk 0.1 mile to road's end, and then turn right (south) on gravel Rim Drive. When this road ends near a house, continue south on an old jeep track, and then follow a foot trail that winds downhill to Highway 14. From there, it is a short walk to the west to connect with the trail to Cape Horn Falls (see Trip 1).

TRIP 3 Beacon Rock

Distance	1.8 miles, Out-and-back
Elevation Gain	600 feet
Hiking Time	1 hour
Optional Map	Green Trails *Bridal Veil*
Usually Open	All year (except during winter storms)
Best Time	March to November
Trail Use	Dogs OK
Agency	Beacon Rock State Park
Difficulty	Easy

HIGHLIGHTS By far the most recognizable landmark in the Columbia River Gorge is Beacon Rock, an enormous basalt monolith rising above the river. Back on October 31, 1805, William Clark, cocaptain of the Lewis and Clark expedition, wrote of a "remarkable high detached rock" that was "about 800 feet high, [which] we called Beacon Rock." Thanks to a feat of engineering almost as remarkable as the rock itself, visitors today can do something that Lewis and Clark could not: Walk a good trail to the top.

DIRECTIONS Drive east from Vancouver on State Highway 14 for about 34 miles to the unmistakable rock on the south side of the road. Park in the paved lot beside the restrooms just below the rock's eastern cliffs. The trail begins about 50 yards west of the parking lot.

You begin with a gentle climb through a typical Gorge forest of Douglas fir, western hemlock, and bigleaf maple. In late April it also features splashes of the large, white blossoms of Pacific dogwood trees. The trail gradually works its way around the west side of Beacon Rock, first in forest, then above a talus slope, and finally onto the sheer basalt cliffs of the rock itself.

You are bound to be awed by the engineering of the trail, especially when you come to a plaque informing you that the trail was built from 1915 to 1918 by just two men, Henry J. Biddle and his assistant, Chas Johnson. Most of the path is blasted out of the rock face with wooden catwalks across the airiest places. Dozens of tiny switchbacks are carved into the rock, some across places that are so steep the trail has to loop around on top of itself to make its way upward. Metal handrails line the entire length of the route to provide a level of safety and comfort for those afraid of heights.

Amazingly, all of this was accomplished while still keeping the uphill grade quite gentle. If this trail was planned for construction today, it would cost millions of dollars. Indeed, it probably wouldn't be permitted at all because it would be considered too dangerous to build.

The trail, which is definitely not for acrophobics, goes through a metal gate, which is closed in winter if the trail is too icy, and then begins a series of switchbacks up the west and south sides of the rock. The views improve as you ascend, but most of the route is open to the afternoon sun, so it can be uncomfortably hot on summer days. Eventually, the path rounds a ridge with fine views to the south and west and then works its way to the summit through open forests on the southeast side of the rock. As you might expect, the views from the top are superb, although some directions are blocked by small trees. You cannot expect to be alone, however, as the trail is very popular and the summit area quite small.

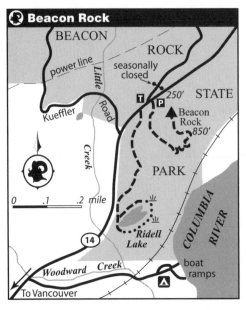

Beacon Rock

BEACON
ROCK
power line
seasonally
closed
Little
Kueffler
Road
Creek
STATE
250'
Beacon
Rock
850'
PARK
COLUMBIA RIVER
Ridell
Lake
14
Woodward Creek
boat
ramps
To Vancouver
0 .1 .2 mile

Hikers who are up for a bit of bushwhacking can extend this outing by taking a much quieter, 0.8-mile, unsigned nature trail that leaves from a parking area about 75 yards west of the Beacon Rock Trailhead. This path drops through the forest beside Highway 14 to Ridell Lake, a marshy pond and then loops around this pool. There are some good views of Beacon Rock from the south shore of the pond, which also has a wealth of frogs, ducks, beavers, and other interesting wildlife. Much of the route around the pond, however, is badly overgrown with blackberry brambles and stinging nettles, so most people will want to skip this adventure.

Beacon Rock Trail

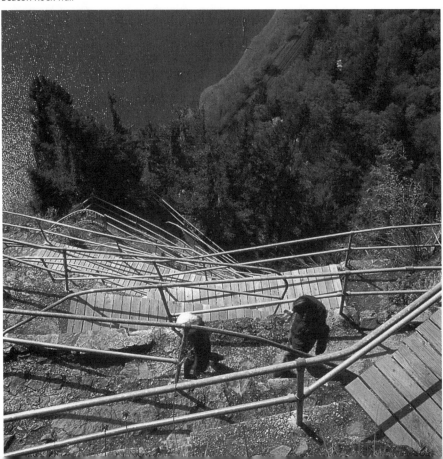

TRIP 4 Hardy Ridge & Phlox Point

Distance	8.4 miles, Out-and-back
Elevation Gain	2300 feet
Hiking Time	4 hours
Optional Map	Green Trails *Bridal Veil* (part of trail not shown)
Usually Open	March to November
Best Time	Mid-April to June
Trail Use	Dogs OK, horseback riding
Agency	Beacon Rock State Park
Difficulty	Difficult

HIGHLIGHTS There are thousands of miles of old logging roads winding through the forests of the Pacific Northwest. Hikers have not traditionally looked at them as a recreational resource, but that may be a mistake. Some of these old roads lead to very worthwhile locations, and they can serve effectively as wide, well-maintained trails with relatively easy grades.

This outing in a little-visited corner of Beacon Rock State Park is an excellent example. The old jeep routes here are intended now to be a playground for mountain bikers and equestrian visitors, but hikers are also welcome, and none of the routes are crowded. Best of all, however, is that this hike's destination is a spectacular open ridge with acres of wildflowers and terrific views.

DIRECTIONS Drive east from Vancouver on State Highway 14 about 34 miles to Beacon Rock, a huge basalt monolith just south of the road. Turn left on Kueffler Road just west of the park headquarters building, and drive uphill on this paved route. After 1.0 mile, turn right on a gravel side road signed for the equestrian trailhead. Drive this route 0.4 mile to the developed turnaround, complete with parking, pit toilets, picnic tables, and horse ramps.

The route from the trailhead begins as a closed gravel road and gradually winds up long switchbacks on a hillside covered with red alder and Douglas fir. About 0.5 mile after the road switches from gravel to rough dirt, you come to a four-way junction. The jeep road to the right makes a 1-mile loop. You go straight and gradually climb for about 0.4 mile to a second four-way junction.

You turn left at this junction and follow an old road overgrown with grasses that makes its way up the east side of a ridge. There are some decent views of Hamilton Mountain to the east, but most of the route is in the trees as you climb for 1.6 miles to where the old road simply ends. Continue the ascent on a good trail that curves off to the left climbing steadily in a dense second-growth, western-hemlock forest.

After a long uphill traverse, you make a switchback and emerge from the trees on an open rocky ridgeline where the views are superb, amply compensating for the long climb. Only the view to the north is blocked by trees, so take some time to look west down the length of the Gorge toward Vancouver, south to the rugged Oregon side of the river, and, best of all, southeast to Hamilton Mountain and down to Bonneville Dam.

The trail continues uphill along the narrow ridge, passing numerous exceptional viewpoints from moss-covered rock outcroppings. The trail gradually becomes sketchier, especially in some rocky and brushy spots, but it remains

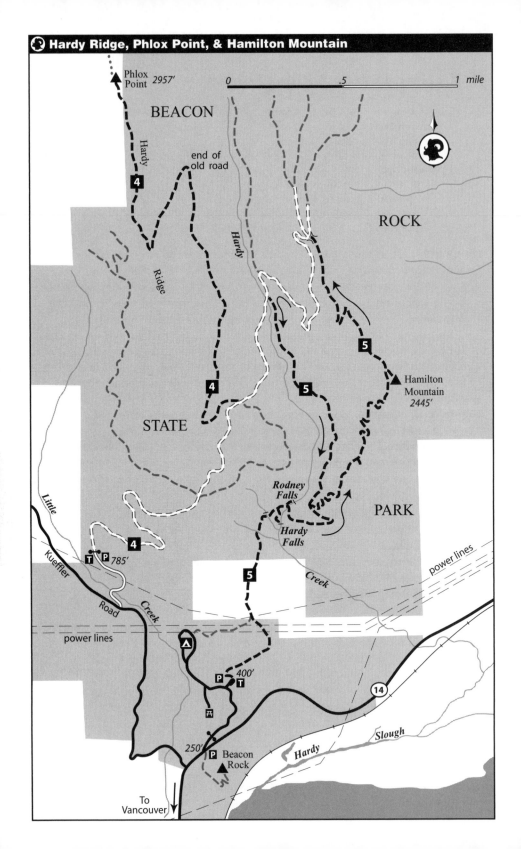

Hardy Ridge, Phlox Point, & Hamilton Mountain

Phlox Point 2957'

BEACON

ROCK

STATE

PARK

end of old road

Hardy

Hardy

Ridge

Hamilton Mountain 2445'

Rodney Falls

Hardy Falls

4

4

4

5

5

5

5

Little

Kueffler

Road

Creek

Creek

power lines

power lines

785'

400'

250'

Beacon Rock

Hardy

Slough

14

To Vancouver

0   .5   1 mile

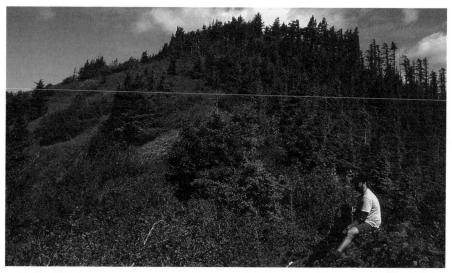

Hardy Ridge

reasonably easy to follow. Your goal is an obvious high point at about 4.2 miles, known unofficially as Phlox Point. Rivaling the abundant flowers (including, not surprisingly, phlox) for your attention is the view, especially east to Hamilton Mountain and south to the Oregon side of the Columbia River. Although rugged cross-country routes go north along the ridge and west down to an abandoned road, it is much easier and safer to return the way you came.

Western Columbia River Gorge

TRIP 5 Hamilton Mountain Loop

Distance	7.6 miles, Semiloop
Elevation Gain	2000 feet
Hiking Time	4 to 5 hours
Optional Map	Green Trails *Bridal Veil*
Usually Open	March to November
Best Time	April
Trail Use	Dogs OK
Agency	Beacon Rock State Park
Difficulty	Difficult

HIGHLIGHTS While its signature basalt monolith is Beacon Rock State Park's primary highlight, the view from atop Hamilton Mountain is a close second. The wildflower-spangled slopes of this peak provide some of the most memorable views in the entire Columbia River Gorge. The trail described here provides a varied and scenic approach to the summit views—visiting waterfalls, skirting impressive cliffs, and passing through meadows that in April are covered with terrific wildflower displays.

DIRECTIONS Drive east from Vancouver on State Highway 14 about 34 miles to Beacon Rock, a huge basalt monolith just south of the road. To reach the Hamilton Mountain Trailhead, bear left on the campground access road, drive 0.3 mile, and then turn right into the marked trailhead parking lot. This access road opens for the season on about April 1, so if you are visiting out of season, you will have to park at the lot beside Beacon Rock and walk up the gated road.

The trail starts in front of the restrooms at the northeast corner of the parking lot. You begin by walking past a sign board and then loop around the back side of the restroom building on a woodsy hillside. The wide path steadily gains elevation for about 0.5 mile, before the forest cover breaks and you cross beneath a set of power lines. From here you'll obtain a decent view of Hamilton Mountain, although the scene is somewhat despoiled by the power lines. At the far end of the clearing, go straight at an unsigned but obvious junction with a trail going back toward the park's campground. Soon after this you reenter the forest, as the trail begins to level off. In early to mid-April, the forest sprouts many woodland wildflowers, chief among them being bleeding heart, trillium, wood violet, and twinflower.

The trail crosses a small side creek on a quaint wooden bridge and then makes a short level traverse to a second tributary creek, below a large waterfall. Just past this, you reach much larger Hardy Creek, which cascades in a series of impressive falls, both above and below the main trail.

Before the route crosses the creek, a short side trail drops off to the right to a mediocre viewpoint of Hardy Falls below the trail. A short distance past this turnoff, a second dead-end trail goes left to visit Pool of Winds, where you'll be blasted by the spray of Rodney Falls—a refreshing experience in summer but uncomfortably cold in winter. These waterfalls are a good low-elevation destination for winter visitors or hikers with children.

The main trail loses about 50 feet of elevation to reach a wooden bridge over rushing Hardy Creek and then begins to go uphill. The next 0.5 mile formerly climbed steeply up a series of short switchbacks, but in late 2001 the path was rerouted. It now ascends gradually in a long switchback with an easier grade and better views to a possibly unsigned junction with the return route of this loop. For the most direct route to the summit, turn right and switchback 23 times through increasingly open and attractive terrain. The switchbacks end temporarily at a major highlight of the trip, where a short side trail goes out to a dizzying

Cliffs below summit of Hamilton Mountain

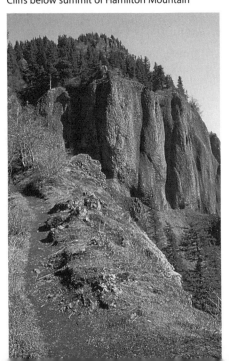

viewpoint atop a rock outcropping. From here, there are first-rate views of Beacon Rock, which looks surprisingly small from up here. The view also takes in high points on the opposite side of the Gorge, such as Tanner Butte and Nesmith Point. Circling in the air both above and below you are violet-green swallows and graceful turkey vultures, effortlessly soaring on the thermals. If you are getting tired, you can turn around here, already amply rewarded for your efforts so far.

From this viewpoint the trail traverses a partly forested hillside with nice views to the northwest of the alder-choked valley containing Hardy Creek. You pass a great view of the lichen-covered cliffs below the summit of Hamilton Mountain and then make a final push up a couple dozen often very short switchbacks to a junction on the windy summit ridge. To the right, there is a short dead-end trail to a brushy viewpoint, but that view is no better than the one you already enjoy. The best part of this view is looking east to Table Mountain and Aldrich Butte.

You can make a loop on a trail that has a more gradual descent and is easier on the knees than the one you just completed. Turn left (north) at the ridgetop junction and follow the path along the top of the view-packed but breezy ridge. After 0.2 mile, the trail drops down the west side of the ridge on two long switchbacks, traverses a forested hillside, and comes to an open, wind-whipped saddle. At this saddle you meet a road that is closed to cars, except for the occasional park maintenance vehicle. The road forks at the saddle. To return to your car, follow the leftmost branch and hike downhill, as the road uses two long switchbacks to make its way down into the canyon of Hardy Creek. Just above the creek at a final switchback is a junction where you turn left (downstream) and soon come to a tiny meadow, where a road culvert crosses the stream.

To complete the loop, leave the road just before it crosses the culvert, and pick up a trail paralleling the creek. This virtually level route contours for 1.1 miles along the alder-covered hillside above the creek and then rejoins the Hamilton Mountain Trail at the junction 0.5 mile above Hardy and Rodney Falls.

TRIP 6 Aldrich Butte

Distance	4.2 miles, Out-and-back
Elevation Gain	1350 feet
Hiking Time	2½ hours
Optional Map	Green Trails *Bonneville Dam*
Usually Open	All year (except during winter storms)
Best Time	April
Trail Use	Good for kids, Dogs OK
Agency	Columbia River Gorge National Scenic Area
Difficulty	Difficult

HIGHLIGHTS Aldrich Butte is an easier alternate destination for hikers who don't want to tackle the difficult trip to the top of Table Mountain (Trip 7). Aldrich is neither as high as its neighbor to the north, nor is its view as expansive, but you'll still find it well worth a visit, especially in early spring when other trails are still covered by snow.

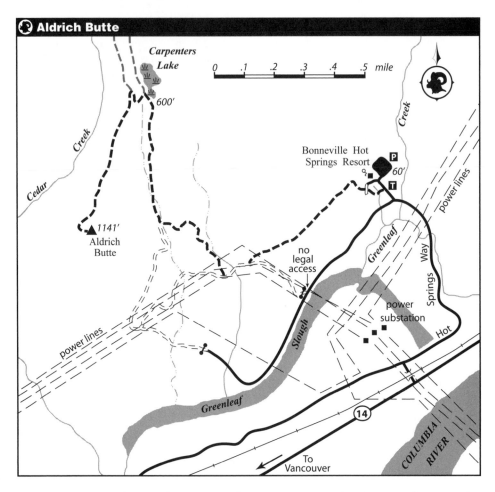

Aldrich Butte

Carpenters Lake

600'

Creek

Cedar
Creek

1141'
Aldrich
Butte

Bonneville Hot
Springs Resort

60'

no
legal
access

Greenleaf

Springs Way

Hot
Springs Way

power
substation

power lines

power lines

Slough

Greenleaf

Greenleaf

14

To
Vancouver

COLUMBIA RIVER

DIRECTIONS Drive State Highway 14 east from Vancouver to a junction near the town of North Bonneville at milepost 38.5. Turn left (north) on Hot Springs Way, immediately go through a narrow tunnel under a set of railroad tracks, and come to a T-junction. Turn right, go 0.8 mile, and then turn right into the Bonneville Hot Springs Resort. Drive 0.1 mile and park in the enormous lot on the east side of the hotel. This is private property, but hikers are allowed to park here and hike through.

Walk 100 yards back along the resort's access road, turn right (west), and cross a trail bridge over a creek in the middle of a miniature golf course. Stay on this paved trail for 0.1 mile, and then go straight across a gravel road near a group of out buildings. You go steeply uphill for 0.1 mile to where the trail turns left (west) and the pavement ends. The route now follows a primitive jeep track that goes up and down for 0.2 mile to a four-way junction in a clearing beneath a power line. Go straight on a somewhat better jeep road, drop briefly to a culvert over a small creek, and then, 80 yards later, come a second unsigned junction.

You veer right (slightly uphill), walk 100 yards to the base of a power line

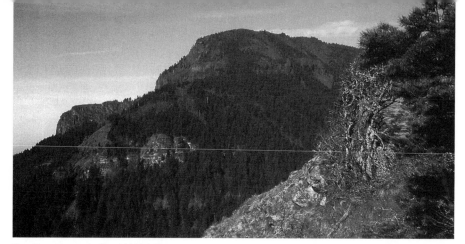
Hamilton Mountain from Aldrich Butte

tower, and then continue straight on an unsigned but obvious foot trail that goes north into the forest. This trail winds through an attractive Douglas-fir forest for 0.4 mile to a junction with a long abandoned road. Turn right and ascend this sometimes muddy ATV route for 0.5 mile to a junction beside a large scenic meadow called Carpenters Lake. Turn left and ascend two quick switchbacks to an unsigned junction.

Turn left on a closed jeep road (still used by ATVs), and climb steadily but moderately around the west side of Aldrich Butte to a flat turnaround just below the summit. From the top, there are fine views of the Columbia River, the town of North Bonneville, high points on the Oregon side of the Gorge, and nearby Table and Hamilton mountains. In addition to the views, there are usually violet-green swallows and ravens circling overhead. In the first half of April, colorful purple grass widows grace the open south-facing slopes below the top. There are some nice picnic spots at the summit with the old concrete foundations of a building providing welcome stools.

TRIP 7 Table Mountain

Distance	9.6 miles, Out-and-back
Elevation Gain	3650 feet
Hiking Time	5 to 6 hours
Optional Map	Green Trails *Bonneville Dam*
Usually Open	Late March to November
Best Time	May to June
Trail Use	Dogs are allowed, but the trail is too rough and difficult for most.
Agency	Columbia River Gorge National Scenic Area
Difficulty	Strenuous

HIGHLIGHTS The climb to the top of Table Mountain, one of the most distinctive landmarks in the Columbia River Gorge, is not for the faint of heart (or of legs or lungs, for that matter). The elevation gain and the distance are both significant, making this a challenge for hikers no matter what their ability level. Adding to the difficulties is that fully half the elevation gain is concentrated in just the last 1.2 miles, making for a very steep stretch, which must be tackled after you complete the long approach. A new trailhead has taken almost 6 miles off the round-trip distance of this climb, so while it is still very challenging it is a little more reasonable.

Because it opens early in the year, mountain climbers often use this route to get in shape for the climbing season. For ordinary hikers, the prize for this tough hike is the outstanding view from the flat top of the peak, one of the most far-ranging anywhere in the Columbia River Gorge.

DIRECTIONS Drive State Highway 14 east from Vancouver to a junction near the town of North Bonneville at milepost 38.5. Turn left (north) on Hot Springs Way, immediately go through a narrow tunnel under a set of railroad tracks, and come to a T-junction. Turn right, go 0.8 mile, and then turn right into the Bonneville Hot Springs Resort. Drive 0.1 mile and park in the enormous lot on the east side of the hotel. This is private property, but hikers are allowed to park here and hike through.

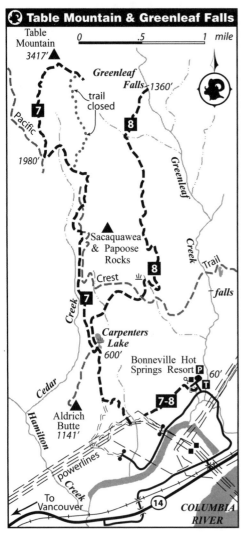

Table Mountain & Greenleaf Falls

Walk 100 yards back along the resort's access road, turn right (west), and cross a trail bridge over a creek in the middle of a miniature golf course. Stay on this paved trail for 0.1 mile, and then go straight across a gravel road near a group of outbuildings. You go steeply uphill for 0.1 mile to where the trail turns left (west) and the pavement ends. The route now follows a primitive jeep track that goes up and down for 0.2 mile to a four-way junction in a clearing beneath a power line. Go straight on a somewhat better jeep road, drop briefly to a culvert over a small creek, and then, 80 yards later, come a second unsigned junction.

You veer right (slightly uphill) at this junction, walk 100 yards to the base of a power line tower, and then continue straight on an unsigned but obvious foot trail that goes north into the forest. This trail winds through an attractive Douglas-fir forest for 0.4 mile to a junction with a long abandoned road. Turn right and ascend this sometimes muddy ATV route for 0.5 mile to a junction beside a large scenic meadow called Carpenters Lake. Turn left and ascend two quick switchbacks to an unsigned junction.

Keep straight on the old road and walk north for 1 mile to where the Pacific Crest Trail (PCT) crosses your route. Turn onto

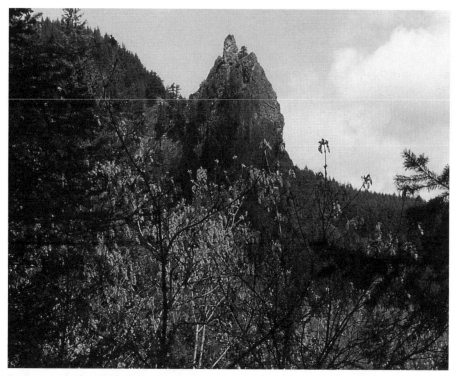

Sacaquawea Rock on Table Mountain

that trail, soon cross the road a second time, and ascend to a junction. The trail to the right was once the wickedly steep east side of a loop to the top of Table Mountain. That trail is now closed, so continue straight on the PCT, cross a dry gully, and contour to a four-way junction on a ridgetop.

The PCT goes straight, but to reach the summit and its grand views, turn right and begin climbing. In the next 1.1 miles, you ascend fully 1700 feet and, since much of the way is exposed to the sun, you'll pour out gallons of sweat on a hot day. The route is rocky, but if you take it slow, which the steepness forces you to do in any event, it's not overly dangerous. At the frequent rest stops demanded by the grade, you enjoy ever-improving views, so at least your effort is continuously well compensated.

Once you reach the flat summit of Table Mountain, turn right (east) and wander on a boot path along the partly forested top to any of several outstanding viewpoints. Directly below you, the Gorge extends both west and east in all of its awesome beauty.

Rising majestically over the hills on the Oregon side is pointed Mt. Hood, covered by its year-round mantle of snow. If you take the trail all the way to its end, you will look down from dizzying cliffs on Table Mountain's precipitous eastern face and see the entire route of your hike. Bring a windbreaker for protection against the almost constant winds. You will also want a lunch to replace some of those calories you just burned up and a camera with plenty of film or digital memory chips. Once you've rested and soaked in all the views, return the way you came.

TRIP 8 Greenleaf Falls

see map on p.198

Distance	8.8 miles, Out-and-back
Elevation Gain	1550 feet
Hiking Time	4 hours
Optional Map	Green Trails *Bonneville Dam*
Usually Open	All year (except during winter storms)
Best Time	April
Trail Use	Dogs OK
Agency	Columbia River Gorge National Scenic Area
Difficulty	Difficult
Note	Good in cloudy weather

HIGHLIGHTS If you are in the Table Mountain area and find that the weather has turned gloomy, skip the viewpoint destinations at Aldrich Butte and Table Mountain, and head instead for Greenleaf Falls. The trip is even better in the sunshine, of course, but the pleasant forests, together with the little-known twisting cascade at trail's end, are equally impressive under a layer of clouds. Really adventurous hikers can combine this destination with a trip to Aldrich Butte for the best of both worlds.

DIRECTIONS Drive State Highway 14 east from Vancouver to a junction near the town of North Bonneville at milepost 38.5. Turn left (north) on Hot Springs Way, immediately go through a narrow tunnel under a set of railroad tracks, and come to a T-junction. Turn right, go 0.8 mile, and then turn right into the Bonneville Hot Springs Resort. Drive 0.1 mile and park in the enormous lot on the east side of the hotel. This is private property, but hikers are allowed to park here and hike through.

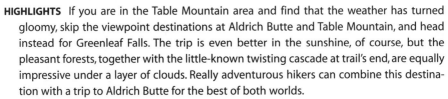

Walk 100 yards back along the resort's access road, turn right (west), and cross a trail bridge over a creek in the middle of a miniature golf course. Stay on this paved trail for 0.1 mile, and then go straight across a gravel road near a group of outbuildings. You go steeply uphill for 0.1 mile to where the trail turns left (west) and the pavement ends. The route now follows a primitive jeep track that goes up and down for 0.2 mile to a four-way junction in a clearing beneath a power line. Go straight on a somewhat better jeep road, drop briefly to a culvert over a small creek, and then, 80 yards later, come a second unsigned junction.

You veer right (slightly uphill) at this junction, walk 100 yards to the base of a power line tower, and then continue straight on an unsigned but obvious foot

trail that goes north into the forest. This trail winds through an attractive Douglas-fir forest for 0.4 mile to a junction with a long abandoned road. Turn right and ascend this sometimes muddy ATV route for 0.5 mile to a junction beside a large scenic meadow called Carpenters Lake. Bear right, skirt the west side of the frog-filled "lake," and then wind uphill for 0.8 mile in deciduous woods, crossing two seasonal creeks along the way, to an obvious but unsigned four-way junction with the Pacific Crest Trail.

Go straight (a little uphill) at this junction, and follow a route that used to be a logging road, but, since it has been closed for so long many decades, is now barely a trail. The path soon skirts the right side of a tiny marsh, where there are tantalizing views of Table Mountain's impressive cliffs and the pointed pinnacles called Sacaquawea and Papoose rocks. The route now heads north and climbs steadily, but never too steeply, through pleasant second-growth forests. The trail tops a minor ridge with rather disappointing views, loses elevation for about 0.2 mile, and makes two short, rounded switchbacks, before resuming its very gradual ascent.

The next major highlight is about 0.8 mile past the switchbacks, where you cross a large, moss-covered talus slope. The opening here is directly beneath the cliffs of Table Mountain, a neck-craning 1800 feet above you. The sheer cliffs are the result of a massive landslide that fell away from Table Mountain about 700 years ago. The debris from this slide, over which you have been hiking for the entire trip, changed the course of the Columbia River and even temporarily blocked the stream. Many scholars believe that this is the source of the Native American legend about a natural "Bridge of the Gods" over the Columbia River. If you can tear your eyes away from the close-up views, try shifting your gaze southward to the top third of Mt. Hood, poking over Tanner Ridge on the Oregon side of the Gorge.

From the talus slope you should be able to hear the sound of multitiered Greenleaf Falls just a short distance northeast. This cataract is actually several smaller waterfalls that are formed where good-sized Greenleaf Creek tumbles down a series of twisting cascades. It is hard to get a good view of the entire falls, but the two-pronged cataract right above the trail is worth the hike all by itself. Really athletic hikers may be tempted to scramble up the slopes beside the falls, hoping to get a better look. This effort is not only dangerous but it doesn't result in any improvement in the view and so is not worth it.

Cliffs of Table Mountain from the southeast

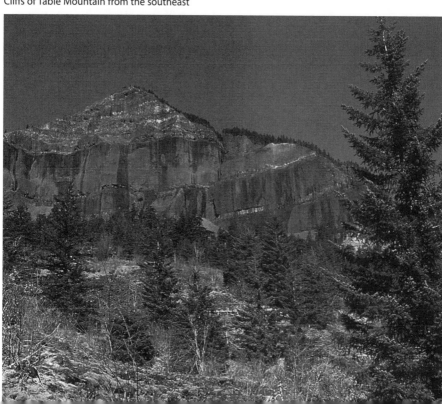

TRIP 9 Gillette Lake & Greenleaf Overlook

Distance	7.6 miles, Out-and-back
Elevation Gain	650 feet
Hiking Time	4 hours
Optional Map	Green Trails *Bridal Veil*
Usually Open	All year
Best Times	April and May
Trail Use	Good for kids, dogs OK, backpacking option
Agency	Columbia River Gorge National Scenic Area
Difficulty	Moderate

HIGHLIGHTS This low-elevation section of the Pacific Crest Trail (PCT) explores a unique, jumbled landscape with an interesting geologic history. About 700 years ago a huge landslide tumbled off the north sides of Table Mountain and Greenleaf Peak. This landslide not only left behind the distinctive towering cliffs seen on those mountains today but dumped an enormous amount of rock and debris at their base. That debris covered several square miles and even temporarily blocked the Columbia River. The river broke through, but the remaining rocks and boulders created a major rapids that eventually gave the city of "Cascade" Locks (and the entire "Cascade" Mountain Range, for that matter) its name. The rapids are now flooded under the slack water behind Bonneville Dam, but the cliffs and landslide material are still there and worth investigating. Nestled neatly amid this now forest-covered chaos are this hike's two principal destinations—Gillette Lake, an attractive pool suitable for year-round backpacking, and Greenleaf Overlook, a nice viewpoint where you can see Bonneville Dam and many landmarks on the Oregon side of the Columbia River.

View from Greenleaf Overlook

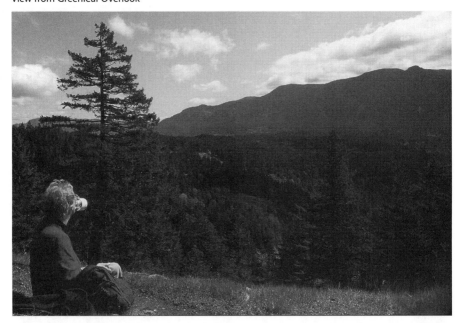

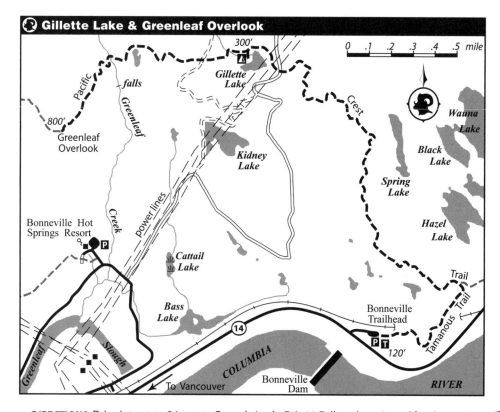

Gillette Lake & Greenleaf Overlook

Pacific

falls

Greenleaf

300'

Gillette
Lake

Crest

0 .1 .2 .3 .4 .5 mile

*Wauna
Lake*

800'

Greenleaf
Overlook

Kidney
Lake

*Black
Lake*

Spring
Lake

Creek

power lines

Bonneville Hot
Springs Resort

Cattail
Lake

*Hazel
Lake*

Trail

Bass
Lake

14

Bonneville
Trailhead

120'

Tamanous Trail

Greenleaf

Slough

COLUMBIA

Bonneville
Dam

RIVER

To Vancouver

DIRECTIONS Drive Interstate 84 east to Cascade Locks Exit 44. Follow the exit road for about 0.3 mile, and then turn right (uphill) on a cloverleaf that takes you over the Bridge of the Gods (a $1 toll applies, as of 2007). Turn left at the junction with State Highway 14, drive 2 miles, and then turn right into the spacious and well-marked Bonneville Trailhead parking lot.

The trail, signed as the TAMANOUS TRAIL, begins as a gravel-covered path that departs from the northeast end of the parking area. After climbing a hillside covered with second-growth Douglas firs, the winding trail goes up and down to a junction with the PCT at 0.6 mile. Turn left (northbound) on this famous path, and for the next 0.5 mile follow an undulating course in a rather unattractive human-made clearing that looks like it was intended for a power line, although no such line is in place today. The clearing does provide some decent views of Table Mountain to the northwest and Oregon's Wauna Point and Eagle Creek Canyon to the south.

Upon finally reentering forest, the trail begins to noticeably traverse the old landslide material. This contorted landscape is peculiar because it completely lacks any recognizable ridges and ravines that are usually left behind by years of erosion. Instead you find disconnected hills and hollows, huge moss-covered boulders, and rocky depressions that strangely have no water since all the precipitation soon percolates below the surface. Although forests now cover the debris, it remains fascinating, especially once you realize what caused this jumble.

The trail crosses a gravel road and then descends to Gillette Lake at 2.5 miles. There are nice camps near the inlet of this green-tinged lake, which features excellent swimming from late spring to early fall.

If you are continuing to Greenleaf Overlook, keep right at an unsigned junction with the spur trail that goes to Gillette Lake, and then ascend a bit to cross a primitive dirt road. The trail then passes above a pond—look for rare western pond turtles sunning themselves on logs—and comes to a bridge over clear-flowing Greenleaf Creek. Another 0.5 mile of gentle uphill takes you to a break in the trees at Greenleaf Overlook, a rocky viewpoint with fine views to the south of Bonneville Dam and the rugged Oregon side of the river. The trail continues past this point to Table Mountain and beyond, but that area is more easily accessed by a new and much shorter route. See Trip 7 for details.

TRIP 10 Rooster Rock State Park Loop

Distance	2.7 miles, Loop
Elevation Gain	300 feet
Hiking Time	2 hours
Optional Map	Green Trails *Bridal Veil*
Usually Open	All year
Best Times	April to May and late October to November
Trail Use	Good for kids, dogs OK
Agency	Oregon State Parks, Columbia Gorge Region
Difficulty	Easy

HIGHLIGHTS Although probably best known for its officially sanctioned nude beach, Rooster Rock State Park offers delights for those who prefer to remain clothed (in hiking boots at least) as well. The views are excellent (and we will have no crude jokes about what you are "viewing") and the loop trail in the park's eastern section is a real delight. The park's other "exposure" issue is that it is quite open and has rather sparse tree cover, so the trails are frequently cold and windy. Come prepared.

DIRECTIONS Drive east from Portland on Interstate 84 to Exit 25 for Rooster Rock State Park. Loop around to the fee collection booth (a $3 daily fee is charged, as of 2007), and then come to a T-junction. Turn right and proceed 0.4 mile to the huge parking lot at the east end of the road.

Access to the clothing-optional beach descends from the northeast end of the parking lot. Unless that is your goal, skip that heavily used path, and go directly east from the restroom building, across a mowed area, and then pick up an unsigned but obvious foot trail heading into the forest. This pleasant route goes up and down on a wooded bench about 50 to 100 feet above a paralleling beach-access trail on your left. Look for several short side paths branching off to the left that provide views across the river to Washington. Other unmarked side trails go to the right and lead to picnic sites and a disc golf course or connect with the official loop trail farther up the ridge. The vegetation is dominated by a relatively low, wind-stunted forest of Oregon white oaks and Douglas firs.

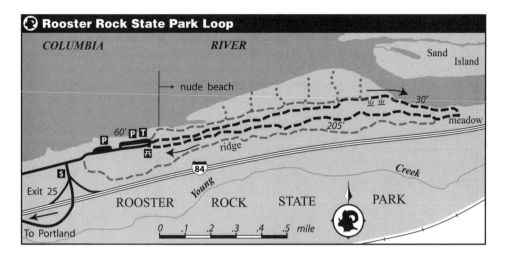

Rooster Rock State Park Loop

COLUMBIA   RIVER

Sand Island

nude beach

30'

meadow

205'

60' P T

P

ridge

Creek

84

S

Young

Exit 25

ROOSTER   ROCK   STATE   PARK

To Portland

0   .1   .2   .3   .4   .5 mile

After about 0.7 mile the trail drops to the left and connects with the paralleling beach-access trail. Nude bathers sometimes make it this far, but by hiking in winter and the cool days of spring you will dramatically diminish or maybe even eliminate the flesh quotient. Turn right (east) and continue mostly on the level beside a lowland area of seasonal wetlands covered with willows, bulrushes, and grasses. Unmarked spur trails go left to isolated all-over-tan sunbathing locations, but your route stays straight and after some 0.2 mile comes to a channel of the Columbia River separating you from

aptly named Sand Island, which features large sand dunes at its western end. Keep going east on a sometimes eroded trail that follows the water's edge. In the mud near the water look for the tracks of deer, raccoons, foxes, and other animals that, unlike many local *Homo sapiens*, have the decency to wear fur coats.

At about 1.4 miles, where the ridge on your right peters out, veer right and make a short climb up a sandy gulch to a large meadow. From here there are good views east to Angels Rest and other landmarks in the Gorge. Unfortunately, you can also see and hear Interstate 84, across the

Western Columbia
River Gorge

View east from ridge trail

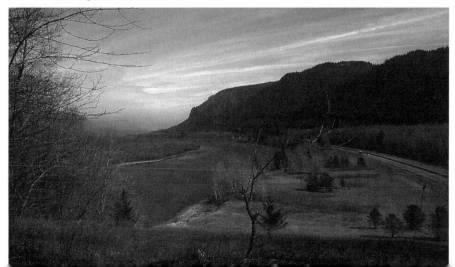

meadow to the south. Turn right (west) and climb a steep boot path through a sloping meadow for 200 yards to the top of the ridge where the oak trees resume. Follow the boot path another 10 yards into the forest to reach the end of the park's official loop trail and a choice of return routes.

The trail to the right is more private because it stays in the trees on the north side of the ridge, away from the sights and sounds of Interstate 84. The paralleling trail on the left stays near the top of the ridge, which provides better views, but keeps you in sight of the freeway. The two routes are rarely far apart, and at a couple of locations you can easily walk from one to the other to check out a different hiking experience. By either route the trail rolls up and down mostly in the woods, often passing magnificent old oak trees liberally festooned with mosses and licorice ferns. Both trails eventually take you back to the parking area, although the upper trail is a little longer because it comes out at a parking lot farther to the west.

TRIP 11 Latourell Falls Loop

Distance	2.3 miles, Loop
Elevation Gain	300 feet
Hiking Time	2 hours
Optional Map	Green Trails *Bridal Veil*
Usually Open	All year (except during winter storms)
Best Times	April and May
Trail Use	Good for kids, dogs OK
Agency	Oregon State Parks, Columbia Gorge Region
Difficulty	Moderate
Note	Good in cloudy weather

HIGHLIGHTS The Columbia River Gorge is justifiably famous for its waterfalls. From the west, the first major waterfall you encounter is Lower Latourell Falls, and it provides one whale of an introduction! Plunging 249 feet in a single sheer drop, this falls is a very impressive sight. The awe-inspiring scene is far from private, however, since there is a developed viewpoint just 150 yards from the road. For more privacy, hikers can make a highly enjoyable loop to beautiful Upper Latourell Falls, a great place to quietly enjoy the Gorge's two best attributes—waterfalls and lush vegetation.

DIRECTIONS Take Interstate 84 east from Portland to Bridal Veil Exit 28, and then follow the 0.4-mile access road to the Old Columbia River Highway. You turn right (west) and drive 2.9 miles to the good-sized parking area on the left.

From the Latourell Falls parking lot, a wide, paved trail goes rather steeply uphill to a smashing view of Lower Latourell Falls. The spot is so photogenic that countless travelers have gone back to their cars for additional film. To escape the tourist hordes, you bear left, away from the developed viewpoint, and immediately leave the paved trail behind. The footpath ascends a lush, green hillside, especially appealing in April and May when it bursts with spring greenery,

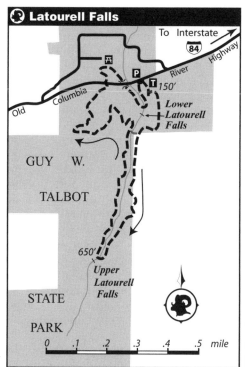

Latourell Falls

Columbia River. From here, you make a lazy descent back to the road, which you cross, and then go down some stairs on the north side of the road. The trail goes through a picnic area, turns right, and travels under a tall, arcing highway bridge. You cross the creek one last time and emerge at the base of Lower Latourell Falls. Schedule plenty of time for gawking here, not only at the falls, but at the almost perfect displays of columnar basalt in the surrounding amphitheater. A wide-angle lens is essential to do the scene justice with your camera. The last couple of hundred yards of trail back to the parking lot are gently uphill.

Upper Latourell Falls

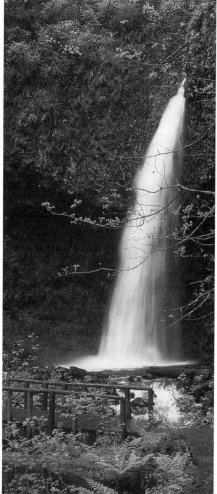

and in early November, when the big-leaf-maple leaves turn bright yellow. The path splits just after you climb to a less photogenic viewpoint at the top of Lower Latourell Falls.

For a short loop that skips the upper falls, turn right; but for the rewards of the full loop trip, go left. This trail goes upstream 0.5 mile in a lovely woodsy canyon, crossing several quaint wooden footbridges on its way to a bridge just below twisting Upper Latourell Falls. The last fall of this cascade is short but perfectly suited for great pictures; the scenic bridge and overhanging tree limbs create an excellent foreground.

The downstream return route follows the path on the west side of the creek, back to the junction with the shortcut trail mentioned above. You go left here and make two quick switchbacks, gaining about 150 feet, to an attractive pair of viewpoints looking up and down the

TRIP 12 Bridal Veil & Shepperds Dell Falls

Distance	1.2 miles (combined), Out-and-back
Elevation Gain	200 feet
Hiking Time	1 to 2 hours
Optional Map	Green Trails *Bridal Veil* (some trails not shown)
Usually Open	All year
Best Times	April and May
Trail Use	Good for kids, dogs OK
Agency	Oregon State Parks, Columbia Gorge Region
Difficulty	Easy
Note	Good in cloudy weather

HIGHLIGHTS These two outstanding adjacent destinations in the western Columbia River Gorge combine to make an easy and fun family outing. Although more adventurous types often combine this trip with a visit to Latourell Falls (Trip 11) or Multnomah Falls (Trip 15), these beautiful and dramatic falls, in combination with the nearby fields of wildflowers, make the drive more than worthwhile.

DIRECTIONS Take Interstate 84 east from Portland to Bridal Veil Exit 28, and then follow the 0.4-mile access road to the Old Columbia River Highway. Turn right (west) and drive 0.9 mile to Bridal Veil Falls State Park and its large parking lot on the right. To reach Shepperds Dell go west another 0.9 mile on the Old Columbia River Highway and park in the very limited space just before a tall bridge over the deep chasm of Young Creek.

From the east end of the parking lot the trail wanders under a shady canopy of bigleaf maple and Douglas fir. On either side of the wide gravel path are masses of tall thimbleberry, vine maple, and other shrubs. The 0.3-mile trail drops in one long switchback to a bridge over Bridal Veil Creek. You turn right here and climb a flight of stairs to a stunning overlook of two-tiered Bridal Veil Falls. The scene is most impressive when the creek is running high after spring rains.

If you are up for still more exploring, take the Overlook Trail loop, which heads north from the restroom building near the parking lot. True to its name, this paved nature trail passes several good viewpoints. It is especially attractive in late April and early May, when the meadows along the way are carpeted with the beautiful blue blossoms of camas. This small state park, in fact, has Ore-

Bridal Veil Falls

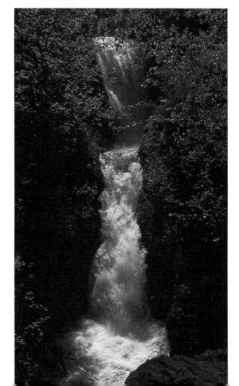

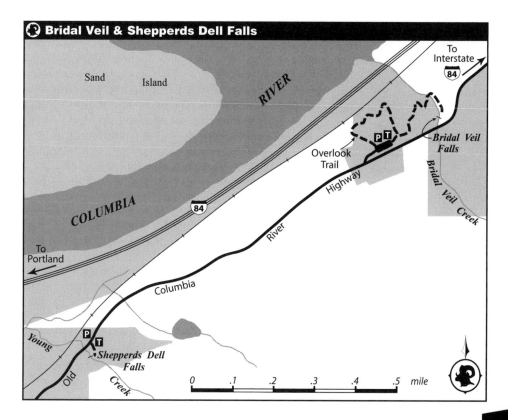

Bridal Veil & Shepperds Dell Falls

Sand   Island

RIVER

To
Interstate
84

Overlook
Trail

Bridal Veil
Falls

Highway

Bridal Veil Creek

COLUMBIA

84

River

To
Portland

Columbia

Young

Shepperds Dell
Falls

Old

Creek

0   .1   .2   .3   .4   .5   mile

gon's largest surviving camas fields in the Columbia River Gorge. Please stay on the trails because these plants are very sensitive and cannot survive being trampled. After 0.4 mile, the trail returns you to the west end of the parking lot.

To explore dramatic Shepperds Dell, drive to that destination and look for an unsigned but obvious trail that descends a flight of stone stairs from the east side of the road bridge. The paved trail is separated from the cliffs below by a stone guardrail, so hikers can feel safe while they gawk at the gorgeous multitiered falls that twists down into the fern-filled grotto of Shepperds Dell. The 150-yard dead-end trail stops right next to the spraying falls, but the best views are actually back near the trailhead, where twisted trees frame the scene.

TRIP **13** Angels Rest

Distance	5.8 miles, Out-and-back
Elevation Gain	1650 feet
Hiking Time	2½ to 3 hours
Optional Map	Green Trails *Bridal Veil*
Usually Open	February to December
Best Time	Mid-April to June
Trail Use	Dogs OK
Agency	Columbia River Gorge National Scenic Area
Difficulty	Difficult

HIGHLIGHTS Like some ancient castle battlement, the rocky fortress of Angels Rest rises dramatically above the forested ridges of the western Columbia River Gorge. The trail to the top is justifiably one of the most popular in the Gorge because it has a classic mix of good exercise, easy access, and outstanding scenery. In mid-April, the forests along the trail support some of the finest displays of beautiful white trillium in the region.

DIRECTIONS Take Interstate 84 east from Portland to Bridal Veil Exit 28, and then drive the exit road 0.4 mile to the junction with the Old Columbia River Highway. The large parking lot for the Angels Rest Trail is on your right.

The trail leaves from the south side of the road and then goes uphill through a lovely Douglas-fir forest. If you are visiting in mid-April, expect to be delighted by thousands of trillium filling the forest with their spectacular three-petaled white flowers. The trail goes up a couple of switchbacks and then traverses to a mediocre viewpoint before moving into a creek canyon. You'll get only a partial look at Coopey Falls below you on the left, but when you come to the bridged creek crossing, there is a good view of a smaller, but attractive, 30-foot waterfall.

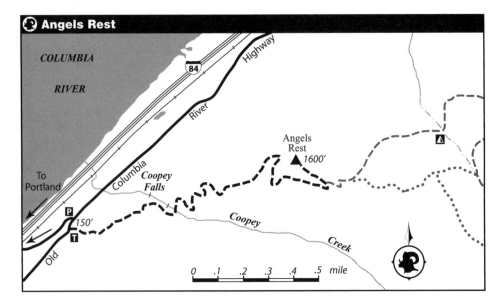

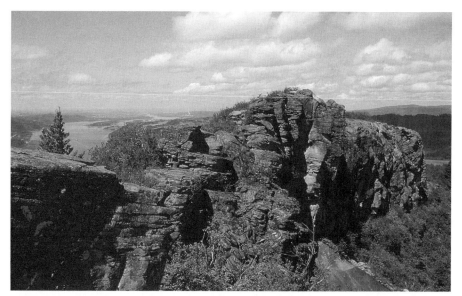

Angels Rest

After the creek, the uphill begins in earnest, as you traverse a hillside covered with bigleaf maples and red alders whose mossy trunks sprout licorice ferns by the hundred. On the forest floor are bracken and sword fern, as well as some poison oak, especially in the rocky areas. A series of short switchbacks takes you through forests and finally up a rocky slope to a ridgetop junction with the side trail that leads out to imposing Angels Rest. Turn left on this rather rugged trail and follow it out to the end of the flat-topped rock formation, where a confusion of side trails leads to stunning viewpoints up and down the Gorge.

This entire area was burned in a 1991 wildfire, leaving behind weathered snags both on the summit and on many of the surrounding hillsides. It is interesting to observe how some stands of trees were left untouched by the flames, while others were totally obliterated, and how the flowers and shrubs have benefited from the increase in available light. Near the summit, you can expect to see pink wild rose, blue iris, white carrot, yarrow, daisy,

yellow wallflower, red columbine, and tall blue larkspur—all taking advantage of the nearly treeless slopes. Peak flower time is usually in May.

Angels Rest is a very exposed location, which makes it particularly susceptible to the famous Gorge winds. It is not uncommon for the winds to be blowing so strongly that you are literally unable to stand up at the summit. If the howling gales are such that you can't eat your lunch in comfort, or if you just want more exercise, you might consider extending this hike to include a visit to the more protected forests nearby. To do so, return to the main trail and follow it up the ridge for 0.1 mile to a junction. Go left on the trail toward Wahkeena Falls, and travel nearly on the level into a shady forest. Here the ground is covered with white-blooming plants like vanilla leaf, star-flowered smilacina, and false lily-of-the-valley. After about 0.4 mile, you will reach a small creek and a nice site for a picnic or camp that is protected from wind by big Douglas firs and western hemlocks.

TRIP 14 Devils Rest Loop

Distance	7.9 miles, Semiloop
Elevation Gain	2300 feet
Hiking Time	4 to 5 hours
Optional Map	Green Trails *Bridal Veil* (part of route not shown)
Usually Open	Late March to December
Best Time	April to June
Trail Use	Dogs OK
Agency	Columbia River Gorge National Scenic Area
Difficulty	Difficult
Note	Good in cloudy weather

HIGHLIGHTS Other than a similar name, Devils Rest shares little in common with its better known neighbor, Angels Rest (Trip 13). While the latter is a dramatic viewpoint on a towering rock abutment, the former is an unassuming forested knoll, with little in the way of views. While the trail to Angels Rest ascends a burned-over hillside, the path up Devils Rest climbs a densely forested realm of waterfalls and lush vegetation. The two locations can be combined into one hike, but it is better to do them on separate trips tailored to enjoying their individual charms and attributes. The author usually selects his destination based on the weather. If the skies are clear and promise outstanding views, head for Angels Rest. If the clouds are low and threatening, then Devils Rest is the better choice because the forests and waterfalls on this trail are just as impressive under overcast skies as sunny ones.

DIRECTIONS Take Interstate 84 east from Portland to Bridal Veil Exit 28, and then drive the exit road 0.4 mile to the junction with the Old Columbia River Highway. Go left (east) on the old highway, and drive 2.6 miles to the roadside parking lot for Wahkeena Falls.

The initially paved trail starts at the bridge over cascading Wahkeena Creek and climbs in one long switchback to an upper bridge, right in the spray of the falls. From here, you climb a hillside covered with luxuriant gorge vegetation on a switchbacking gravel trail to a ridge crest where a 30-yard side trail leads to a good viewpoint. The main trail goes steeply upstream beside loudly cascading Wahkeena Creek until it crosses a tributary creek beside Fairy Falls. From here, you climb a series of short switchbacks to a junction.

Either route from this junction will work as the first part of this loop, but the views are better if you take the one to the left and hike out to a ridge crest, where another short spur trail leads to a good viewpoint. From this junction, the route ascends seven quick switchbacks to another ridgetop junction, this one with the alternate route from Fairy Falls. Turn left and in 50 feet bear right (uphill) on a possibly unsigned, but obvious, trail that makes a series of evenly spaced and moderately graded switchbacks up a woodsy hillside. At the top of the climb, the trail curves to the right to follow the edge of a ridgeline. Although it stays close to a steep drop-off, the trail is surprisingly gentle with only very gradual uphill sections. The forest floor along this high ridge is dominated by common flowering plants like bunchberry, false Solomon's seal, twisted stalk, anemone, wild iris, and yellow wood violet.

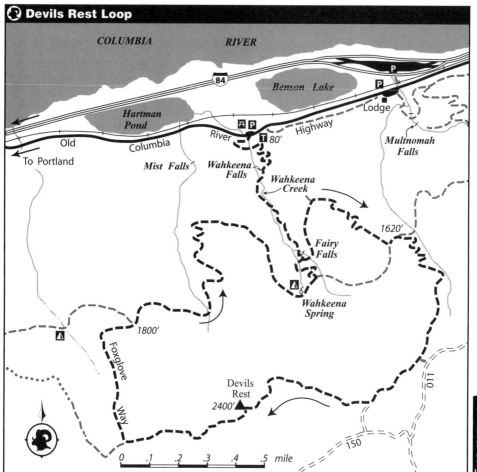

Devils Rest Loop

COLUMBIA   RIVER

Benson Lake

Hartman Pond

Old   Columbia   River   Highway

To Portland

Mist Falls   Wahkeena Falls

Lodge

Multnomah Falls

80'

Wahkeena Creek

1620'

Fairy Falls

Wahkeena Spring

1800'

Foxglove Way

Devils Rest 2400'

0   .1   .2   .3   .4   .5   mile

150

011

As you make your way south and west along the ridge, ignore an unsigned path to the left leading to an unseen forest road, but do take advantage of two short side trails to the right, which lead to nice viewpoints. After a final climb, you come to a junction just a few yards below the top of Devils Rest. The forested summit has lots of large, moss-covered boulders and is quite lovely despite its ominous name.

To continue the loop trip, go back to the junction with the path just below the summit, and then turn west onto the trail signed FOXGLOVE WAY. This boot path is not shown on any official maps and isn't maintained by the U.S. Forest Service, but it's easy to follow as it descends steeply through dense, head-high shrubbery to an unsigned junction. Turn right and descend for 0.5 mile through forest and some brushy areas to a junction. The trail to the left goes west to Angels Rest (Trip 13).

You turn right (east) on a well-maintained path that immediately leaves the burned area and descends a series of switchbacks. This trail drops from the top of a rocky slope and then down a forested hillside, where the vegetation tells a story about the benefits of natural fire. A huge fire swept through this forest in 1991, and evidence of this blaze can still be seen, in the form of several burned snags and lots of charred bark on the living trees. But this fire had benefits as well, as you can see from the dense ground vegetation, which has taken advantage of the increased sunshine to produce a profusion of greenery. The most conspicuous of the sun-loving plants here is a spectacular and unusual 4-foot-tall species of larkspur that boasts striking blue flowers in early June.

At the bottom of the switchbacks, the trail does an up-and-down traverse of a hillside to reach a camp beside large Wahkeena Spring, where a full stream gushes directly out of the ground. Just 100 yards beyond the spring is a trail junction. Turn left and descend a series of switchbacks that in 0.4 mile takes you back to the junction above Fairy Falls.

TRIP 15 Multnomah & Wahkeena Falls Loop

Distance	5.4 miles, Loop
Elevation Gain	1700 feet
Hiking Time	2½ to 4 hours
Optional Map	Green Trails *Bridal Veil*
Usually Open	All year
Best Time	April to June
Trail Use	Good for kids, dogs OK
Agency	Columbia River Gorge National Scenic Area
Difficulty	Moderate
Note	Good in cloudy weather

HIGHLIGHTS Even without the waterfalls, this magnificent loop trip would be worthwhile. The western Columbia River Gorge is famous for its lush greenery, and probably the most beautiful forests of all are found in the canyons and hillsides near Multnomah Falls. The dense forest canopy and the luxuriant tangle of ferns, mosses, and other plants make for a verdant rain forest of stunning beauty. But despite the lovely forests, it is the waterfalls that are the star attraction of any hike in this area.

In addition to famous Multnomah Falls, which at 542 feet is one of the highest falls in North America, the loop trip includes visits to at least a half dozen other falls on upper Multnomah Creek and neighboring Wahkeena Creek. The downside of hiking here is crowds. With its wide fame, enormous parking lot, and even its own exit off a busy interstate freeway, Multnomah Falls is said to be the most visited tourist attraction in the entire state of Oregon. For crowd control purposes, especially on weekends, it is probably best to start this loop at quieter Wahkeena Falls.

DIRECTIONS Take Interstate 84 east from Portland to Bridal Veil Exit 28, and then drive the exit road 0.4 mile to the junction with the Old Columbia River Highway. Go left (east) on the old highway, and drive 2.6 miles to the roadside parking lot for Wahkeena Falls.

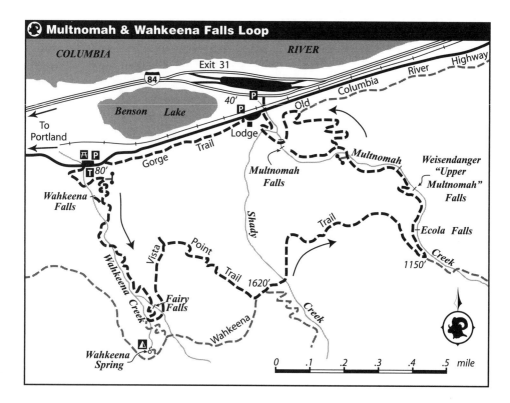

The trail starts at the bridge over loudly cascading Wahkeena Creek, where you can look straight up at 242-foot-high Wahkeena Falls, a twisting cascade of water in a narrow chute. The paved trail makes one switchback and then comes to a bridge over Wahkeena Creek, in a grotto beside the falling water. You can expect to get showered with spray when making this crossing, which will be welcome on hot summer days and bone-chilling in the winter months.

After the bridge, the trail turns to gravel and comes to a second switchback, where a wire gate blocks access to the closed Perdition Trail. Past this junction, your trail keeps climbing, often beside mossy rock walls, up a hillside covered with luxuriant vegetation, including thimbleberry, goatsbeard, cow parsnip, maidenhair fern, columbine, beardtongue, and poison oak. Ten uphill switchbacks weed

out most of the tourists and take you up to a ridge just above the top of Wahkeena Falls. From this ridge, a short dead-end side trail to your right leads to a fine viewpoint.

The main trail goes upstream steeply, climbing beside loudly cascading Wahkeena Creek and then crossing the flow twice on wooden plank bridges. With dense thickets of lady and maidenhair fern covering the canyon walls, and a shady canopy of western red cedar and western hemlock, this area has a jungle-like feel. Past the second bridge, a few short, steep switchbacks take you to a split in the creek and up to the base of lacy Fairy Falls. A wooden bench here allows hikers to relax and enjoy the sight and sound of falling water. Five more short switchbacks lead up to a junction with the Vista Point Trail. You can turn either right or left here, as the trails meet again in about 0.5 mile. The left route goes by a nice viewpoint and switchbacks up a ridge to the junction where the two trails reunite. The route to the right goes through lush greenery to a junction near Wahkeena Spring, where you turn left and climb a wooded hillside to the same ridgetop junction.

From this point, you turn east on the Wahkeena Trail and immediately pass an unsigned trail that goes to the right up to Devils Rest (Trip 14). Go straight on the Wahkeena Trail, which takes you over tiny Shady Creek and contours across a heavily wooded north-facing slope, before descending into the canyon of Multnomah Creek. You turn left (downstream) at the junction with the Multnomah Creek Trail and closely follow this beautiful stream past Ecola Falls to a switchback that takes you down to the base of Weisendanger or "Upper Multnomah" Falls. This almost perfect falls is neither as tall nor as famous as its lower namesake but still commands the attention of hikers and their cameras.

Continue downstream 0.5 mile, past a succession of waterfalls of various heights, to a junction with the other end of the closed Perdition Trail and a huge culvert over Multnomah Creek. Just past this crossing, you meet a very popular side trail that bears left and leads to the viewpoint at the top of Multnomah Falls. Don't expect to be alone here, as virtually all the occupants of the hundreds of cars you can see parked below seem to make this spot their hiking goal. From here, you descend a series of switchbacks on a paved trail that has been pounded by countless thousands of pairs of tennis shoes, to a much photographed bridge between the two tiers of Multnomah Falls. You then follow this busy trail downhill, partly on stone steps, to the historic lodge at the base of the falls.

To return to your car, you can either walk west on the Old Columbia River Highway or follow the parallel, poison-oak-lined Gorge Trail, which starts a few hundred feet west of the lodge. It is only 0.8 mile by either route to Wahkeena Creek.

Weisendanger "Upper Multnomah" Falls

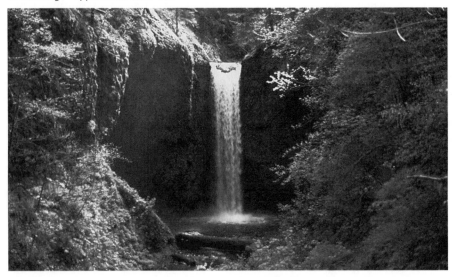

TRIP *16* Larch Mountain Upper Loop

Distance	6.0 miles, Loop
Elevation Gain	1300 feet
Hiking Time	2½ to 4 hours
Optional Map	Green Trails *Bridal Veil*
Usually Open	Late May to October
Best Time	June
Trail Use	Dogs OK, backpacking option
Agency	Columbia River Gorge National Scenic Area
Difficulty	Moderate

HIGHLIGHTS Except for the major volcanic snow peaks, Larch Mountain is probably the most recognizable landmark on the Portland skyline. This hike allows you the opportunity to get a close look at the features that give this mountain its distinctive profile, especially the high rock outcropping called Sherrard Point, right at the summit. And while this relatively easy outing won't give you the same sense of accomplishment you get from climbing to the summit from Multnomah Falls (Trip 17), it also won't give you the sore muscles and blisters that come with the longer hike.

DIRECTIONS From Interstate 84, take Corbett Exit 22 and drive 1.4 miles up the steep access road to the south. Turn left on the Old Columbia River Highway, and after 1.9 miles bear right at a fork onto East Larch Mountain Road. Follow this good paved road, which eventually becomes Forest Road 15, for 14.5 miles to the large parking lot and turnaround just below the summit of Larch Mountain.

The Multnomah Creek Trail leaves from the southwest corner of the parking lot and follows a gravel path past several widely spaced picnic tables. After 0.1 mile, you go left at an unsigned junction and gradually descend through a cool, shady forest of Pacific silver fir and western hemlock. Initially, there is virtually no ground cover, only a few scattered huckleberry bushes and beargrass plants, but as you descend these are joined by increasing numbers of oxalis, star-flowered smilacina, trillium, vanilla leaf, and bunchberry. The gently graded trail gradually loses elevation, following a wide but viewless ridge, on a trail covered with needles and soft dirt that provide excellent cushioning for every footfall.

After 1.5 miles, you cross a closed dirt road and immediately thereafter pass a good, but waterless, campsite. Below this, the trail loses elevation more quickly on a gravel path for 0.5 mile to a junction. The main trail goes straight, but for this loop you turn right and wind downhill for 0.2 mile to an excellent camp and a log bridge over the softly trickling headwaters of Multnomah Creek.

You are now at the bottom of a basin that 4 million years ago was part of a fiery volcano and, more recently, was carved out by Ice Age glaciers. Both fire and ice are long gone now, but they have been replaced by equally impressive old-growth forests. The trees here may not be quite as big as those at lower elevations, but they are splendid nonetheless.

On the other side of the log bridge is a junction, where you turn right, climb past some massive old-growth trees, and then skirt the left side of a lovely meadow that features great views up to craggy Sherrard Point. This meadow used to be a lake sitting in a glacial cirque. Over thousands of

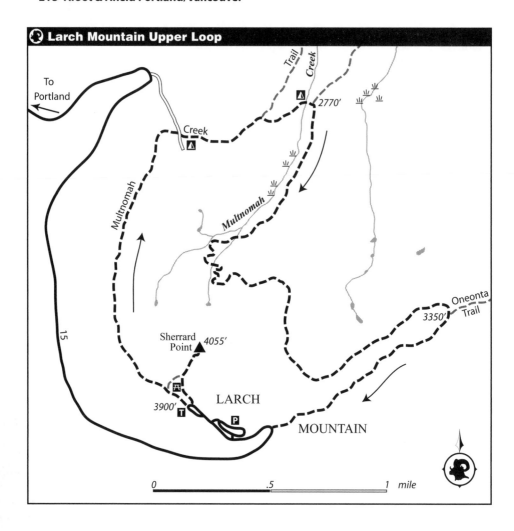

⊙ Larch Mountain Upper Loop

To Portland

Trail
Creek
2770'

Creek

Multnomah

Multnomah

Oneonta
3350' Trail

15

Sherrard
Point 4055'

LARCH

3900'

MOUNTAIN

0   .5   1 mile

years, the lake gradually filled with sediment, becoming a meadow. In time, the meadow too will disappear, to be replaced by forest. For now, this marshy paradise is home to lots of water-loving wildflowers, especially marsh marigold and shooting star. Mosquitoes also like this habitat, so be sure to bring repellent.

Beyond the meadow, the trail climbs in fits and starts through dense forest. As you climb, take a break from time to time to appreciate the birds. You may see or hear winter wrens, dark-eyed juncos, or either of two types of thrush. The varied thrush looks like a slimmed down robin that got all dressed up with an extra orange eye stripe and a black breast band. The hermit thrush looks rather drab but has a fascinating, almost metallic, buzzing call. If the birds don't interest you, try examining the vegetation. The old-growth forests here have lots of Pacific silver and grand fir, Douglas fir, and western hemlock. Many of the oldest trees have fallen and now serve as nurse logs for young trees. Beneath the shade of these big trees grow ground-cover species, like queen's cup, false lily-of-the-valley, and a high concentration of deer fern.

The trail turns left and keeps wandering uphill. You go over an indistinct ridge and then join an ancient roadbed that is noticeable only because it allows you to travel at a perfectly level grade for the next mile. During this time, you cross several tiny trickles and then make a long traverse to meet the Oneonta Trail on a wooded ridgeline. You turn right here and follow the trail up a gently sloping ridge 0.8 mile, meeting the East Larch Mountain Road at a switchback just 0.3 mile below the parking lot. Simply walk the road shoulder from here up to your car.

Before leaving for the day, be sure to take the easy but crowded 0.2-mile trail that goes to the top of Sherrard Point. The paved path leaves from the northwest

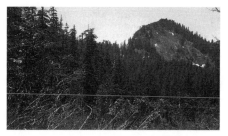
Larch Mountain from a meadow to the north

corner of the parking lot and traverses a heavily wooded hillside, before climbing a series of steps to the rocky overlook. From this exceptional grandstand you can see five towering volcanic snow peaks (Mounts Rainier, St. Helens, Adams, Jefferson, and, of course, nearby Hood), as well as countless lower summits that you could spend hours identifying.

TRIP 17 Larch Mountain from Multnomah Falls Loop

Distance	16.3 miles, Semiloop
Elevation Gain	4300 feet
Hiking Time	9 to 12 hours
Optional Map	Green Trails *Bridal Veil*
Usually Open	Late May to October
Best Time	June
Trail Use	Dogs OK, backpacking option
Agency	Columbia River Gorge National Scenic Area
Difficulty	Strenuous

Western Columbia River Gorge

HIGHLIGHTS With good paved roads providing access to both ends of this hike, it's not surprising that both Multnomah Falls and Larch Mountain are very crowded. The trails connecting these two locations, however, are amazingly quiet. Well, perhaps it isn't all that amazing, when you consider that it takes a lot of sweat to get from one to the other. Although not overly steep, it is a very long way up, from nearly sea level at the base of Multnomah Falls to over 4000 feet at the top of Larch Mountain. If you can arrange a car shuttle, the best plan is to start from the top and hike downhill, but starting from the bottom, it's best to plan on doing a long, scenic loop. From a crowd-control standpoint, one advantage of this approach is that, in order to complete this hike in one day, you have to start out very early in the morning, which means that few tourists will be around to distract you from the views of Multnomah Falls at the trailhead.

DIRECTIONS From Interstate 84, take Multnomah Falls Exit 31 and park in the enormous lot built to accommodate the millions of tourists who come to visit this famous falls.

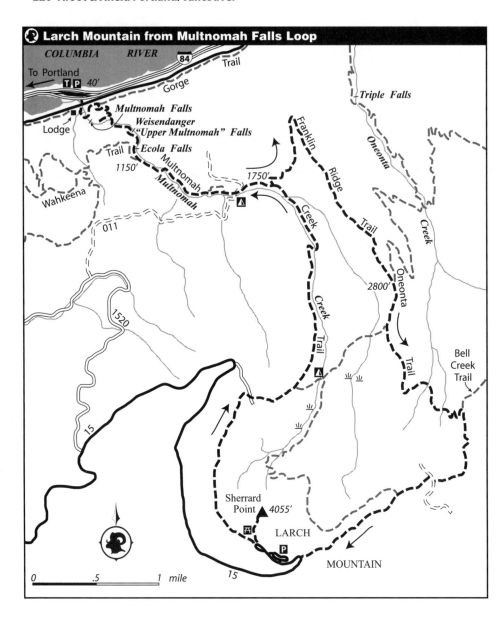

Larch Mountain from Multnomah Falls Loop

Follow the crowds through the tunnel under the eastbound lanes of Interstate 84 and to the historic log Multnomah Falls Lodge. After elbowing aside your fellow visitors and snapping a few pictures from the stonework viewing area at the bottom of the falls, turn right on the wide trail that heads uphill on stone stairs.

This paved trail climbs in a long switchback up to the much-photographed bridge that spans the flow below the tall upper part of Multnomah Falls and above the shorter lower cascade. You cross the bridge, making sure to smile for the dozens of photographers snapping pictures from below, and climb a little more to a junction with the Gorge Trail. You stay on the main paved route and ascend a series of switchbacks all the way to the short side trail that goes to the viewing platform at the top of the 542-foot falls.

After admiring the view, you leave the tourist hordes behind and begin hiking up the Multnomah Creek Trail. You quickly cross the creek on a huge culvert and come to a junction with the closed Perdition Trail. Keep left and climb beside the cascading stream, in a wet canyon of lush vegetation. On your left, the creek drops over a series of hard-to-view falls of varying heights. A little after crossing under a massive rock overhang that will often shower you with water, you come to photogenic Weisendanger "Upper Multnomah" Falls, switchback away from this lovely falls, and traverse to a junction with the Wahkeena Trail (see Trip 15).

Keep straight on the main trail, and about 0.2 mile later cross Multnomah Creek on a bridge, then go lazily uphill along the banks of the creek about 0.3 mile to a trail split. To the left is a short but rugged high-water route that bypasses a creekside section of trail that is usually flooded during spring snow melt. If the lower route is feasible, take that one, as it is both easier and more attractive. After a few hundred yards, the two routes reunite and soon come to an old dirt road and a possible camp. You cross the road and continue upstream about 0.2 mile to a junction.

The shortest route to Larch Mountain goes straight on the Multnomah Creek Trail, but for a longer, more scenic route, turn left on the Franklin Ridge Trail. This path goes over a low ridge and then gradually climbs a forested hillside to an open clearing on top of Franklin Ridge. The best views are to the east, over the depths of Oneonta Creek Canyon, and west, over Multnomah Basin.

The trail turns right here and goes back into the trees on the ridge crest. For the next mile or so, the trail goes up in stair-step fashion, with some steep uphill pitches and some relatively level sections. Most of the way, you are among the trees, but there are also frequent breaks that provide excellent views to the east. When you reach a junction with the Oneonta Trail, which drops steeply to the left, you go straight through an area of extensive blowdown and lose some elevation. After just 0.3 mile, you come to the next junction, where you turn left on the Oneonta Trail.

Walk through attractive mid-elevation forests, up a sloping ridge, lose some elevation, and make an easy crossing of Oneonta Creek, which should get your feet wet only during high water. Then go over a low ridge and splash through an even smaller creek before climbing rather steeply up a half dozen short switchbacks to a junction with the Bell Creek Trail. You turn right and travel mostly on the level to the south and west.

The trail comes to a dirt jeep road, where you walk a short distance to your right to pick up the continuation of the trail. After another 0.4 mile, go straight at a final junction, and climb 0.8 mile up a gently sloping ridge to where the trail ends at a switchback on paved East Larch Mountain Road. To reach the top of the mountain, you veer right and walk the shoulder of the road 0.3 mile to the parking lot just below the summit.

Having come this far, you won't want to miss the opportunity to take in the view from Sherrard Point. To reach it, take a crowded, 0.2-mile paved trail from the northwest corner of the parking area up to the developed viewpoint. Signs point you to the five major volcanic peaks you can see from the summit (Mounts Rainier, Adams, St. Helens, Hood, and

Jefferson), but you will have to rely on either experience or a good map to pick out the hundreds of lower summits visible in every direction.

To return to Multnomah Falls, pick up the Multnomah Creek Trail from the southwest corner of the parking lot, and walk through a cool forest, past a dispersed picnic area. The trail gradually descends a sloping ridgeline for 1.5 miles and then crosses a closed dirt road. You walk downward for another 0.5 mile and go straight at a junction, staying on the main Multnomah Creek Trail. This path descends at a steady grade on a wooded hillside, crosses a scree slope, and makes a short switchback down to Multnomah Creek. After crossing the main creek, you go downstream for 0.3 mile, make a couple of more very short switchbacks, and cross a tributary creek. A short distance past this ford is the junction with the Franklin Ridge Trail.

TRIP 18 Oneonta Gorge

Distance	1.2 miles, Out-and-back
Elevation Gain	50 feet
Hiking Time	1 to 2 hours
Optional Map	USFS *Trails of the Columbia Gorge*
Usually Open	July to September
Best Times	August and September
Trail Use	No dogs
Agency	Columbia River Gorge National Scenic Area
Difficulty	Moderate
Note	Good in cloudy weather

HIGHLIGHTS This trip is only for adventurous souls who don't mind getting wet. There is no trail up Oneonta Gorge, although the route is never in doubt. In lieu of a trail, you simply wade up the bed of Oneonta Creek, through a spectacular slot canyon. It is best to wait until late summer to do this outing because the water level will be lower then and, with the hot temperatures, you will actually welcome getting soaked. The standard hiking clothing doesn't apply to this adventure. Your best options are ratty old tennis shoes with good tread for wading, and either shorts or a swimsuit. It is also advised that you have a dry change of clothes in the car for when you return. Oneonta Gorge is a special botanical area with a unique ecosystem of delicate ferns and mosses. In deference to this special status, visitors must be extremely careful to avoid disturbing the plant life.

DIRECTIONS Drive Interstate 84 east from Portland and take Bridal Veil Exit 28. At the end of the 0.4-mile exit road, turn east on the Old Columbia River Highway. After 3.1 miles, slow down to pass the crowds at Multnomah Falls Lodge and, 2.0 miles later, park in any of the small lots near the bridge over Oneonta Creek.

An unsigned and sometimes rugged trail goes down a series of stone steps from the west side of the bridge to water level, and then goes steeply up and down beside the creek for about 150 yards to a log jam. Crawl over the jam, and then make your way upstream, sometimes walking on rocks and sometimes simply

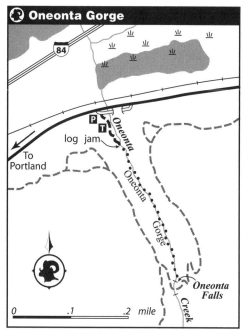

Oneonta Gorge

To Portland

log jam

84

0   .1   .2 mile

Oneonta

Oneonta Gorge

Oneonta Creek

Oneonta Falls

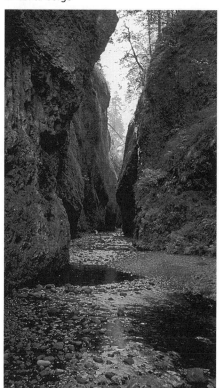

Oneonta Gorge

wading up the creek itself. The canyon narrows very quickly, so within just a few short yards you are already squeezing into the 15- to 20-foot-wide slot canyon. You'll need to crane your neck to see up the 200 or so feet of vertical walls rising to the top of the canyon. The walls are covered with an array of ferns, giving this cool grotto a junglelike feeling. Although they look lush and hardy, these ferns are actually quite delicate and barely manage to hang onto the vertical walls. Please avoid touching these plants whenever possible. While looking up and around, be sure to also look *down* at your footing because it is easy to turn an ankle on the slippery rocks.

In places the creek bends and you can walk on gravel bars, but the creek also has some deep pools that you must wade into or try to scramble around. Some of these pools can be waist deep, depending on the water level in the creek. After about 0.6 mile of twists and turns in the gorge, you arrive at the head of the gorge, where spectacular 100-foot Oneonta Falls drops over a sheer cliff.

There is very little light in this slot canyon, so photographers must use a tripod and fast film to get pictures. They also will want to protect their gear in plastic bags as they hike to avoid getting everything wet should they slip on a rock while wading. The vertical canyon walls are impressive, but they absolutely preclude any exit other than going back the way you came.

TRIP 19 Horsetail Falls to Triple Falls Loop

Distance	4.5 miles, Semiloop
Elevation Gain	700 feet
Hiking Time	2 hours
Optional Map	USFS *Trails of the Columbia Gorge*
Usually Open	All year (except during winter storms)
Best Times	April to June and late October to early November
Trail Use	Good for kids, dogs OK (but the trail is dangerous for them in places)
Agency	Columbia River Gorge National Scenic Area
Difficulty	Moderate
Note	Good in cloudy weather

HIGHLIGHTS Everything that makes the Columbia River Gorge so special is on spectacular display on this easy hike. There are lush forests, fern-lined grottos, deep slot canyons, excellent viewpoints, and, of course, lots of impressive waterfalls. Not surprisingly, all of these features have made this hike extremely popular. The large parking lot at Horsetail Falls overflows on summer weekends, so try to arrive early in the day or visit on a week-day.

DIRECTIONS Drive Interstate 84 east from Portland and take Bridal Veil Exit 28. At the end of the 0.4-mile exit road, turn east on the Old Columbia River Highway. After 3.1 miles, slow down to pass the crowds at Multnomah Falls Lodge, and 2.5 miles later turn left into the large parking lot on the north side of the highway, directly across from Horsetail Falls.

The well-signed trailhead is just a few yards east of 176-foot Horsetail Falls, a beautiful, twisting, roadside cataract that is as far as most carbound tourists ever get. Hikers can take the wide, well-graded, gravel path, as it slowly switchbacks up a densely vegetated slope with lots of bleeding heart and maidenhair fern growing under some impressive examples of bigleaf maple and Douglas fir. At the fourth switchback is a junction with the Gorge Trail.

Turn sharply right and take two more switchbacks before making a level traverse at the base of a basalt cliff curving to the left into the canyon above Horsetail Falls. Immediately in front of you is an impressive falls that is officially given the rather prosaic name of Upper Horsetail Falls, but for decades hikers have given it the more colorful moniker of Ponytail Falls. In deference to this tradition, some

U.S. Forest Service trail signs even use this name.

Not that you will need any encouragement, but take some time to admire this falls as it plunges down a slot in a basalt

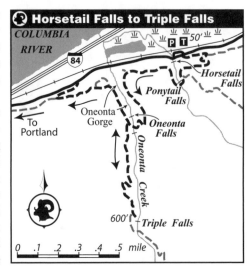

cliff and shoots out over an overhanging ledge. The trail goes behind the falls, taking advantage of the dry grotto under the ledge to give visitors a unique perspective of standing under a wild waterfall.

After leaving the amphitheater holding Ponytail Falls, the trail contours across a steep hillside with several mossy rockslides. Just as the trail begins to curve left into the canyon of Oneonta Creek, two unsigned trails go right to visit dramatic viewpoints. The best views are to the east, to such landmarks as Nesmith Point, Beacon Rock, Aldrich Butte, and Hamilton Mountain. Back on the main trail, you walk south, staying on the level past a dripping overhanging rock, and then begin a series of six downhill switchbacks. At the second switchback, there is a signed viewpoint where you can look directly down into the depths of Oneonta Gorge. This amazing, fern-lined slot canyon is only about 20 feet wide and often has fallen trees spanning the chasm as much as 200 feet above the creek at the bottom.

At the bottom of the switchbacks a metal bridge spans Oneonta Creek just below a lovely 60-foot falls. Just downstream and out of sight is the even more impressive, 100-foot Oneonta Falls, where the creek drops into the slot canyon. Once across the bridge, you climb two switchbacks and come to a junction. If you only want a short trip, bear right. But if you want to visit one of the finest waterfalls in the Columbia River Gorge (or anywhere else, for that matter), turn sharply left and make a long gradual uphill traverse on the cliffs above the deep canyon of Oneonta Creek. After about 0.2 mile, you make two uphill switchbacks and then walk on the level across almost vertical slopes, before dropping slightly to an unsigned junction. Bear left and drop 50 feet to a dramatic viewpoint of Triple Falls.

This magnificent falls is especially appealing because the creek splits into three almost perfectly, and each part cascades over the cliff in twisting falls. Individually, these falls are works of art, but together they are a masterpiece. A visit here is worthwhile during any season, but one of the nicest times to visit is in the autumn when the bigleaf maples turn yellow and sprinkle the canyon with color.

To close out the trip, return along the Oneonta Trail to the junction above the bridge. Instead of going back the way you came, go straight at this junction and climb gradually to a junction with a spur trail to the right, which leads to some fine viewpoints. The main trail curves to the left, going across a rockslide with an

Horsetail Falls

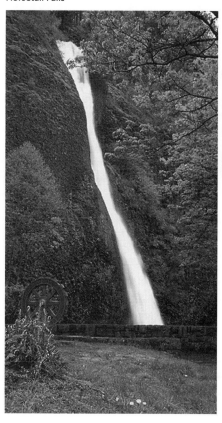

abundant population of pikas that like to peep at passing hikers. From here, you descend gradually through dense forests to a junction at a switchback.

The Gorge Trail goes straight, but you turn right and descend in a long traverse to the Old Columbia River Highway. To return to your car, simply walk along this road for 0.5 mile, past the bottom of Oneonta Gorge and back to Horsetail Falls and your starting point. There is no sidewalk, and almost no shoulder, so be very alert for traffic as you walk along on this narrow road.

TRIP 20 Rock of Ages & Horsetail Creek Loop

Distance	9.4 miles, Loop
Elevation Gain	3300 feet
Hiking Time	5 to 7 hours
Optional Map	USFS *Trails of the Columbia Gorge*
Usually Open	Mid-April to October
Best Time	Mid-April to June
Trail Use	No dogs (too dangerous)
Agency	Columbia River Gorge National Scenic Area
Difficulty	Strenuous

HIGHLIGHTS The hike up Rock of Ages Ridge is not for the faint of heart. Every time I take this route, I envision mountain goats getting together around the campfire to tell horror stories about how steep it is. There are compensations, however. Chief among these are the terrific views from a rocky ridge called the Devils Backbone, together with the fun loops this route accesses on rarely hiked trails in the backcountry of the Gorge. One of the best of those loops follows the quiet Horsetail Creek Trail down to Oneonta Creek and past great waterfalls back to your car.

DIRECTIONS Drive Interstate 84 east from Portland and take Bridal Veil Exit 28. At the end of the 0.4-mile exit road, turn east on the Old Columbia River Highway. After 3.1 miles, slow down to pass the crowds at Multnomah Falls Lodge, and 2.5 miles later turn left into the large parking lot on the north side of the highway, directly across from Horsetail Falls. This trailhead gets very busy on summer weekends, so arrive as early as possible.

This popular trail starts just east of Horsetail Falls and climbs four switchbacks to a junction with the Gorge Trail. You turn sharply right, climb two more switchbacks, and then make a short traverse to where the trail curves to the left into the canyon holding Ponytail Falls.

Just 20 yards after turning this corner, look for an unsigned use path veering uphill to the left over the roots of a large Douglas fir. You turn onto this trail and in a few yards pass one of those small, ominous signs you see from time to time in the Gorge saying TRAIL NOT MAINTAINED, which always means that the path will be steep and difficult. True to this rule, the ridiculously steep trail crawls over roots and rocks and charges up slopes where the trail is quite slippery when wet. A sturdy hiking pole will help to keep you steady, and you'll feel better from time to time using your hands to help pull yourself up. Adding to the difficulties are lots

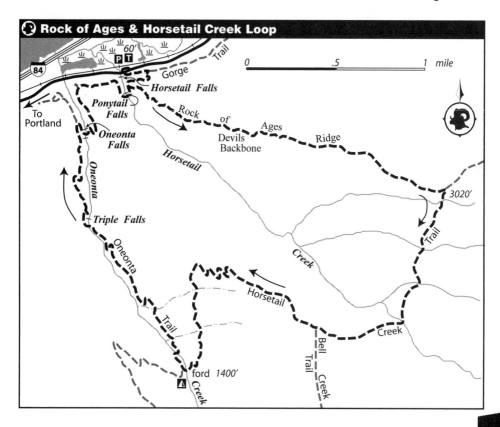

Rock of Ages & Horsetail Creek Loop

of poison oak plants, although they are usually easy to avoid.

In order to go around trees and rocks, the path makes lots of small dips and turns, but it is always very steep as you ascend the slopes east of Ponytail Falls. After about 0.4 mile, there is a split in the trail. The path to the left looks like the main route, but it actually dead-ends after about 75 yards at a good viewpoint on a rocky overlook. The main trail goes to the right and contours for 100 yards across a steep, mostly open hillside with lots of oak trees, before climbing steeply once again. The trail makes several twists and turns before curving left and reaching a narrow slot in the ridgecrest. You turn right here and keep climbing at an extremely steep grade up to a grassy ledge perched on the spine of the ridge.

This narrow rock crest is called the Devils Backbone, and the trail goes right along its spine. Sometimes this spine is only a few inches wide, and it drops off very steeply on both sides, so be very careful. For acrophobics, a safer but less spectacular path skirts around the left side of Devils Backbone. If your shaky nerves allow you the luxury of looking around, you will be delighted with the terrific views of the forested ridges to the south, as well as across the river all the way to Mt. Adams. Flowers abound, especially yarrow, yellow daisy, stonecrop, buckwheat, blue bellflower, and onion.

Once past this dramatic section, the trail becomes somewhat easier, as you climb at a more moderate grade in deep woods, always on or near the ridge crest. There are still some very steep sections, but the trail here is not as rugged or as

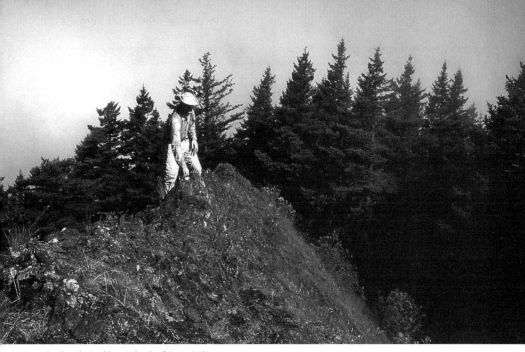

On Devils Backbone, Rock of Ages Ridge

difficult as it was below. You will get occasional glimpses through the trees on the left of the towering rock buttress called Rock of Ages, for which this ridge was named, but mostly you stay in viewless forests. A little past a short section where you actually lose some elevation, the steep climbing begins again on a final push to the top of the rim. You will know when you reach the top, because the ridge widens rather abruptly, and the trail's grade becomes remarkably gentle. The forests here feature lots of perky little wildflowers, like starflower, star-flowered smilacina, and pipsissewa, whose cute little pink blossoms turn downward. Once on top of the rim, the path gently winds along for about 1 mile, staying near a steep drop-off on your left, before coming to a junction with the Horsetail Creek Trail.

To make the loop, turn right (downhill) on the quiet Horsetail Creek Trail and very quickly come to a tiny splashing tributary of Horsetail Creek, amid dense riparian vegetation that is dominated by

devil's club, salmonberry, lady fern, and baneberry. Over the next mile, you cross three larger branches of the creek, each separated by a rounded woodsy ridge. None of the crossings have bridges, but the creeks can all be crossed with simple rock hops. After the final crossing, you gradually climb for about 0.5 mile to a junction with the rarely traveled Bell Creek Trail, where you turn right.

It's pretty much all downhill from here, but most of it is gradual. First, you go down a gentle wooded slope, and then, just as the slope ends at a steep drop-off, you switchback to the left on what is only the first of 15 remarkably well-graded switchbacks. After six switchbacks, look for a 50-foot spur trail to the left that goes to a small rocky overlook with nice views of Sherrard Point on Larch Mountain, peeking over Franklin Ridge.

After the last of the 15 switchbacks, you make a long descending traverse to the south, crossing two tiny tributaries of Oneonta Creek along the way, and then make six short, but quite steep, downhill switchbacks to an unbridged crossing of Oneonta Creek. There are lots of boulders in the creek that appear to invite a dry-footed crossing. But these smooth rocks are dangerously slippery, so it is much safer either to search for a log crossing or simply ford the creek. It is an easy ford, and your feet will appreciate the cool water.

A short distance up the opposite bank is an excellent campsite and a junction with the Oneonta Trail. You turn right and drop quickly to another crossing of Oneonta Creek, this time on a nice, safe log bridge. From here, you descend along the east bank of the stream, as the trail drops rapidly to keep pace with the cascading creek. This section of trail is very attractive because the forest is dense, mossy, and elegant, and the creek is a constant joy for both visiting humans and the resident dippers, who dive under the water in search of food.

After about 0.7 mile, you cross the creek on a wide plank bridge and, just downstream, come to a short side trail on the right that leads to an overlook of gorgeous Triple Falls. This is the usual turnaround point for hikers coming up Oneonta Creek, so from here on the trail is very crowded.

You follow the Oneonta Trail as it works along the steep slopes above the deep canyon of Oneonta Creek for 0.9 mile and then turn sharply right at a junction. You drop to a crossing of the creek just above one waterfall and just below another before climbing a set of six switchbacks past a dramatic view of Oneonta Gorge. From here, you contour around a ridge and finally return to Ponytail Falls, closing the loop.

TRIP 21 Nesmith Point

Distance	9.8 miles, Out-and-back
Elevation Gain	3800 feet
Hiking Time	5 to 6 hours
Optional Map	Green Trails *Bonneville Dam & Bridal Veil*
Usually Open	Late April to early November
Best Time	Mid-May to mid-June
Trail Use	Dogs OK
Agency	Columbia River Gorge National Scenic Area
Difficulty	Strenuous

HIGHLIGHTS When hikers new to our region drive Interstate 84 through the Columbia River Gorge, they often crane their necks to see the tops of the towering cliffs and think, "Wow, the view up there must be great, but, man, it looks like a long way up!" Well, they're right on both counts, and Nesmith Point is the place to prove it. As one of the highest points directly overlooking the river, Nesmith Point provides excellent, if partially obstructed, views over much of the scenic masterpiece that is the Gorge. Be prepared, however, to pay a stiff physical admission fee to enjoy the show. Just as it appears from the bottom, it is a long way up.

DIRECTIONS Coming from the west on Interstate 84, take Ainsworth Park Exit 35 and turn left, following signs for Dodson. After just 150 feet, turn right on Frontage Road, and drive 2.2 miles to the large parking lot on the right for John B. Yeon State Park.

The trail starts at the west end of the parking lot and makes one quick switchback past a leaky wooden water tank to a junction. You turn right and walk gradually uphill for 0.9 mile, through dense forests to a junction with the Gorge Trail, just before a rocky slope and gully. Turn left here and you soon begin the promised long, hard climb. There is no shortage of switchbacks, far too many to count, but they don't prevent the route from being relentlessly steep. At first, you make your way out to a small ridge crest viewpoint and then climb up a gully, with switchbacks taking you back and forth across the usually waterless bottom. There is lush vegetation here beneath the trees: ferns, false Solomon's seal, thimbleberry, and other species crowd the gully.

The route leaves the gully, traverses a nearly vertical slope to round a ridge, and then makes several short switchbacks up the ridge's west side, where you can expect to crawl around logs and washouts. The trail recrosses the ridge and then also crosses the slopes of a large basin. Here you will get your first good views of the nearby cliffs and, across the river, of Beacon Rock and Mt. Adams in Washington. You make your way over to the head of the basin, before once again switchbacking back and forth

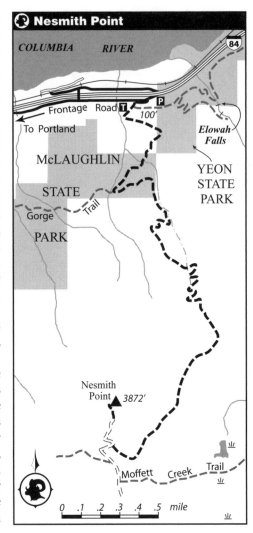

View of Mt. Adams from the Nesmith Point Trail

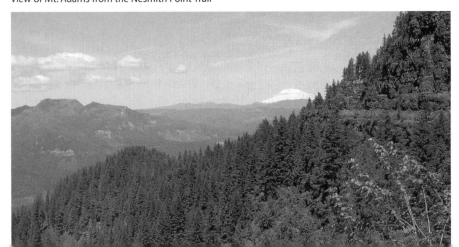

across a cedar-filled gully, and then finally reach a narrow ridgeline, where you can look down into McCord Creek Canyon to the east. You meet your first beargrass and huckleberry plants here too, which, as usual in the Gorge, means that the worst of the climb is over.

The trail turns up the ridge, staying on its east side, to pass through lovely mid-elevation woods of Douglas fir, Pacific silver fir, and hemlock. The grade is considerably less severe than it was below but still ascends steadily uphill, as the trail curves to the right and gently climbs a final section to a junction with an abandoned road.

To reach the summit, turn right and follow this curving road for 0.3 mile to the old lookout site atop Nesmith Point. Views here are excellent to the west,

but trees block every other direction. For better vistas, continue past the high point, and drop about 200 yards to a larger opening, where you can look not only west but also north to Beacon Rock, Hamilton Mountain, and Mt. Adams, and even straight down to the area near the trailhead.

The trail to the top of Nesmith Point is about as much as any reasonable dayhiker can handle, but backpackers can use this trail as the jumping-off point for longer trips. The most logical options are west to Oneonta Creek via the Horsetail Creek Trail and east to Tanner Creek on the recently reopened Moffett Creek Trail. Car shuttles to the trailheads at Horsetail Falls or Tanner Creek make these long trips more manageable.

TRIP 22 Elowah Falls

Distance	3.0 miles, Out-and-back
Elevation Gain	600 feet
Hiking Time	1½ to 2 hours
Optional Map	Green Trails *Bonneville Dam*
Usually Open	February to December
Best Time	Mid-April to June
Trail Use	Good for kids, dogs OK (but the trail is dangerous for them in places)
Agency	John B. Yeon State Park
Difficulty	Easy
Note	Good in cloudy weather

HIGHLIGHTS Several factors come together to ensure that Elowah Falls is an exceptional waterfall, even in an area with so many to choose from. First it's tall, plunging 289 feet in a single shooting fall. Second, the setting is incredibly dramatic: a circular amphitheater of basalt cliffs, sprinkled with green mosses and lichens. Third, you get two falls for the price of one, with a second impressive drop of water tucked away above the famous lower falls. Finally, the two trails exploring the falls are both spectacular and of very different character. The higher trail is perched on a rock ledge blasted out of the cliffs beside the falls, while the lower trail explores the mossy canyon at the falls' base.

DIRECTIONS Coming from the west on Interstate 84, take Ainsworth Park Exit 35 and turn left, following signs for Dodson. After just 150 feet, turn right on Frontage Road and drive 2.2 miles to the large parking lot on the right for John B. Yeon State Park.

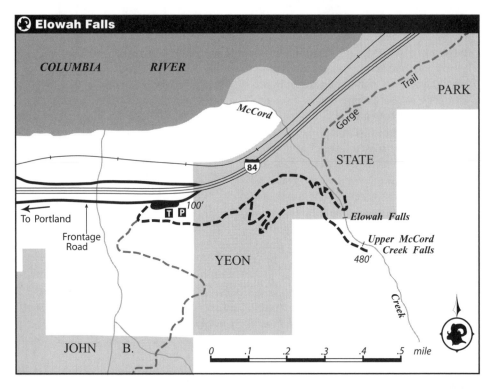

Elowah Falls

COLUMBIA   RIVER

McCord

Gorge   Trail

PARK

84

STATE

100'

T P

← To Portland

Elowah Falls

Frontage
Road

*Upper McCord
Creek Falls*

YEON

480'

Creek

JOHN   B.

0   .1   .2   .3   .4   .5   mile

The trail leaves from the west side of the lot and climbs in one switchback past a leaky water tank, to a junction with the trail to Nesmith Point. Stay on the wide main trail to the left, walking through lovely woods, first of bigleaf maple then of Douglas fir, to a junction of the two trails that explore the falls. The upper trail goes sharply right and climbs moderately, on five increasingly short switchbacks, up a mostly open slope with lots of wildflowers. Look for stonecrop, tiger lily, columbine, penstemon, and a host of others amid the rocks and mosses.

You pass the remains of an old water diversion pipe and then travel a dramatic section of trail that has been blasted out of the sheer basalt cliffs. Metal guardrails have been installed here to help acrophobics feel safe. Views from this airy perch are very good, featuring distant looks at Table Mountain and Mt. Adams in

Elowah Falls

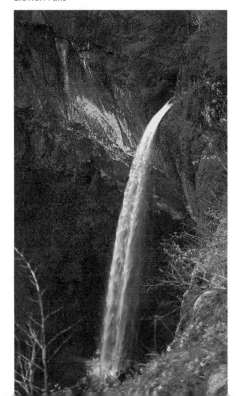

Washington, but these are quickly forgotten as you round the corner to be confronted with the magnificent sheer drop of Elowah Falls in a huge, cliff-walled basin below you. Photographers should note that this steep, north-facing cliff gets very little sunlight, so you may need fast film and a tripod to take pictures in the low light. Stop to gawk as long as you like, snap a few dozen pictures, and then walk the level trail up to the canyon above the falls, to where pleasant Upper McCord Creek Falls hides. For most of the year, this waterfall is actually a pair of side-by-side flows. In high water, it is a three-part cascade. The trail ends at the creek just above this falls.

To explore the lower trail, retrace your steps to the junction and turn east on a trail that goes past a rockslide and then drops in six quick switchbacks to a bridge over McCord Creek, in a bouldery glen below the towering lower falls. Late October to early November is the ideal time to visit because the bigleaf maple trees will be bright yellow, adding a distinct autumnal ambiance to the scene. From the bridge, the trail continues east to Munra Point and Wahclella Falls, as part of the low-elevation Gorge Trail. Although noisy and not very wild, due to the proximity of Interstate 84, this is a pleasant walk for those seeking additional exercise.

TRIP 23 Munra Point

Distance	2.8 miles, Out-and-back
Elevation Gain	1800 feet
Hiking Time	2 to 4 hours
Optional Map	Green Trails *Bonneville Dam*
Usually Open	April to November
Best Time	May to June
Trail Use	No dogs (too dangerous)
Agency	Columbia River Gorge National Scenic Area
Difficulty	Difficult

HIGHLIGHTS Munra Point is one of the most recognizable landmarks in the western Columbia River Gorge. The narrow, bald-topped ridge, with its distinctive pointed top, is an irresistible destination for adventurous hikers. But, to get there, you'd better be really adventurous! The trail, using that term loosely, is definitely not for everyone. Although the lower reaches have been improved in recent years to include some switchbacks, the trail remains so steep in places that you will have to use your hands to grab onto roots and limbs to help pull yourself up. On the lower part of the hike, the poison oak is so abundant that it's practically impossible to avoid it. Near the top, the old trail is now gone, forcing hikers to make a dangerously steep rock climb for the last 100 feet. Finally, when the tread is wet, it can be dangerously slippery, so try to save this hike for a dry spell. The great views and abundant wildflowers at the summit are worth the effort, but don't be misled by the short distance.

DIRECTIONS The only parking near the trailhead is along the westbound lanes of Interstate 84, so if you are coming from Portland, drive the freeway to Bonneville Dam Exit 40 and circle around to the westbound lanes. Drive 1.1 miles and park in an unsigned gravel lot on the right.

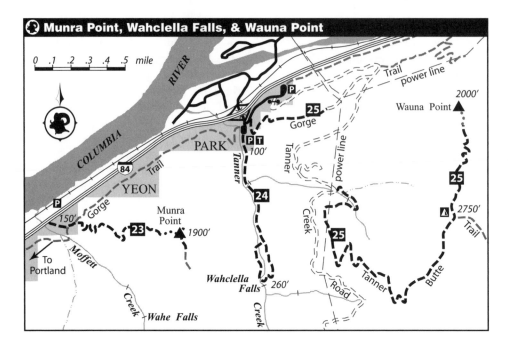

Munra Point, Wahclella Falls, & Wauna Point

Walk west along the freeway shoulder 0.1 mile until just before the bridge over Moffett Creek. From here, look for and follow a faint path, going south through a small grassy area, that leads you under the tall highway bridge for the eastbound lanes of Interstate 84. You then go up a brushy little slope for about 50 feet and intersect the Gorge Trail. Turn left and walk about 70 yards to an unsigned junction with an obvious boot path going up to the right. You turn onto this path and, a few yards later, pass a small sign tacked to a tree that states simply TRAIL NOT MAINTAINED—an understatement worthy of some kind of award.

The first 0.1 mile is moderately steep, but this will soon seem tame, as the path gets quite rocky and climbs rapidly through woods. You work your way up the south side of a steep ridge and then turn to the left and climb very steeply for about 0.2 mile, before reaching a ridgetop junction with a short downhill spur trail to a viewpoint. This makes a good excuse for a stop, but really the views are better at the top. Above the viewpoint, you generally stay close to the narrow crest, crawling over rock outcroppings, pulling yourself up beside trees and bushes, and dodging poison oak. Although steep and rugged, the path is reasonably obvious

Top of Munra Point

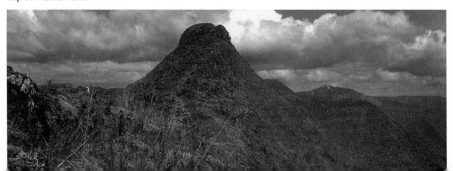

and easy to follow. Nonetheless, it is wise to look back from time to time, especially at any confusing spots, to ensure you can find the proper route to get back down. The trail becomes increasingly exposed, with fewer trees and better views, as you climb. At about 1.1 miles the trail levels off briefly at a view-packed ridge crest, which makes a good turnaround point for most hikers.

If you are an experienced and confident scrambler, continue climbing 0.1 mile to the base of a rocky cliff. Ascending this cliff requires shimmying up a narrow chute with tiny footholds and lots of exposure. It is definitely not for the faint of heart, especially since coming back down the chute is even more difficult. At the top of this climb you reach the views and grassy slopes of the summit area.

The most notable of the many flowers here is the wild onion, which carpets the area in early spring. Another notable feature is the wind, which often blows very hard at this exposed location. Narrow and exposed paths explore the open ridge and offer outstanding views for those who made it this far. The best views are straight down to Bonneville Dam and Tanner Creek, but you can also see Mt. Adams, Table Mountain, Hamilton Mountain, and, rather surprisingly, a snippet of Mt. Rainier. Stay as long as you want to enjoy the view—you've earned it.

TRIP 24 Wahclella Falls

Distance	1.8 miles, Out-and-back
Elevation Gain	300 feet
Hiking Time	1 hour
Optional Map	Green Trails *Bonneville Dam*
Usually Open	February to December
Best Time	Mid-April to June
Trail Use	Good for kids, dogs OK
Agency	Columbia River Gorge National Scenic Area
Difficulty	Easy
Note	Good in cloudy weather

see map on p.234

Western Columbia River Gorge

HIGHLIGHTS With such a wealth of waterfalls in the Columbia River Gorge, it strains an author's vocabulary to find enough different superlatives to cover each one. If any of the dozens of towering falls here were moved almost anywhere else in the country, it would draw millions of admirers. But here, with such an embarrassment of riches, people become a bit blasé. Still, no matter how jaded you may be, you won't want to miss this short trail to spectacular, two-tiered Wahclella Falls. The name, which rolls so nicely off the tongue, was suggested in 1915 by the Mazamas, a Portland hiking and climbing club, to honor the Native American name for a locality near Beacon Rock. For a while, the name was changed to the rather prosaic "Tanner Creek Falls," but in an unusual display of governmental good sense, the original name was restored and is now firmly established.

DIRECTIONS Leave Interstate 84 at Exit 40 and turn right (south) at the bottom of the exit ramp. You immediately come to a T-junction and bear right for about 100 yards to reach the parking lot for the Wahclella Falls Trail.

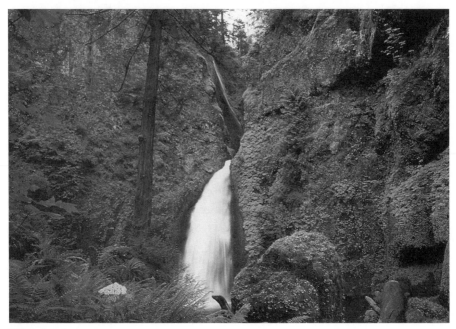

Wahclella Falls

The first 0.2 mile of this hike follows an old gravel road beside the splashing waters of Tanner Creek to a small concrete dam that diverts water for a fish hatchery downstream. Just past this dam, the footpath crosses a side creek right below a waterfall, where you might get a bit of a shower during high water. The well-constructed route then climbs gradually away from the creek, up a series of steps, for about 0.5 mile, to a fork in the trail that is the starting point of a small loop. Bear right, descend to a bridged crossing of the creek, and then follow the west bank upstream to another bridge just below impressive Wahclella Falls. Near this spot, you may be intrigued by the enormous boulders that litter the bottom of the canyon. These came from a massive 1973 landslide that fell from the steep west wall of the canyon, temporarily damming the creek's flow. Today, the boulders are covered with mosses and ferns, and they make interesting foregrounds for pictures of the falls.

The falls is made up of two parts—a long, wispy stream of water from the east side of the canyon, and a shorter, but more boisterous, 60-foot horsetail falls that shoots out of the slot canyon at the bottom. You'll need at least half an hour to snap pictures and just soak in the scene. Once you've had your fill of the view, climb a couple of tiny switchbacks and return along the loop trail on the east side of the canyon back to the trail split.

TRIP 25 Wauna Point

Distance	10.4 miles, Out-and-back
Elevation Gain	3200 feet
Hiking Time	5 to 6 hours
Optional Map	Green Trails *Bonneville Dam*
Usually Open	Late March to November
Best Time	Mid-April to early June
Trail Use	No dogs (too dangerous)
Agency	Columbia River Gorge National Scenic Area
Difficulty	Difficult

see map on p.234

HIGHLIGHTS   Until recently, the trail to the excellent viewpoint at Wauna Point was a straightforward, not-too-difficult, 6-mile round-trip, starting from the quiet Tanner Creek Road. That hike has now been made into a much longer and more strenuous adventure because Tanner Creek Road is now closed to motor vehicles, adding 4.4 miles and more than 1000 feet of elevation gain and loss to the round-trip hike. The advantage of this closure is that it significantly increases the chances of solitude for those hikers willing to make the extra effort. And Wauna Point is worth the effort. With a mountain bike, you can shorten the walking distance by riding the closed Tanner Creek Road to the old trailhead. The name *Wauna*, which is used for several features in this area, is believed to be a Klickitat word for a mythological being who represents the Columbia River.

DIRECTIONS   Leave Interstate 84 at Exit 40, and turn right (south) at the bottom of the exit ramp. You immediately come to a T-junction and bear right for about 100 yards to reach the parking lot for the Wahclella Falls Trail.

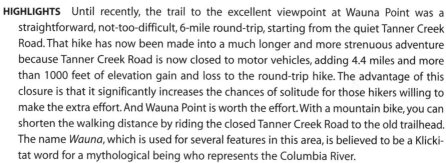

Pick up the eastbound Gorge Trail at a sign directly opposite the T-junction, and follow it up a switchback. You then traverse a forested hillside, where the sounds of traffic on Interstate 84 disturb the natural quiet, but at least the forest is attractive. You make two short switchbacks and then a long traverse to a junction with a power line access road, about 0.8 mile from the trailhead. Follow this route for 0.2 mile to a junction with the closed Tanner Creek Road, where you turn right and walk uphill as the road rounds a ridge and enters the canyon of Tanner Creek. The signed Tanner Butte Trail leaves from the left side of the road, just before you cross a small creek in a side canyon.

Having reached a true foot trail, you follow the rocky Tanner Butte Trail as it climbs beside a splashing creek that tumbles over a series of small but attractive waterfalls. Water-loving plants, like maidenhair fern, monkeyflower, and bleeding heart thrive in this environment. Overhead, drooping western hemlock and western red cedar are the dominant tree species. The fairly steep trail crosses two branches of the creek, traverses a hillside, and then twice passes under a set of power lines in forest openings that provide excellent views, both north toward Table Mountain and west to Munra Point.

After crossing a rocky power line access road at a diagonal, you slowly climb a hillside above the power line, in a Douglas-fir forest that comes alive in May with the white blossoms of Pacific dogwood trees. From here, six long switchbacks steadily, but not too steeply, lead you uphill. Five more short, steep switchbacks take you up to a viewpoint spur trail. The open area at this viewpoint provides good views to the west. A few hardy wildflowers, like larkspur, columbine, and onion, brighten the foreground.

After this viewpoint, you make a fairly long uphill traverse to the northeast on a heavily wooded slope. Along the way you cross a tiny seeping trickle of water, continuing to a possibly unsigned junction near a dry campsite shortly before the main trail turns sharply right.

For Wauna Point, you turn left, soon passing a sign that says TRAIL NOT MAIN-TAINED. The path descends gradually at first and then much more steeply as it winds down the rocky spine of Wauna Point. After a series of very short switchbacks, you crawl carefully down a dangerously narrow rocky ridge to a small flat spot just above a steep drop-off. From here, you can enjoy a terrific view of steep-sided Eagle Creek Canyon to the east, Table Mountain to the north, Beacon Rock downriver to the west, and Bonneville Dam and the mighty Columbia River almost directly below you.

Daredevil hikers sometimes look at the map and see that Wauna Viewpoint (Trip 27) is directly below Wauna Point, and they dream of somehow connecting the two into a loop trip. Forget it! There is no trail, not even a remotely reasonable cross-country route, between the two. Trying it is a recipe for disaster. Go back the way you came.

TRIP 26 Tanner Butte

Distance	20.8 miles, Out-and-back
Elevation Gain	4700 feet
Hiking Time	10 to 12 hours
Optional Map	Green Trails Bonneville Dam
Usually Open	Late May to October
Best Time	June
Trail Use	Dogs OK, backpacking option
Agency	Columbia River Gorge National Scenic Area
Difficulty	Strenuous

HIGHLIGHTS The rounded summit of Tanner Butte, with its gouged-out eastern face, is a well-known landmark in the central Columbia River Gorge, visible from viewpoints more than 50 miles away. Since the line of sight goes in both directions, you might deduce that the views from Tanner Butte are also mighty impressive. And you'd be correct.

The view alone would be worth the hike, but in addition, the area around the mountain features wide, sloping wildflower meadows and scenic talus slopes, which are delightful even without the view. It's no wonder that hardy hikers have long enjoyed this outing, some making it a treasured annual trip.

That annual trip, however, must be rethought or at least planned differently now. Although it was never an easy hike, the trip to Tanner Butte was made even more difficult recently when the old Tanner Creek Road was closed to motor vehicles, making the hike a challenge that is probably best left to backpackers. But a handful of the most athletic dayhikers can still visit this classic destination. If you have a mountain bike, you can shorten the round-trip walking distance by 4.4 miles, which makes things a little more reasonable.

DIRECTIONS Leave Interstate 84 at Exit 40, and turn right (south) at the bottom of the exit ramp. You immediately come to a T-junction and bear right for about 100 yards to reach the parking lot for the Wahclella Falls Trail.

Follow the eastbound Gorge Trail that starts opposite the T-junction, climbs in switchbacks, and traverses a forested hillside. After about 0.8 mile, the trail follows a power line access road for 0.2 mile to a junction with the closed Tanner Creek Road, where you turn right. Walk this road uphill as it rounds a ridge and enters the canyon of Tanner Creek. The signed Tanner Butte Trail leaves from the left side of the road, just before you cross a small creek in a side canyon.

The footpath goes up a lush little canyon with several small waterfalls, crossing two branches of the creek before climbing and twice going under a power line. You cross the power line access road at a diagonal and go up a series of six long and five short switchbacks on a heavily forested hillside. After the switchbacks, you make a long traverse to a ridge crest junction where the unofficial Wauna Point Trail goes off to the left.

You turn right, staying on the Tanner Butte Trail, and begin a long, moderately graded ascent of a wide ridge. There are no views along the way, but the hiking is never tedious, as the forest is open and attractive. As you gain elevation, the forests gradually change to typical higher-elevation woods, dominated by Douglas fir and Pacific silver fir, with lots of beargrass and huckleberries on the forest floor.

After 2.1 miles of climbing, you hit a possibly unsigned junction with the Tanner Cutoff Trail, heading downhill to the right. Go straight and, about 150 yards later, reach the junction with the 0.4-mile spur trail to Dublin Lake. If you are backpacking, this is a logical place to spend the night. The trail to the lake begins gently, but after 100 yards it drops quite steeply to the northwest corner of this small, forest-rimmed pool. The best place to set up your tent is at a camp on the southwest shore.

Back on the Tanner Butte Trail, you walk a short distance before dropping to an old jeep road. Look carefully here

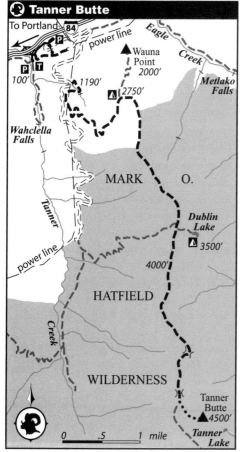

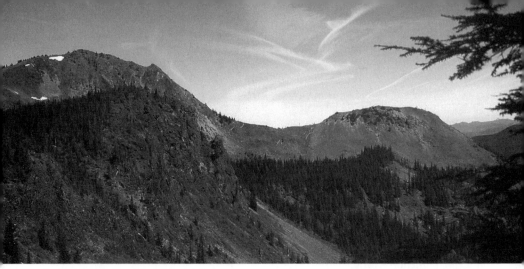

Tanner Butte from a ridge to the southeast

to note where you meet the road, as the trail turnoff is poorly signed on the way back. Walk south on this overgrown road 1.0 mile, staying on the west side of the wooded ridgeline, and then descend slightly to a little saddle where the forest breaks up and the scenery abruptly improves. To the east, you can look down into the green depths of Eagle Creek Canyon, while due south is the steep northeast face of massive Tanner Butte. All around your feet are lots of colorful wildflowers, especially beargrass, lupine, paintbrush, and larkspur. The road is overgrown with huckleberries and foot-tripping beargrass, but the scenery is so good you won't have any complaints.

Still on the old road, continue south through increasingly open and attractive meadows and rocky slopes. Then go over a view-packed knoll and down to a wide saddle on the north side of Tanner Butte. The road works uphill from here and curves around the brushy west slopes of the butte, but if you want to reach the top of Tanner Butte, leave the road at the saddle, and scramble cross-country up the northwest side of the peak. Try not to get too close to the steep drop-off on your left, as the rocks can be unstable. The first few hundred yards are rather difficult, as you have to fight through some brush, but then the going improves as the country opens up. From the top, those promised views extend to Mounts St. Helens, Adams, and Rainier in Washington, as well as Mt. Hood in Oregon. Hikers familiar with the area can also pick out shorter but no less attractive landmarks, like Washington's Silver Star Mountain, and Oregon's Larch and Chinidere mountains.

Backpackers can enjoy this view at leisure and have the time to take in some additional nearby scenery. One option is to scramble east from a saddle just south of Tanner Butte to the cirque basin which holds scenic little Tanner Lake. You can also walk cross-country, out a small ridge southeast of Tanner Butte, for some dramatic photos of the scenic butte, with snowy Mt. Adams in the distance.

Finally, if you want to make a grand three-day loop, you can descend into the Eagle Creek drainage on the rarely used Eagle-Tanner Trail, past Big Cedar Spring (another possible campsite), and then hike down the Eagle Creek Trail (Trip 28) back to civilization. A 3.0-mile section of the Gorge Trail connects the Eagle Creek Trailhead with the Wahclella Falls trailhead to close out this magnificent 28-mile loop.

TRIP 27 Wauna Viewpoint

Distance	3.6 miles, Out-and-back
Elevation Gain	950 feet
Hiking Time	2 hours
Optional Map	Green Trails *Bonneville Dam*
Usually Open	February to December
Best Time	Mid-April to May
Trail Use	Good for kids, dogs OK
Agency	Columbia River Gorge National Scenic Area
Difficulty	Moderate

HIGHLIGHTS The Gorge Trail is a relatively new hiking option in the Portland/Vancouver region. It manages to remain open practically all winter by keeping to low elevations near the Columbia River. It is also useful in other seasons for creating loop trips out of longer hikes in the backcountry of the Gorge. Taken separately, however, most sections of the route are so close to either the Old Columbia River Highway or Interstate 84 that they are just too noisy to be considered "wild," and, therefore, do not qualify for inclusion in this book. But where the trail follows older routes farther away from the traffic, there are some very scenic hiking opportunities. One such segment is the trail up to Wauna Viewpoint, a little west of Eagle Creek.

DIRECTIONS Leave the eastbound lanes of Interstate 84 at Eagle Creek Recreation Area Exit 41. At the bottom of the exit road, turn right, drive about 0.1 mile, and then park in the small lot on the left, across from a prominent hiker's bridge over Eagle Creek. Parking is very limited here on summer weekends, so arrive early in the morning.

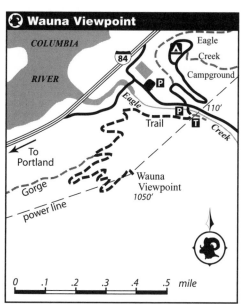

You begin by going west across the impressive hiker's bridge over Eagle Creek. This arcing wooden structure is supported by cables and sways a little as you walk across, but it provides a nice look down at the creek's clear waters. Immediately on the other side of the bridge are a wooden bench and a junction. Turn right on the wide, gently graded trail, which climbs two short switchbacks under the shade of tall fir and hemlock trees and then traverses a wet hillside with lots of mossy overhangs that support an abundance of maidenhair and lady ferns. The traverse ends at a fenced overlook, about 200 feet above Interstate 84 and Bonneville Dam.

The trail switchbacks to the left at this overlook and takes you uphill to three more switchbacks to a brushy opening with lots of thimbleberry, whose bright red berries look and taste like strong, tart raspberries and ripen in midsummer. Before eating too many berries, however, consider that the fruit will stain your skin, so you are likely to get caught red-handed.

Still climbing gradually, you come to a junction marked with one of the old stone signs still occasionally found in the western Gorge. These markers were permanently cemented into the rock at trail intersections, with destinations and distances chiseled into the stone. Changes to the trails over the decades have made the mileages suspect, but the signs still have a quaintly historical appeal.

To reach Wauna Viewpoint, you turn sharply left and climb six long switchbacks in a relatively open forest. One reason the forest is so open is that a fire burned through here in the 1990s, killing many smaller trees and leaving singed bark on the bigger ones that survived the blaze. One plant that has grown back abundantly is poison oak. Fortunately, unlike so many other trails in the Gorge, this path is wide enough to make it easy to avoid the plant.

The trail ends at a spectacular rocky overlook beside a power line tower. To the west, you can see Munra Point, Beacon Rock, and long distances down the Columbia River. To the east are Bridge of the Gods, Cascade Locks, and the cliffs of Ruckel Ridge, across the canyon of Eagle Creek. Most impressive is the view directly across the river, to flat-topped Table Mountain and down to Bonneville Dam.

TRIP 28 Eagle Creek Trail

Distance	4.2 to 12.0 miles, Out-and-back
Elevation Gain	400 to 1200 feet
Hiking Time	2 to 7 hours
Optional Map	Green Trails *Bonneville Dam*
Usually Open	March to December
Best Time	Mid-April to June
Trail Use	No dogs (dangerous), backpacking option
Agency	Columbia River Gorge National Scenic Area
Difficulty	Easy to difficult
Note	Good in cloudy weather

HIGHLIGHTS The famous Eagle Creek Trail has been a favorite of local hikers since it was first built in 1915. The trail opened at the same time as the Old Columbia River Scenic Highway, providing a spectacular hiking destination for visitors just discovering the area. Today, it remains one of the most spectacular trails in the region. It leads hikers through a verdant canyon, beside waterfalls in every shape and size, along a creek that is almost unbelievably beautiful. Of course, lots of other people think this is a great hike too, so don't expect to be alone. To protect the resource, the U.S. Forest Service requires that backpackers camp only in designated sites, and they ask that you leave your dog at home.

DIRECTIONS Leave the eastbound lanes of Interstate 84 at Eagle Creek Recreation Area Exit 41. At the bottom of the exit road, turn right and drive about 0.6 mile on a narrow paved road to the parking lot at the end of the road. Parking is very limited here on summer weekends, so arrive early in the morning.

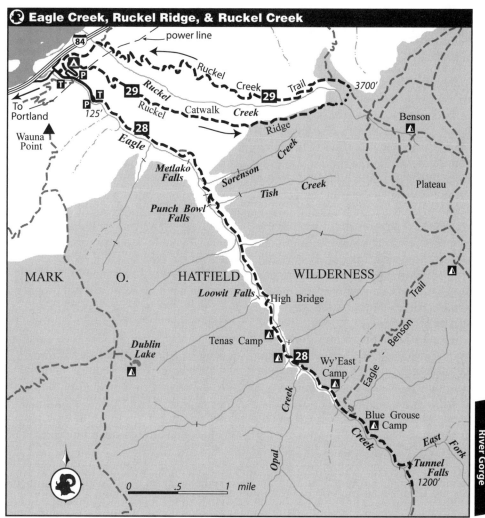

⊙ Eagle Creek, Ruckel Ridge, & Ruckel Creek

power line

Ruckel Creek Trail

29   3700'

Ruckel Creek

29

Ruckel   Catwalk   *Creek*

28   125'

To Portland

Wauna Point

Eagle

Ridge

Benson

Sorenson   Creek

Metlako Falls

Tish   *Creek*

Plateau

Punch Bowl Falls

MARK   O.   HATFIELD   WILDERNESS

Loowit Falls   High Bridge

Benson   Trail

Tenas Camp

28   Wy'East Camp

Eagle

Dublin Lake

Creek

Blue Grouse Camp

Opal   *Creek*

Creek

East   Fork

0   .5   1 mile

Tunnel Falls 1200'

The trail is paved for the first 0.3 mile, as it wanders gradually uphill along the wooded hillsides, above the cascading stream. The path eventually climbs to some very steep slopes a few hundred feet above the creek, with nice views down into the canyon, and crosses several small, unnamed side creeks along the way, which add variety to the lush forest scenery. Poison oak is part of that lush vegetation, but the wide, heavily used trail makes avoiding the plant easy.

After 1.5 miles, you come to the first waterfall. A short side trail to the right makes a loop past a fenced overlook, where you can look up a narrow canyon to the impressive drop of Metlako Falls. Not long after this marvelous taste of things to come, you cross Sorenson Creek on a bridge and come to a junction with the side trail to the bottom of Punch Bowl Falls. Don't miss the chance to visit this spot as the trail drops to a world-famous view of this short, but spectacular, falls. For decades, calendars have featured this outstanding scene of a glassy creek, winding through a fern-lined grotto, with a perfect bowl-shaped falls that drops to a pool at the head of the canyon. This is a rewarding turnaround point for those who want an easy hike.

Back on the main trail, you traverse heavily wooded slopes to a viewpoint directly above Punch Bowl Falls, giving you a different perspective on this classic cascade. Above this point, the scenery grows even more dramatic, as you are forced to cross vertical basalt cliffs where the trail has simply been blasted into the side of the rock. The trail is wide enough so that those afraid of heights shouldn't have a problem, but parents will want to keep a close eye on their children. In fact, young children probably shouldn't take this trail at all.

Along one of these steep slopes you get a terrific view of wispy Loowit Falls, on a side creek across the canyon. Shortly after this, you cross appropriately named High Bridge, which spans a slot canyon about 90 feet above the clear waters of Eagle Creek.

After the bridge, the slopes are less steep and are covered with dense forests. At Tenas Camp, the first legal campsite along the creek, you may want to take a

Lower Punch Bowl Falls

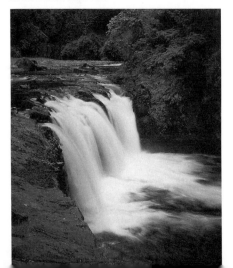

side trip to the creek to visit a lovely two-stage waterfall, which has very nice pools that invite a cold dip in the water. Above Tenas Camp, you recross the creek on a much shorter bridge and then work your way upstream to Wy'East Camp.

A short distance past this camp is a junction with the little-used Eagle-Benson Trail. If you are up for a steep side trip, follow this narrow trail for about 0.5 mile to an open, rocky overlook, with a perspective on Eagle Creek Canyon not available from the lower trail.

Resuming the main trail, you travel gradually uphill in partial forest, past Blue Grouse Camp, and then traverse through forests and over talus slopes well above the creek. A steep side trail drops down one of these talus slopes, visiting an impressive waterfall on the creek, but most people skip this attraction and head straight for Tunnel Falls, in the side canyon just ahead. This colossal 120-foot-high falls on East Fork Eagle Creek drops over a sheer cliff in a shady side canyon. To get past this falls, the trail doesn't go around it but behind it in a tunnel that was dynamited out of the cliff about halfway up the falls. You can still expect to get wet, but it's an exhilarating walk. Just past the falls, you round a ridge where the trail once again takes an exposed course blasted out of vertical basalt cliffs, right beside another tall falls, on the main branch of the creek. Metal cables here give acrophobic hikers something to hang onto and a greater sense of security. There is a terrific lunch spot on the flat creekside rocks, just above this falls.

The trail continues past this point all the way to Wahtum Lake. Unlike the route so far, the trail ahead gains a great deal of elevation and lacks the compensation of waterfalls. Most hikers have already had their fill of great scenery, and they turn back near Tunnel Falls.

TRIP 29 Ruckel Ridge & Ruckel Creek Loop

Distance	9.6 miles, Loop
Elevation Gain	3700 feet
Hiking Time	5 to 7 hours
Optional Map	Green Trails *Bonneville Dam* (part of route not shown)
Usually Open	Late April to early November
Best Time	Late April to May
Trail Use	No dogs (too dangerous for them)
Agency	Columbia River Gorge National Scenic Area
Difficulty	Strenuous

see map on p.243

HIGHLIGHTS This classic but demanding loop features some of the best views and wildflower displays in the Columbia River Gorge. The views are outstanding, especially those of the deep canyon of Eagle Creek, while the wildflower displays in the meadows partway down the Ruckel Creek Trail are exceptional. But you have to work very hard if you want to enjoy these attributes. The unofficial route up Ruckel Ridge is often extremely steep and should be attempted only by confident hikers in top condition. Even on the downhill, you will pay a hefty price in abused knees and jammed toes, so come prepared for both the good and the bad offered by this hike.

DIRECTIONS Leave the eastbound lanes of Interstate 84 at Eagle Creek Recreation Area Exit 41, and turn right at the bottom of the exit road. You can either park in the lot immediately on your left, or drive about 0.1 mile and then park in the small lot on the left, across from a prominent hiker's bridge over Eagle Creek. Parking is very limited on summer weekends, so arrive early in the morning.

From the lot next to the hiker's bridge, turn east and walk through a comfortable little picnic area, up the campground access road about 200 yards, to a large sign on your right that identifies the Gorge Trail. Turn onto this route and climb gradually through lush vegetation of skunk cabbage, ferns, and some menacing stinging nettles that hang over the trail. You go straight at an unsigned four-way junction after just 80 yards and then wind up to a fence line that keeps hikers back from a drop-off above Interstate 84. Walk east along the fence line, past campsites in Eagle Creek Campground. Just as the trail begins to go downhill, you turn right to pick up the campground loop road. When you reach camp 5, you will see a large sign for the Buck Point Trail.

This trail ascends six well-graded switchbacks and then comes to an unsigned junction. The official Buck Point Trail goes straight, but you turn left and soon pass a small sign saying TRAIL NOT MAINTAINED. You are now on the unofficial Ruckel Ridge Trail, and the difficult character of this route soon becomes apparent.

The first hazard, which will be with you for the first mile or so, is poison oak. It is quite prevalent beside the trail, so be sure to wear long pants. The really substantial obstacle of this hike, however, is the steep, rugged grade.

At first things are deceptively easy. You ascend six short switchbacks to a viewpoint beneath some power lines. Then you wander on a gentle, forested path to a rocky area that features hardy wildflowers

Western Columbia River Gorge

and a population of pikas who squeak loudly at passing hikers. From here, the trail switchbacks to the left and crawls over an area of boulders and sloping rocks to an open spot on the ridgeline. The route now gets a lot more difficult, as it turns right and climbs the crest of the ridge, making occasional detours to avoid cliffs and rock outcroppings.

Much of this very steep route keeps exactly to the spine of the ridge, often on a rocky tread that is only a foot or two wide, so acrophobics won't enjoy it much, but those who like exhilarating views will love it. A little over halfway up the ridge is a particularly narrow and dangerous section called the Catwalk. You can skirt it by way of a rough scramble path on the right-hand side. About 0.1 mile later, traverse the right side of a very steep, open, rocky slope and then go back into the forest and descend to a small saddle.

From the saddle, you again crawl up the spine of the ridge, with one detour to the left before the final, very steep push to the rim of Benson Plateau. You know you have reached the plateau when the uphill grade abruptly ends and you enter deep woods. The correct route becomes indistinct from here, but you generally go east, carefully looking out for cut logs, old blazes, or survey tapes tied to tree limbs to help with navigation. The path leads you to a rock-hop or log crossing of Ruckel Creek and then goes on about 100 yards to an unsigned junction with the Ruckel Creek Trail.

To do the loop, you turn left on the Ruckel Creek Trail, as it descends very steeply from the lip of Benson Plateau—although not as steeply as the Ruckel Ridge Trail ascended it. Nearby, Ruckel Creek remains out of sight, but not out of sound, as it rollicks along in one long cascade. The trail can be slick when wet and hard on the knees at any time, so I

recommend that you use hiking poles. Just as you encounter the first bushes of poison oak, the downhill abates, and you contour across a series of large, sloping meadows that are separated by stands of Douglas fir.

From late April to mid-May, these meadows are ablaze with color from the yellows of monkeyflower, lomatium, and groundsel, to the purples of cluster lilies and onion, the blue of lupine, the white of yarrow, and numerous other species. It is truly a spectacle you won't want to miss. There are also good views from the meadows, especially looking west to Ruckel and Tanner ridges.

The steep downhill resumes after the meadows end, as you descend 14 quick switchbacks. At the fifth, you hit a terrific

Ferns and moss-covered trees and rocks along Ruckel Creek

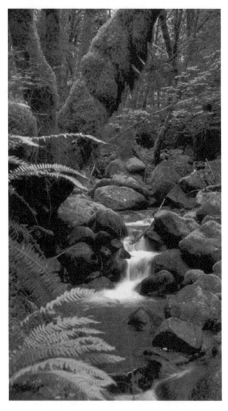

clifftop overlook, where you can see Bonneville Dam and the Bridge of the Gods, as well as Wauna Lake and Table Mountain in Washington.

The rest of the way down is a mix of short switchbacks, traverses, and ridge crest walking. Eventually you reach a moss-covered rockslide, where you will notice rock pits built by Native Americans for ceremonial purposes. As always, it is important that hikers respect the integrity of this site and not disturb even

one rock. From here, you pass beneath a set of power lines and then drop to the lovely banks of cascading Ruckel Creek and a junction with a paved bike trail.

Turn left and walk about 0.3 mile on this bike route to a junction with the Gorge Trail, bearing uphill and to the left. You can stay on the bike path, which soon takes you back to the lower parking area, or you can hike the Gorge Trail past the campground and to the upper parking area near the hiker's bridge.

TRIP 30 Dry Creek Falls

Distance	4.2 miles, Out-and-back
Elevation Gain	600 feet
Hiking Time	2 to 3 hours
Optional Map	Green Trails *Bonneville Dam*
Usually Open	All year (except during winter storms)
Best Times	April and May
Trail Use	Good for kids, dogs OK
Agency	Columbia River Gorge National Scenic Area
Difficulty	Moderate
Note	Good in cloudy weather

HIGHLIGHTS The Columbia River Gorge is a waterfall lover's paradise. There are hundreds, perhaps thousands of falls, ranging from towering cataracts right beside the freeway to hidden cascades miles from the nearest trail. Somewhere between these two extremes are the countless waterfalls reachable along the Gorge's hundreds of miles of trails.

One of the most attractive, but least visited, of this middle group is Dry Creek Falls. Perhaps this falls' scant popularity is due to the fact that no signs direct hikers to it. Or it may be the result of hikers wrongly assuming, from the creek's name, that it has no water. Whatever the reason, Dry Creek Falls remains on the list of falls enjoyed by only a small group of hikers who are "in the know," a group that now includes you!

DIRECTIONS From Interstate 84 east of Portland, take Cascade Locks Exit 44. Follow the exit road for about 0.3 mile and then turn right on a cloverleaf that takes you up toward Bridge of the Gods. Park in the Pacific Crest Trail parking lot, on your right in the middle of the cloverleaf. This trailhead is closed throughout the winter and early spring. During these months you will have to leave your car in front of the concrete blocks that bar access to the parking lot.

The Pacific Crest Trail (PCT) starts on the south side of the bridge-access road and then goes up the wooded road-side bank. After a short traverse you hook up briefly with a paved road that runs under the freeway and then bear right

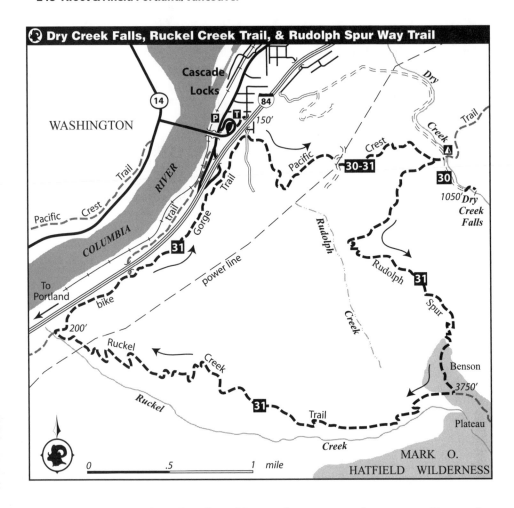

onto a narrow gravel road. Follow this road for 75 yards to a trail junction where you turn left onto a pleasant section of the PCT that gradually climbs through lush forests, dominated at first by bigleaf and vine maple and later by Douglas fir. The forest floor is equally green with vanilla leaf, twisted stalk, fringecup, northern inside-out flower, and sword, bracken, and maidenhair fern, among many others. In May and June, one of the showiest inhabitants of this forest is the tiger lily, with its tall stalks and gorgeous orange flowers.

After about 0.6 mile of gradual uphill, the trail joins a jeep road for about 50 yards, crosses under a power line, and then veers left back onto a true footpath. The PCT then crosses a series of steep hillsides and benches, with lots of impressively straight and tall Douglas firs. Despite the uneven terrain, the trail remains remarkably level all the way to a jeep road, just before a crossing of Dry Creek. There is a camp here and a bridge over the creek—something that would obviously not be necessary if the creek were indeed dry.

To visit Dry Creek Falls, you turn right (uphill) on the jeep road and follow it for 0.2 mile to the base of the falls. The concrete dam and catch basin just below it do nothing to diminish the beauty of this waterfall, a narrow chute of water that drops some 50 feet over a basalt cliff. The scene is exceptionally photogenic, so don't forget your camera.

If you want more exercise, continue east on the PCT for about 1.3 miles to visit a pair of interesting rock pinnacles on the north side of the trail (see Chapter 5, Trip 12).

Dry Creek Falls

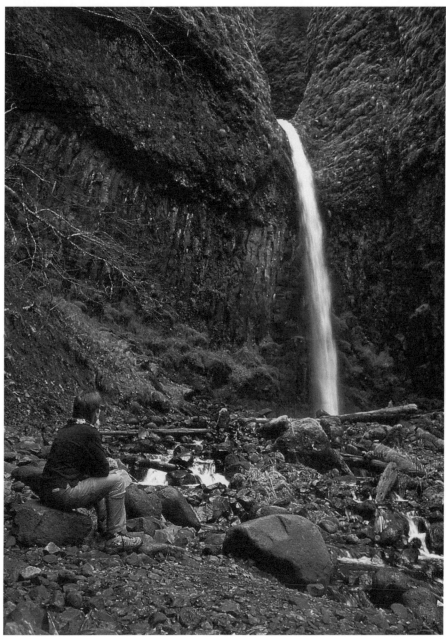

TRIP 31 Rudolph Spur Way Trail Loop

see map on p.248

Distance	10.4 miles, Loop
Elevation Gain	4000 feet
Hiking Time	7 to 10 hours
Optional Map	Green Trails *Bonneville Dam*
Usually Open	May to November
Best Time	May to early June
Trail Use	No dogs (trail is too rough and difficult)
Agency	Columbia River Gorge National Scenic Area
Difficulty	Strenuous

HIGHLIGHTS Many trails reach the top of Benson Plateau, and since they all involve an elevation gain of 3800 feet or more, none of them are easy. Among that group of challenging outings, the most strenuous is the unmaintained route up Rudolph Spur. The trip is difficult, not only because it is one heck of a long way up, but also because it is very steep and requires scrambling over several downed logs. It also challenges you mentally, as this unofficial trail is often sketchy and requires some route-finding ability. In short, this trip is strictly for that group of hard-core hikers who relish exploring little-known routes and don't mind paying the physical price that these trails demand.

DIRECTIONS From Interstate 84 east of Portland, take Cascade Locks Exit 44. Follow the exit road for about 0.3 mile and then turn right on a cloverleaf that takes you up toward Bridge of the Gods. Park in the Pacific Crest Trail parking lot, on your right in the middle of the cloverleaf.

Follow the Pacific Crest Trail (PCT) from the south side of the bridge-access road, as it crosses a forested hillside and then links up with a paved road to travel under the freeway. From here you veer right on a gravel road for 75 yards, turn left on the PCT, and walk this pleasant route for another 1.5 miles to the crossing of misnamed Dry Creek.

About 12 feet before you meet the jeep road that parallels the west bank of Dry Creek, look carefully for the unsigned Rudolph Spur Way Trail that veers south. Hikers should wear long pants on this rather overgrown route, as it climbs steeply on a densely forested hillside, gradually working away from the sound of cascading water in Dry Creek. Try not to step on the banana slugs that live here in incredible abundance, both for their sake and your own—the squishing sensation rates very high on the disgusting

scale. More pleasant are the loud staccato calls of pileated woodpeckers, the rattle of their smaller hairy woodpecker cousins, or the imitation of red-tailed hawks performed by Steller's jays.

The trail climbs quite steeply—this trail does everything steeply—to the top of a forested gully and then traverses a little before rapidly losing about 100 feet of elevation. The trail then goes straight across a small talus slope, whose mossy rocks support lots of yellow stonecrop, as well as a population of pikas. Shortly after reentering the trees, this rugged hike significantly increases its challenge as the trail charges almost directly up a super-steep slope. Adding to the difficulties is the fact that you need to dodge sprigs of bothersome poison oak. Fortunately, the rewards increase, as you climb past forest openings with increasingly good views of Table Mountain and Wauna Lake in

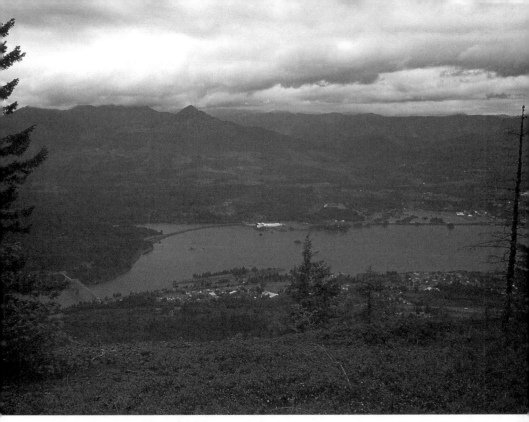

View to Cascade Locks from Rudolph Spur Way Trail

Washington, the Columbia River, and the Bridge of the Gods at Cascade Locks.

The path comes to the top of a minor ridge and then turns onto the spine of this ridge and goes very steeply uphill. The route is often sketchy, so route-finding skills are helpful, but the main requirements for hiking this section are strong thighs and determination. You will probably lose the route from time to time, but red survey tapes that have been tied to some of the rocks and trees provide excellent guidance. Lacking these, you can usually relocate the proper route just by sticking to the crest of the ridge.

You will eventually come to a perfect rest stop, in a good-sized opening on the ridge, with fine views and lots of wildflowers, like yellow daisies, lupine, lomatium, and stonecrop. This spot also tends to catch the constant Gorge breezes, which are welcome on this long climb.

The unrelentingly steep ascent continues as you come to a rocky meadow, with outstanding views down to Cascade Locks and lots of higher-elevation flowers like wallflower, phlox, and cliff penstemon. Just above this meadow is a second open area with reddish rocks and almost no vegetation. The trail disappears briefly here, but you can find it easily enough by looking for the point where it heads into the trees on the left, about 50 feet after you start the climb up the reddish rocks.

Beyond this point, the trail improves considerably; the route is generally well defined and no longer as steep. You also begin to encounter tufts of beargrass—a sure sign that most of the climbing is over. The trail now makes a long, gradual eastward up-and-down traverse on a steep hillside. The biggest obstacle along this section is having to crawl over lots of small downed trees on this unmaintained trail.

After about 0.5 mile, you begin a series of six fairly steep switchbacks and then traverse below a ridge. Just as the trail curves around a minor ridgeline, it turns sharply uphill to the right. The trail here is rather indistinct, but you are aided by occasional yellow paint spots on the trees marking the trail. It is often a good idea to look behind you from time to time, to ensure that the paint spots mark the route in that direction as well. The final 0.1 mile crosses a corner of Benson Plateau and is basically flat until the trail ends at an unsigned junction with the well-maintained Ruckel Creek Trail.

You could return the way you came, but it is easier on the knees to make a loop out of this hike by following the Ruckel Creek Trail on the way down. For this option, turn right and descend steeply from the lip of Benson Plateau to a series of spectacular hanging meadows. Once the meadows end, you switchback down to an outstanding clifftop viewpoint and then continue through more fairly steep switchbacks to a set of power lines and a junction with a paved bike path.

To close out the loop, you turn right on the 12-foot-wide bike path and walk through a tunnel of trees, following the route of the historic Old Columbia River Highway. The walk is pleasant, except for the overwhelming noise pollution from Interstate 84 just a few yards to your left. After 0.7 mile, the bike route passes under the freeway through a tunnel, while the Gorge Trail for hikers veers off to the right, staying on the south side of the divided highway. By either route, it is 1.2 miles back to your car.

Chapter 5

Eastern Columbia River Gorge

Although there is virtually no change in the elevation at river level, everything else about the eastern, or "rain shadow," end of the Columbia River Gorge is radically different from its counterpart to the west. Instead of a lush, near rain forest environment, you find yourself in a semidesert dominated by dry grasslands, scattered ponderosa pines, and sun-baked rock formations. Most streams are intermittent, there are few waterfalls, and sunshine is the rule rather than the exception. Common wildlife includes such dry-land specialists as rattlesnakes, badgers, and ground squirrels, all of which are virtually unknown in the western Gorge. The transition between these two life zones occurs around Dog Mountain on the Washington side and Hood River on the Oregon side. It is in this relatively narrow area, sometimes referred to as the "middle Gorge," where the clouds rapidly dissipate and, in just 10 or 15 miles, the dominant vegetation changes from dense forest to open grassland.

All of the "middle Gorge" is covered in these pages, but only a small sampling of the eastern Gorge is accessible within

View west from Gorge Trail #400 near Wyeth Trail (Trip 17)

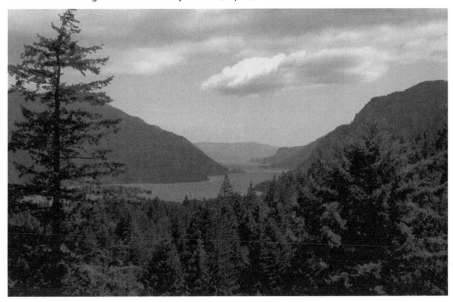

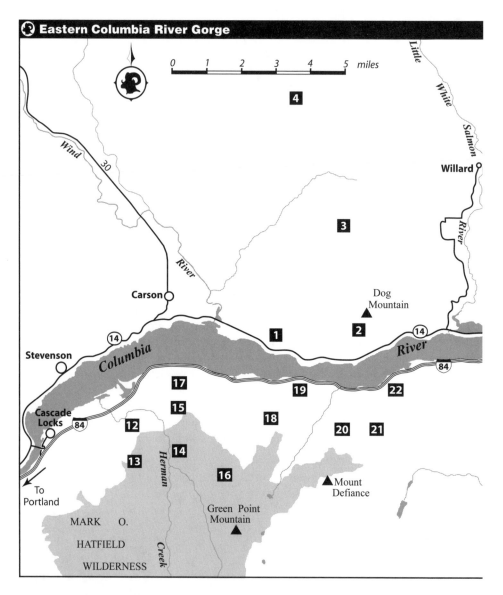

Eastern Columbia River Gorge

0 1 2 3 4 5 miles

a one-hour drive of Portland. Still, as always, every featured trail is worth taking and is likely to inspire you to seek out other routes even farther east. Some excellent recommended hiking trails in the far eastern Gorge include those up Stacker Butte in Washington's Columbia Hills, around Rowena Plateau and the Memaloose Hills near Mosier, and along the Deschutes River east of the Dalles.

The best time to hike the trails in the eastern Gorge is from March to early

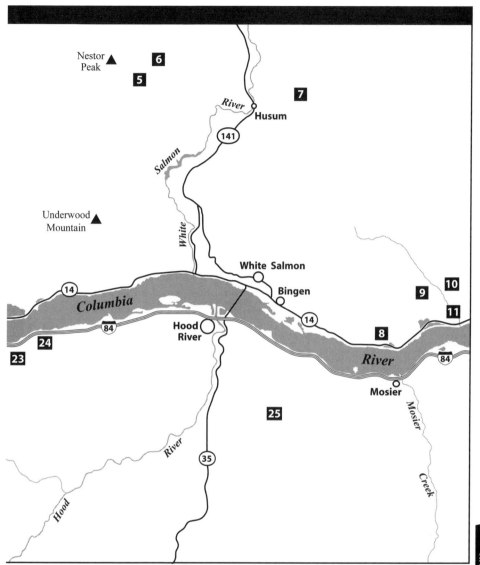

May, when the open slopes are tinged with green, the wildflower displays are truly outstanding, and you can escape the incessant dampness back in Portland or Vancouver. Avoid this area, however, in midsummer, because the temperatures can be well over 100°F and the vegetation will be parched brown. Two other hazards of note here, which you are unlikely to encounter west of the Cascades, are ticks and rattlesnakes. Be careful where you step, and take appropriate precautions.

TRIP 1 Wind Mountain

Distance	2.7 miles, Out-and-back
Elevation Gain	1100 feet
Hiking Time	2 hours
Optional Map	Green Trails *Bonneville Dam & Hood River* (trail not shown)
Usually Open	All year (except during winter storms)
Best Time	All year
Trail Use	Dogs OK
Agency	Columbia River Gorge National Scenic Area
Difficulty	Moderate

HIGHLIGHTS Almost any high point in the Columbia River Gorge could accurately be named "Wind Mountain." This prominent landmark is no windier than neighboring peaks, but a windbreaker is still mandatory, especially if you want to spend some time at the top taking in the view. The well-graded path up Wind Mountain is not on any map but, rest assured, it's there. The trail is neither as spectacular nor as crowded as the one up adjacent Dog Mountain, but this hike does include some interesting Native American history, which the trip up Dog Mountain does not.

Good trail manners are always important, but that is especially true for hiking on Wind Mountain. A short section of the lower trail crosses private land, and while the owners have not traditionally barred public access, it is important that visitors not abuse this privilege. In addition, the sensitive archaeological site at the summit necessitates that hikers exercise the greatest care not to disturb the resource.

DIRECTIONS Drive east on State Highway 14 from the town of Stevenson to milepost 50.7, about 1 mile beyond the bridge over the Wind River. Turn left (north) on Wind Mountain Road, and after 1.0 mile turn right at the junction with Home Valley Road. Just 0.4 mile later, turn right on Girl Scout Camp Road, and in 0.3 mile come to the end of the pavement, where you'll find ample parking space at a rocky saddle. To reach the trailhead, walk 0.1 mile down the rough dirt road that runs downhill from the other side of the pass, and then look for the unsigned footpath going off to the right.

The path ascends steadily, but not terribly steeply, on a hillside covered with the usual Douglas-fir forests; salal, sword fern, and Oregon grape populate the understory. The ever-present Gorge breezes whistle through the tree tops, but they rarely bother the hiker, who is protected by the surrounding big trees. The path rounds a ridge and follows the ridgeline for 0.1 mile, before bearing off to the left and climbing another hillside. Three quick switchbacks take you higher still, and as you approach the summit,

you cross two rockslides with good views east to Augspurger and Dog mountains.

Just before the top of the mountain is a large sign explaining the Wind Mountain Vision Quest Site. Here you learn that Native Americans used this site for as many as 1000 years in a traditional, religious rite of passage for young men. The youngsters came here in solitude to fast and seek guidance from their animal gods. Some tribal members still come here for this purpose. To protect this important archaeological and cultural site, it is crucial that hikers not stray

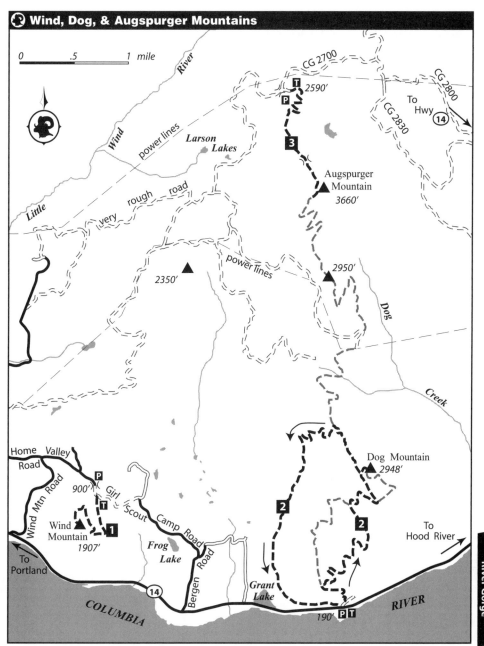

Wind, Dog, & Augspurger Mountains

0   .5   1 mile

Wind River

CG 2700

CG 2800

T 2590'

P

To Hwy

CG 2830

14

power lines

Larson Lakes

Little

Wind

3

very rough road

Augspurger Mountain
3660'

2350'

power lines

2950'

Dog

Creek

Home Valley Road

P

900'

T

Girl Scout Camp Road

Wind Mtn Road

Wind Mountain
1907'

1

Frog Lake

Bergen Road

Grant Lake

To Portland

14

COLUMBIA

Dog Mountain
2948'

2

2

To Hood River

190' P T

RIVER

even one foot from the trail so as not to disturb any of the rock pits built by Native Americans. Restrain your pets and children too.

The view from the top is partly obstructed by trees, but it is still excel-lent. The best views are to the west toward the town of Carson, Table Mountain, and distant Silver Star Mountain. To the south are the cliffs and peaks on the Oregon side of the Gorge, Mt. Defiance being the tallest of many high points.

TRIP 2 Dog Mountain Loop

see map on p.257

Distance	7.2 miles, Loop
Elevation Gain	2900 feet
Hiking Time	3 to 5 hours
Optional Map	Green Trails *Hood River*
Usually Open	Late February to December
Best Time	Mid- to late May
Trail Use	Dogs OK
Agency	Columbia River Gorge National Scenic Area
Difficulty	Difficult

HIGHLIGHTS The secret of Dog Mountain's charms got out generations ago because it was a secret that would be impossible to keep. The bulky mountain is prominently in view to tens of thousands of drivers zipping back and forth on Interstate 84 and Washington State Highway 14. For hikers, the huge, open meadows covering the mountain's upper slopes are an irresistible attraction because they hold a promise of both views and flowers. Once you actually hike the trail, that promise is spectacularly fulfilled with some of the Gorge's most stunning views and the best flower displays in the area covered by this book.

DIRECTIONS Cross the Columbia River on the Bridge of the Gods at Cascade Locks, and drive east on State Highway 14 for 12 miles to the huge lot for the Dog Mountain Trail on your left.

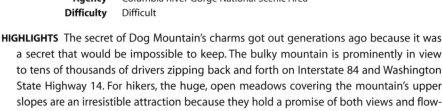

From the trailhead parking lot, you are faced with an immediate decision. Your choice of trails will be dictated primarily by which is stronger, your knees or your lungs. If your lungs and cardiovascular system are strong, then opt for the much steeper old trail that begins from the east side of the lot. If your lungs aren't up for this tiring ascent, but your knees are strong enough to handle the steep descent when you return on the old trail, then climb the longer, gentler, new trail that takes off from the west end of the lot. Photographers will want to select the steeper route to get to those famous meadows as quickly as possible because the best pictures are looking west down the Gorge in the early morning.

If the steeper old trail is your choice, you will begin on an abandoned road. After just 100 yards, leave the road on a foot trail that goes left. You'll have no real opportunity to celebrate this change to wilder country, however, because you immediately face a series of steep switchbacks. In the first 0.5 mile you gain almost 700 feet under a canopy of big old Douglas firs and Oregon white oaks. The most common lower-growing plant is poison oak; in the heat of late spring and summer, careful hikers are kept on their toes as poison oak teams up with rattlesnakes to create a dual hazard.

At a fork in the trail after 0.5 mile, the older, less scenic trail veers left. You'll want to turn right, a choice made easy in spring by the appeal of a sign saying TO THE FLOWERING INFERNO, which is both a charming name and an accurate description. This path is more gradual than what you've already endured, but there are still lots of switchbacks and few breaks in the relentless ascent. After about 1 mile, the trail leaves the trees in favor of an open, grassy viewpoint. Flowers here give a taste of what is to come, lupine, paintbrush, and balsamroot being the star attractions. The only disappointing thing about this view is how far you still must look up to see the higher meadows and viewpoints near the top of Dog Mountain.

Filled with the hope of great scenery and a determination not to give up, you trudge uphill away from this viewpoint, foregoing switchbacks in favor of a straightforward woodsy ascent. About 0.5 mile later, you go right at a junction with the old trail and continue climbing, now at a wickedly steep grade. Just 0.5 mile (and several rest stops) later, you are rewarded with the start of the summit meadows. Some of the most photogenic views and best flowers are near the lower edge of the meadows. Looking west down the Gorge is especially appealing, as distinctive Wind Mountain makes for an impressive landmark, with the large, yellow blossoms of arrowleaf balsamroot providing colorful foregrounds for photographs. While the uphill is not over yet, from now on the scenery is so good you will hardly notice the exertion. Something you probably will notice is that like most Gorge hikes, chilly winds often sweep across these meadows, so bring a windbreaker.

At an open ridge crest is a possibly unsigned junction with two trails that form a 1.1-mile loop around the summit of Dog Mountain. The easier, but much less scenic, route goes straight from this junction and loops mostly through forests. The shorter, steeper, more spectacular route goes left and crawls up the view-packed ridgeline.

A little before the more scenic route reaches the summit, the return trail of this hike veers off to the left. After absorbing all of the views up and down the Gorge that you can handle, turn onto this path and hike north, staying in the gorgeous sloping meadows for another 0.7 mile, before you reach a junction. To return to your car, turn left and make five long, downhill switchbacks in open forests and meadows. Views to the west aren't comparable to those from the top of Dog Mountain, but they are still very good. After the switchbacks end, you make a long, gradual descent across the woodsy western slopes of Dog Mountain. Occasional views through the trees allow you to see lots of wild country near Wind Mountain as well as a rural road, some homes, and a Girl Scout camp. Eventually, the trail curves slowly to the left (east) above Grant Lake and finishes its descent on a hillside above Highway 14.

View west from slopes of Dog Mountain

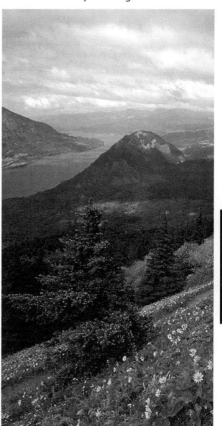

TRIP 3 Augspurger Mountain

Distance	3.6 miles, Out-and-back
Elevation Gain	1200 feet
Hiking Time	2½ hours
Optional Map	Green Trails *Willard*
Usually Open	March to November
Best Time	Mid- to late May
Trail Use	Dogs OK (but dangerous for them in places)
Agency	Columbia River Gorge National Scenic Area
Difficulty	Moderate

see map on p.257

HIGHLIGHTS Assuming that your car can reach the trailhead (or at least get reasonably close), the hike up Augspurger Mountain makes an excellent short outing in the eastern Columbia River Gorge. This hike was once a portion of the Pacific Crest Trail, but after that famous trail was rerouted in the 1970s the path up Augspurger Mountain fell off the radar screen of most hikers. Well, it's time to put it back on your "to do" list because this rocky viewpoint features some of the best views in our area.

DIRECTIONS Road access here is rough and complicated. Start by crossing the Bridge of the Gods at Cascade Locks, and then drive 14.5 miles east on State Highway 14 to a junction with Cook-Underwood Road. Turn left, following signs to Willard, and drive 3.7 miles to a junction where the road makes a 90-degree right turn. Turn left on Jessup Road, proceed 0.8 mile, and then turn left on Little Rock Creek Road. Go 1.1 miles to a gravel turnaround, and then bear left on a narrow gravel and dirt road with a sign saying End County Road. Stay on this rough and bumpy road (CG 2800) for 1.8 miles, and then turn right at a junction with CG 2830 under a set of power lines. Proceed 0.2 mile to a junction with CG 2700, turn left on this dirt route, and drive 1.1 miles to the unsigned trailhead at a pass. There is plenty of room to park in a flat area near a borrow pit. This location is also accessible from the west, but the roads are even rougher than those described here.

The start of the trail is obscured by a confusion of roads and gravel pits. You start by walking southeast (slightly uphill) on a rocky road with a small sign identifying it as Road 469. After 100 yards, this road narrows to a foot trail and begins a fairly steep climb. The switchbacking ascent initially goes through an open, wind-whipped forest of Douglas firs and Pacific silver firs, and then, at 0.2 mile, crosses a large talus slope, which provides the first good views north by northeast to snowy Mt. Adams.

Another short uphill stretch in the woods takes you to a ridgeline, where the views really open up. All three of south-ern Washington's major volcanic peaks (Mounts Adams, St. Helens, and Rainier) are visible and there are terrific vistas up and down the Columbia River. For even better views, keep climbing as the trail snakes up a narrow ridge. The route is rather exposed, so it can be a bit frightening if conditions are windy or icy. At 1.2 miles is a rocky high point, where the previous views are joined by a look south to pointed Mt. Hood towering above Oregon's Mt. Defiance. Below you to the southwest is Wind Mountain, which from this angle looks like only a minor bump rising above the Columbia River.

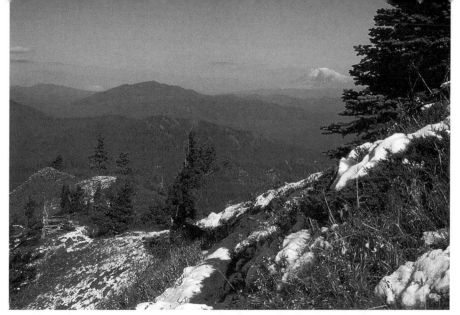

View of Mt. Adams from Augspurger Mountain

This is the trip's best viewpoint, so you might want to turn around here. To reach the actual summit of Augspurger Mountain, however, descend about 80 feet through forest and flower-sprinkled meadows to a woodsy saddle. The sometimes obscure trail then climbs 0.4 mile through forest to a ridgetop just below the summit of Augspurger Mountain. Views are blocked by trees here, but there is a nice open spot a little west of the summit, where the trail drops over the ridge. If you are feeling really ambitious, you can extend the hike south 4 miles to Dog Mountain.

TRIP 4 Grassy Knoll & Big Huckleberry Mountain

Distance	4.4 miles to Grassy Knoll, Out-and-back; 11 miles to Big Huckleberry Mountain, Out-and-back
Elevation Gain	950 feet to Grassy Knoll; 2400 feet to Big Huckleberry Mountain
Hiking Time	2 to 6 hours
Optional Map	Green Trails *Willard, Wind River*
Usually Open	Mid-May to November
Best Times	Late May to mid-June and mid-October
Trail Use	Good for kids, dogs OK, backpacking option
Agency	Mount Adams Ranger District, Gifford Pinchot National Forest
Difficulty	Moderate to Difficult

HIGHLIGHTS Aptly named Grassy Knoll is a bald-topped old lookout site that has everything a hiker could want in a destination—outstanding views, fine wildflower displays, a relatively short trail to the top, and surprisingly few people to share the scenery. The access road is long and bumpy, but the solitude and scenery make it worthwhile. If the hike doesn't provide enough exercise, you can extend the trip along an extremely scenic ridge crest to Big Huckleberry Mountain.

Grassy Knoll & Big Huckleberry Mountain

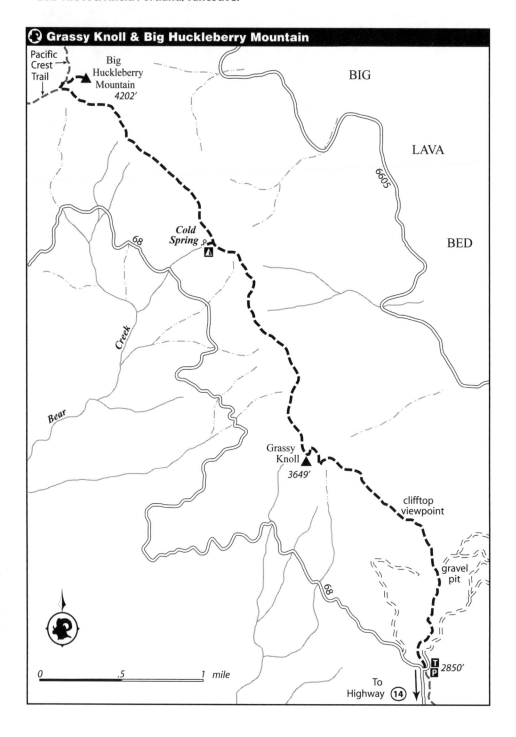

Pacific
Crest
Trail

Big
Huckleberry
Mountain
4202'

BIG

LAVA

6605

68

*Cold
Spring*

BED

Creek

Bear

Grassy
Knoll
3649'

clifftop
viewpoint

gravel
pit

68

0   .5   1 *mile*

2850'

To
Highway (14)

DIRECTIONS Drive Interstate 84 east to Cascade Locks, take Exit 44, and almost immediately veer right to loop around and cross the Columbia River on the Bridge of the Gods (a $1 toll applies, as of 2007). Turn right on State Highway 14, go 6.1 miles, and then turn left (north) on the signed road to Carson. After 0.9 mile you go straight at a junction in the middle of town, proceed 3.2 miles, and then turn right on Bear Creek Road. The pavement ends after 3.7 miles, and then it's 7.4 miles of good gravel to a junction. Turn left on Forest Road 68, and drive 2.1 miles on this pothole-plagued road to a junction. Turn right and almost immediately park in the signed trailhead lot on the right.

The trail starts by climbing through a small meadow alive with color in mid- to late May. Look for prairie star, larkspur, blue-eyed Mary, paintbrush, phlox, lomatium, serviceberry, and many more. After 130 yards you enter forest and begin an uneven but often steep ascent. Growing beneath a canopy of western hemlocks and Douglas firs, the ground cover here is a mix of the usual local shade-tolerant ferns and woodland wildflowers, including twisted stalk, wood violets, false Solomon's seal, star-flowered smilicina, vanilla leaf, and red-flowering currant. Most of the way is in dense forest, although you obtain some decent views to the south at 0.8 mile when you skirt the top of an abandoned gravel pit and at 1 mile when you pass the border of an old burn. At 1.2 miles you reach a dramatic clifftop viewpoint with excellent views of Mt. Adams to the northeast, the peaks of Indian Heaven to the north, and down to the remarkably flat and now forest-covered Big Lava Bed, whose name effectively answers your curiosity about this feature's geologic origins.

From the viewpoint the trail makes a minor descent for 0.3 mile, and then switchbacks twice up an open slope to the old lookout site atop Grassy Knoll at 2.2 miles. In late May the summit is home to a colorful display of seemingly-out-of-place daffodils. In any season there are terrific views of the Columbia River, Mt. Hood, Silver Star Mountain, Augspurger Mountain, Tanner Butte, and pretty much everything else within 25 or 30 miles.

Grassy Knoll makes a very satisfying destination for a relatively short hike, but if you are feeling ambitious there is plenty more excellent scenery awaiting your discovery to the north. Following a section of trail that once served as part of the Pacific Crest Trail, you wander through a mix of forest and rolling meadows that in late May and June are a bonanza of ground-hugging juniper and

Mt. Adams from Big Huckleberry Mountain

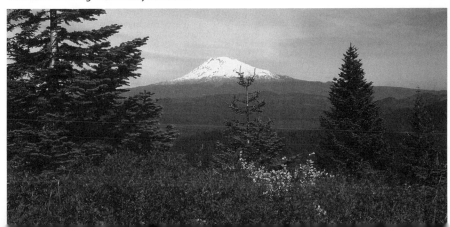

assorted wildflowers. Look especially for glacier lilies, beargrass, spring beauties, and mountain kittentails. The meadows end after about 1 mile (another good turnaround point), but if you still have energy to burn, keep going north, now mostly in forest. You pass a campsite near Cold Spring (down a short side trail to the west) at about 3.7 miles and then come to a junction with the Pacific Crest Trail at 5.3 miles. Turn right here, then right again a few yards later, and walk uphill 0.2 mile to the top of Big Huckleberry Mountain. As the name implies, huckleberries are abundant here, providing a tasty treat in late August and a colorful display of fall color in mid- to late October. Mt. Adams dominates the view to the northeast.

TRIP 5 Nestor Peak

Distance	7.8 miles, Out-and-back
Elevation Gain	2150 feet
Hiking Time	4 hours
Optional Map	USGS *Northwestern Lake*
Usually Open	Mid-April to November
Best Times	Mid-May to June and mid- to late October
Trail Use	Dogs OK, mountain biking, horseback riding
Agency	Washington Department of Natural Resources
Difficulty	Moderate

HIGHLIGHTS This enjoyable hike takes you to a former lookout site with a terrific view that extends from the rolling shrub-steppe of eastern Washington to the glacier-clad peaks of the High Cascades. Although the view would be worth the trip all by itself, the hike also features some unique botany, which adds interest during the long ascent.

DIRECTIONS Drive east on Interstate 84 to Hood River Exit 64, and cross the toll bridge into Washington. Turn left (west) on State Highway 14, drive 1.6 miles to a junction, and then turn right (north) on Highway 141 ALT. Proceed 2.2 miles, turn left on Highway 141, and go 1.9 miles to a junction with paved Northwestern Lake Road. Turn left, and then stay straight at all intersections until the road turns to gravel after 0.8 mile and becomes Road B 1000. Drive another 0.2 mile, turn left on Road N 1000, signed NESTOR PEAK ROAD, and proceed 1.5 sometimes rough miles to a fork. Bear right, go another 0.5 mile, and then turn right on the signed 0.1-mile dirt road to Buck Creek Trailhead #1.

The trail departs from the northwest side of Road N 1000 immediately opposite the turnoff for the trailhead access road. The path climbs, often fairly steeply, in a forest dominated by Douglas firs, but which includes an interesting variety of other species as well. Although this area is east of the Cascade Divide, the close proximity to the Columbia River keeps the elevation low and provides a corridor for westside species to make their way east. Thus, the vegetation here is an interesting mix of drier eastside forest and a much wetter westside environment. As a result this is one of the few places where you will see ponderosa pines, the dominate eastside tree, growing beside Pacific dogwoods, normally a hall-

Nestor Peak & Buck Creek Falls Loop

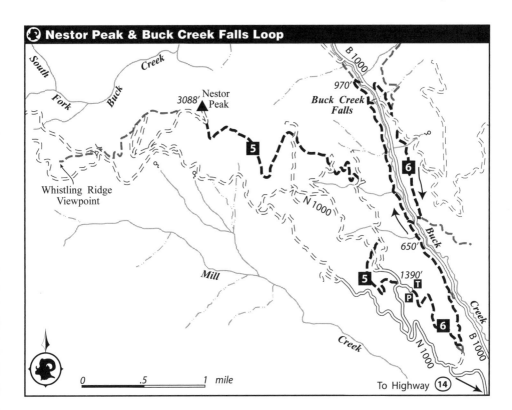

mark of the westside forests. And while there are plenty of rain-loving bigleaf maples around, the environment here is too dry to support the usual tangle of undergrowth that normally accompanies this tree. It is a fascinating area for hikers interested in botany.

After 0.3 mile of uphill, the trail levels out on a minor ridge and then makes a short rolling descent to a crossing of Road N 1000. You then go sharply downhill for 0.1 mile to a junction with a dirt road. Turn left and walk 0.6 mile along this nearly level road before veering left (uphill) onto a poorly marked trail just a few yards after a dead-end spur road branches off to the right. This trail makes six sometimes steep switchbacks, still in viewless forest, to another remote dirt road. Go right, following the road for about 50 yards, and then bear left (uphill) at the resumption of trail.

The uphill immediately resumes as you ascend past a couple of partially logged areas to a crossing of a final logging road at 2.7 miles. The trail now curves to the left, still going steadily upward, although not as steeply. The route finally levels off a bit and then goes northwest as it rolls along near the top of a spur ridge. Here the views begin, intermittent at first, but still excellent, especially to the south of Oregon's Hood River Valley, Mt. Defiance, and Mt. Hood. The open areas that provide these views are also habitat for sun-loving wildflowers. Look for lupine, larkspur, lomatium, prairie star, ballhead waterleaf, wild strawberry, and blue-eyed Mary.

Following another switchback and a brief uphill spur, the trail ends at a rocky jeep road. Straight ahead to the north is the mostly open summit of Nestor Peak, topped with a small metal structure, whose purpose is not apparent. To reach the top, simply climb the jeep road 0.1 mile to the obvious destination. The views are superb, including a terrific look to the north at snowy Mt. Adams added to the previously described vistas to the south. To the east stretch the seemingly endless grasslands and shrub-steppe plains of eastern Washington.

Ambitious hikers who want more views can extend this hike with a visit to Whistling Ridge Viewpoint. To reach it, return 0.1 mile down the jeep road to the trail junction, and then turn right, following the road for 0.25 mile before turning right onto a trail. This path follows a scenic ridgetop for 0.7 mile, passing the ends of two logging roads along the way, and then descends to a saddle. Here you cross another road and follow a dead-end trail to the viewpoint. The views are not as comprehensive as those from Nestor Peak, but they are better to the west of such Gorge landmarks as Dog Mountain.

TRIP 6 Buck Creek Falls Loop

Distance	6.1 miles, Semiloop
Elevation Gain	1350 feet
Hiking Time	3 hours
Optional Map	USGS *Northwestern Lake*
Usually Open	Mid-March to November
Best Time	April to June
Trail Use	Dogs OK, mountain biking, horseback riding
Agency	Washington Department of Natural Resources
Difficulty	Moderate
Note	Good in cloudy weather

HIGHLIGHTS Other than sharing the same trailhead, the hike up Nestor Peak (Trip 5) and this trail to Buck Creek Falls have almost nothing in common. While Nestor Peak affords views that extend for many miles, visitors on the heavily forested Buck Creek Falls Loop will rarely be able to see farther than a few yards. Hikers going to Nestor Peak must climb from the trailhead to their destination, but those who choose to visit Buck Creek start with a descent and won't face any significant uphill until the way back. Finally, while the dominant geography along the Nestor Peak Trail is high ridges, here you spend almost all of your time in a deep canyon. Both trips are highly rewarding and well worth the time. Which one you choose depends on your preferences and mood.

DIRECTIONS Drive east on Interstate 84 to Hood River Exit 64, and cross the toll bridge into Washington. Turn left (west) on State Highway 14, drive 1.6 miles to a junction, and then turn right (north) on Highway 141 ALT. Proceed 2.2 miles, turn left on Highway 141, and go 1.9 miles to a junction with paved Northwestern Lake Road. Turn left, and then stay straight at all intersections until the road turns to gravel after 0.8 mile and becomes Road B 1000. Drive another 0.2 mile, and then turn left on Road N 1000, signed NESTOR PEAK ROAD, and proceed 1.5 sometimes rough miles to a fork. Bear right, go another 0.5 mile, and then turn right on the signed 0.1-mile dirt road to Buck Creek Trailhead #1.

The well-maintained trail starts from the southeast end of the parking loop and descends through a relatively open Douglas-fir forest. With its location east of the Cascade Divide, the forest here is somewhat drier than those to the west, so undergrowth is limited to a few scattered vanilla leaf and Oregon grape. The moderately graded trail, which is marked with white diamonds on trees, descends two switchbacks and then makes a winding traverse to reach a junction at about 0.8 mile. Go left (downhill), and then turn sharply left at another junction just 50 yards later.

The downhill is much less noticeable now as the trail crosses a heavily forested hillside above Buck Creek, which you can hear but not see in the canyon on the right. Gravel Road B 1000 parallels the creek, but it remains unobtrusive and is often gated closed to traffic, so you need not worry about dust or noise from the road. At 1.3 miles is a junction. Go left and gradually ascend in a lush and exceptionally attractive lower-elevation forest that has both grand firs and western red cedars mixed in with the usual Douglas firs. The up-and-down trail stays between 50 and 100 feet above both the creek and Road B 1000 all the way to a junction at 1.8 miles.

The return trail of the recommended loop goes sharply right and downhill. For now, though, go straight and continue traveling up and down, with somewhat more of the former than the latter. With the road now on the other side of Buck Creek, the trail has no obstacles and often closely approaches that stream's beautifully cascading waters. The most noteworthy of these times comes at about 2.8 miles where a small, unsigned footpath goes a few yards to a creekside rock outcropping next to roaring Buck Creek Falls. Although only about 15 feet

tall, this waterfall boasts an exceptionally attractive setting in an open area of moss-covered basalt. It is almost impossible to avoid the temptation to stop for lunch (or at least an extended rest) below this photogenic falls.

The main trail continues upstream from the falls another 0.2 mile to a junction. Turn sharply right, and soon cross the creek on a metal bridge. On the other side you meet the end of a short spur road off Road B 1000. To complete the loop, walk 100 yards down Road B 1000, and then turn sharply left (uphill) onto a signed trail. After making one quick switchback, this trail goes up and down on a hillside for 0.3 mile to a junction. Go straight and soon connect with a primitive dirt road. Follow this road uphill for 0.1 mile, and then veer right back onto a trail.

The trail contours for a while and then descends a partially forested hillside with

Buck Creek Falls

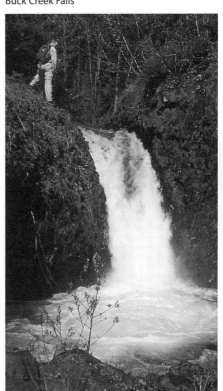

some nice views of the wooded ridge to the west. At 4.2 miles you turn sharply right at a junction and then make two, short, downhill switchbacks to Road B 1000. Cross Buck Creek on the road bridge, and then almost immediately turn right onto a signed trail. This path ascends 80 yards back to the junction at the start of the loop. Turn left and return the way you came.

TRIP 7 Weldon Wagon Road

Distance	4.9 miles, Out-and-back
Elevation Gain	1200 feet
Hiking Time	2 to 3 hours
Optional Map	USGS *Husum* (trail not shown)
Usually Open	All year (except during winter storms)
Best Time	Mid-April to early May
Trail Use	Dogs OK, mountain biking
Agency	Klickitat County Parks
Difficulty	Moderate

HIGHLIGHTS During the White Salmon Valley's "apple boom" in the early 20th century, farmers felt the need for a better transportation route to ship their fruit to distant markets. So in 1911 a pair of local entrepreneurs built a wagon road to connect the valley with the Upper Snowden Road. Apples are still grown in the area, but modern roads long ago put this wagon route out of business. Fortunately, Klickitat County has preserved the trail and keeps it open for hikers and mountain bikers to explore. This is terrific news because, in addition to its historic interest, the trail is a beautiful path featuring open oak-dotted slopes that provide excellent wildflower displays in late April and outstanding views in any season. As usual in the eastern Gorge, keep an eye out for rattlesnakes, ticks, and poison oak, and avoid this hike on hot summer days.

DIRECTIONS Drive east on Interstate 84 to Hood River Exit 64, and cross the toll bridge into Washington. Turn left (west) on State Highway 14, drive 1.6 miles to a junction, and then turn right (north) on Highway 141 ALT. Proceed 2.2 miles, turn left on Highway 141, and go 4.0 miles to an indistinct junction in the tiny town of Husum immediately before a bridge over Rattlesnake Creek. Turn right (east) on gravel Indian Creek Road, and drive 0.6 mile, passing several driveways along the way, to a major fork. Bear left on Indian Cemetery Road, and go 0.3 mile to a junction with a rough jeep road marked with a sign for the WELDON WAGON TRAIL. There is room to park about 4 cars immediately opposite from where the jeep road departs.

Walk about 0.15 mile up the jeep road to the signed trailhead, where you veer right onto a wide foot trail that is part of the old wagon road. The well-graded path climbs at a moderate grade through an open forest of Douglas firs, Oregon white oaks, vine maples, and a few Ponderosa pines. In late April look for blooming Pacific dogwood trees (white blossoms), Oregon grape (yellow blossoms on a low scrub), and blue buttons (small blue flowers on a plant with wide, arrow-shaped leaves). After 0.2 mile the trail leaves the forest and enters a scenic

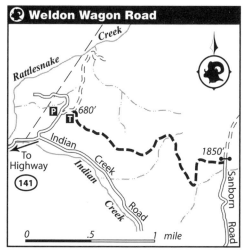

but the public-access trail is only a narrow easement that crosses private land.

As you gain elevation showier wildflowers such as balsamroot, lupine, lomatium, and ballhead waterleaf become more common and the snow-covered summits of Mt. Defiance and Mt. Hood in Oregon become visible over a ridge to the south. At 1.5 miles a sign marks where you enter the White Salmon Oak Natural Resources Conservation Area, which was established in 1993. At 1.9 miles the trail enters a thick forest of Douglas firs and oaks just before it makes a switchback to the left. Soon thereafter you pass below a private residence, loop to the right, and come to a bearing tree boasting several survey markers. From here, the trail goes another 0.1 mile east along the edge of an area replanted with young trees to an isolated trailhead on Sanborn Road. As this trailhead is difficult to reach by car, it is better to make this an out-and back hike and return the way you came.

open hillside sprinkled with picturesque Oregon white oaks. Views here of the White Salmon River Valley are excellent, and they will only improve in the miles to come. Spring wildflowers include prairie star and buttercup. *Despite the temptation to wander the meadows, please stay on the trail.* Not only is poison oak everywhere,

TRIP 8 Coyote Wall Loop

Distance	5.8 miles, Loop
Elevation Gain	1700 feet
Hiking Time	3 hours
Optional Map	USGS *White Salmon* (trail not shown)
Usually Open	All year
Best Times	Mid-March to early May and late October (avoid midsummer's withering heat)
Trail Use	Dogs OK, mountain biking
Agency	Columbia River Gorge National Scenic Area
Difficulty	Difficult

Eastern Columbia River Gorge

HIGHLIGHTS This wildly scenic hike explores a prominent but generally overlooked landmark in the eastern Columbia River Gorge. Coyote Wall is a long cliff that towers above a gently sloping landscape of open forests and wind-whipped grasslands. A little-known loop trail explores all of these landscapes and is one of the most scenic hikes in the Portland/Vancouver area. The unofficial trails here were built and are maintained by volunteers (mostly local mountain bikers), so the routes are unsigned and are not shown on any official map. Still, they are easy to follow and extremely scenic, especially the route along the top of Coyote Wall's dramatic cliffs.

⟳ Coyote Wall Loop

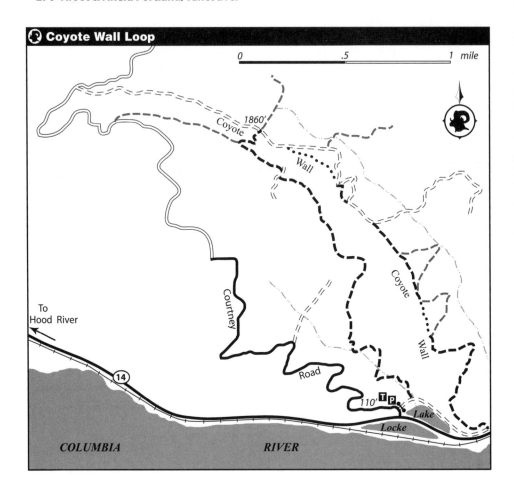

DIRECTIONS Take Exit 64 off Interstate 84 at Hood River, turn left (north), and cross the toll bridge over the Columbia River. Turn right (east) on State Highway 14, and drive 4.7 miles to a junction with Courtney Road. Turn left and almost immediately park where a gated road goes to the right.

Walk around the gate and go 75 yards to a junction at a wooden livestock loading ramp. This is the start of your loop. A clockwise loop is easier to follow, so veer left onto an unsigned but well-worn trail that goes through a gap in a fence. A small brown sign informs visitors that they are entering an area with a mix of public and private property and stresses the importance of good trail etiquette and staying on the trail.

The trail, which is heavily used by mountain bikers, gradually winds uphill over the material of an ancient landslide, which is now covered with grasses, small shrubs (including lots of poison oak), and a woodland of Oregon white oaks and ponderosa pines. From mid-March through April wildflowers such as prairie stars, grass widows, glacier lilies, and western buttercups bring color to the surroundings. The ascending trail crosses an often-dry creek several times as it gradually takes you into a relatively dense forest that includes some Douglas firs. Wildlife, especially birds, is abundant. Look for Steller's jays, pileated woodpeckers, and a wide variety of songbirds. As you climb, occasional openings in the forest provide increasingly good views of Mt. Hood to the southwest.

At about 1.2 miles the trail comes close to the base of Coyote Wall, the line of cliffs that rise to the east, turns left, and then goes under a telephone line at 1.5 miles. This is followed by some irregular uphill that leads to a junction with a faint and long-abandoned skid road. Turn right, briefly following the road, then veer left onto a bike trail, and resume your circuitous climb.

At about 2.2 miles a tiny cairn marks an unsigned and easy-to-miss junction. The more heavily traveled mountain biking trail goes left. You turn sharply right on a faint and rugged foot trail, which soon passes the base of a boulder-strewn slope beneath Coyote Wall. From here the trail follows the undulating top of a small rocky ridge and then makes a short, but very steep climb through a gap in the cliffs to the east.

At the top of the gap is an unsigned but obvious junction with an abandoned road that now serves as a mountain bike trail. You turn right and begin a joyous downhill walk along the grassy top of Coyote Wall's stupendous cliffs. The views are

outstanding, although that word seems woefully inadequate. No single view or direction is better than the rest. Just keep looking around at Mt. Hood, Mt. Defiance, the orchards near Mosier, or the Columbia River, depending on which way you happen to be facing. And don't forget to look back from time to time for impressive views of Coyote Wall's dramatic cliffs. Birders should keep an eye out for prairie falcons, turkey vultures, common ravens, red-tailed hawks, and violet-green swallows, all of which catch the rising thermals and nest on ledges below the trail. Several unofficial trails explore the sloping, grassy tableland to the east, but the best course remains near the top of the cliffs following a winding downhill route that passes numerous great viewpoints, any one of which would make a terrific lunch spot.

At about 3.4 miles you pass under a telephone line and then go through an opening in a fence line. The mountain biking trail makes several long switchbacks as it descends, but hikers often ignore these twists and turns and simply follow the dramatic cliff edge. Eventually, small drop-offs force you to take the last couple of switchbacks, which lead past more unsigned junctions (just ignore them) to the trail's end at an old road. Turn right and follow this road 0.7 mile, passing shallow Locke Lake along the way, back to your car.

Mt. Hood from Coyote Wall Trail

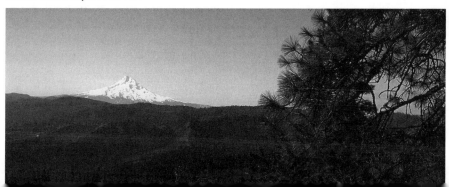

TRIP 9 Catherine Creek West & Rowland Loop

Distance	4.1 miles, Loop
Elevation Gain	1150 feet
Hiking Time	2 to 2½ hours
Optional Map	USGS *Lyle, White Salmon* (trails not shown)
Usually Open	All year
Best Times	April and early May
Trail Use	Dogs OK
Agency	Columbia River Gorge National Scenic Area
Difficulty	Difficult

HIGHLIGHTS Located in the sun-drenched eastern Columbia River Gorge, Catherine Creek is a terrific escape for water-logged westside residents looking for spring hiking opportunities away from the clouds. But this little paradise has more to offer than just its welcoming sunshine. The generally unsigned and unofficial trails here feature excellent scenery, with lovely, oak-dotted grasslands, fabulous views, and impressive basalt ridges. The area is also famous for its wildflowers. Botanists flock here in April and May to see a wide assortment of beautiful and unusual flowers not found in the wetter climates to the west. As with all hikes in the eastern Gorge, beware of poison oak, a few rattlesnakes, ticks in the spring and early summer, and withering heat in midsummer.

DIRECTIONS Take Exit 64 off Interstate 84 at Hood River, turn north, and cross the toll bridge over the Columbia River ($.75 per vehicle as of 2007). Turn east (right) on State Highway 14 and drive 5.9 miles to a junction with Old Highway 8. Turn left, proceed 1.5 miles, and then park in a large gravel lot on the north side of the road.

Two trails start from the north side of the large gate at the trailhead. For this trip go left (northwest) on a trail marked by a small brown post that says simply 015, and travel over a lovely rolling tableland covered with grasses, wildflowers, and scattered ponderosa pines. The way goes gradually uphill on an old rocky roadbed, which soon narrows to a foot trail. The next 0.5 mile goes up and down through a gorgeous mix of pine-oak woodlands, ephemeral ponds, grasslands, and acres of spring wildflowers. Some common species include larkspur, camas, prairie star, western buttercup, blue-eyed Mary, shooting star, and white-blooming serviceberry bushes. April and early May are usually the peak blooming times. Distant views of the top half of Mt. Hood provide an icing on the cake of this lovely landscape.

The rolling terrain ends when you reach the top of Rowland Ridge, where there are excellent views down to Rowland Lake to the west. The main trail goes straight here, crosses over the ridge, and heads for Coyote Wall (see Trip 8). For this trip, however, turn right on an unmarked but obvious footpath that climbs moderately steeply along the top of the short but impressive cliffs of Rowland Ridge. The trail provides excellent views but also has increasing amounts of poison oak, so watch your step. After 0.3 mile another trail forks to the left, but you stay right and continue climbing past dramatic clifftop viewpoints, through gently rolling grasslands, and over occasional rocky areas, all liberally sprinkled with spring

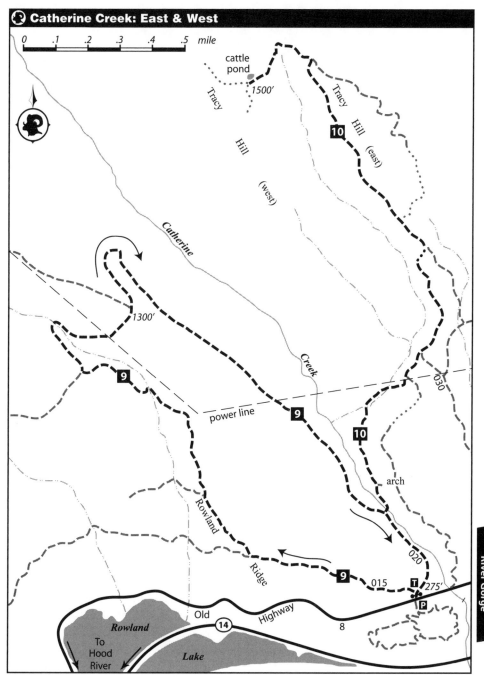

Catherine Creek: East & West

0   .1   .2   .3   .4   .5   mile

cattle pond

1500'

Tracy Hill (west)

Tracy Hill (east)

10

Catherine

Creek

1300'

9

030

power line

9

10

arch

020

Rowland Ridge

9

015

T 275'

P

8

Old Highway

14

Rowland Lake

To Hood River

wildflowers. Shortly after coming close to a power line on your right, the trail dips left, crosses an oak-filled gully, and then steeply climbs a little ridge to a junction with an abandoned jeep road (now just a wide, well-graded trail).

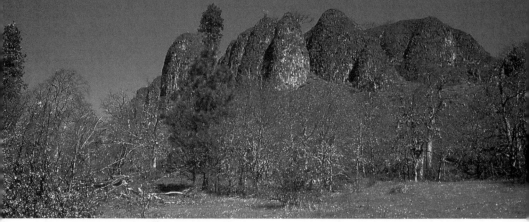

Rock formation above Catherine Creek Trail

Turn right on the trail, which recrosses the woodsy gully and soon reaches a huge sloping grassland. You cross beneath the power lines here and then walk 0.2 mile to a junction at the east side of the grassy slope. The trail to the left goes through the upper part of the grassland and then follows the power lines into a dense forest. The recommended loop continues straight on the abandoned road and soon begins going gradually downhill across a partly forested hillside. The route curves to the right (southeast) and makes a long, steady, moderately graded descent first in a Douglas-fir forest and then through a more open woodland of Oregon white oaks. The downhill ends at a junction beside lovely Catherine Creek. Go straight on a gravel path, which returns to the trailhead in 0.3 mile.

TRIP 10 Catherine Creek East & Tracy Hill

Distance	4.7 miles, Out-and-back
Elevation Gain	1300 feet
Hiking Time	2 to 3 hours
Optional Map	USGS *Lyle* (trails not shown)
Usually Open	All year
Best Times	April and May
Trail Use	Dogs OK
Agency	Columbia River Gorge National Scenic Area
Difficulty	Difficult

see map on p.273

HIGHLIGHTS Like most hikes in the eastern Columbia River Gorge, this trip explores open, view-packed hillsides carpeted with spring wildflowers. You really shouldn't need any further enticement than that to put this outing on your "to do" list, but if that doesn't do the trick, consider that this hike also allows you to get a nice look at the rock arch above Catherine Creek, to walk past some scenic basalt cliffs, and to finish your trip at a high grassy viewpoint that is an ideal lunch spot.

DIRECTIONS Take Exit 64 off Interstate 84 at Hood River, turn north, and cross the toll bridge over the Columbia River (\$.75 per vehicle as of 2007). Turn east (right) on State Highway 14, and drive 5.9 miles to a junction with Old Highway 8. Turn left, proceed 1.5 miles, and then park in an unmarked gravel lot on the north side of the road.

Two trails start from the north side of the large gate at the trailhead. For this hike go right (northeast) on a wide gravel path, signed "020," which starts on a grassy, wildflower-covered tableland but soon drops into the basalt-lined canyon of Catherine Creek. At 0.3 mile is a junction. You veer right and almost immediately cross the creek on a plank bridge. From here you walk 250 yards up an old road/trail to the broken-down remains of a wooden corral and barn. On the basalt cliff just east of the corral is a large rock arch. Since it is hard to see this arch from the trail, look for an unmarked route to the right that climbs about 50 feet to a better viewpoint.

Past the old corral the main trail goes moderately steeply uphill and soon takes you near a power line, which your trail parallels through a wide break in the rimrock. Just after you cross under the power line, an obvious trail angles to the right.

Keep left on the main trail/road, which gradually ascends another 150 yards to a junction with another old road. Route 030 goes sharply right, but for the most direct course to Tracy Hill you should go straight. The old road soon narrows to become an increasingly faint foot trail

that takes you up a minor ridge to the edge of a huge grass-covered slope. The trail peters out here, but if you walk northeast about 80 yards you will intersect an obvious trail. Turn left and steadily ascend the huge rolling grassland that forms the eastern flank of Tracy Hill. To the west you can see across an oak-filled ravine to another grassy slope (the western flank of Tracy Hill) while to the east is the deep but unseen canyon of Major Creek.

The views as you climb are tremendous with the star attraction being a long section of the Columbia River bookended by the high ridge of the Columbia Hills to the east and the snowy, horn-shaped pinnacle of Mt. Hood to the west. The long ascent ends at the top of the grassland where you intersect a faint trail in a lovely woodland of Oregon white oak. Turn left, go around the head of a gully, and then climb through the oak woodland for 0.1 mile to reach the grassy western flank of Tracy Hill. The trail soon peters out near a shallow old cattle pond, but you can explore the open terrain to your heart's content. If you aren't up for exploring, simply sit back in the grass, soak in the sun, and enjoy the view. Once you've had your fill, return the way you came.

Pond on Tracy Hill

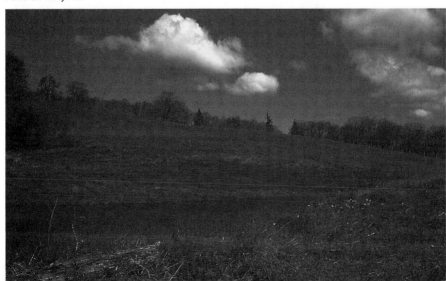

TRIP 11 Catherine Creek: Arch & Lower Loops

Distance	2.9 miles (combined), Loop
Elevation Gain	550 feet
Hiking Time	2 to 2½ hours
Optional Map	USGS _Lyle_ (trails not shown)
Usually Open	All year
Best Times	April and May
Trail Use	Good for kids, dogs OK, partly wheelchair accessible
Agency	Columbia River Gorge National Scenic Area
Difficulty	Moderate

HIGHLIGHTS If the two longer recommended hikes in the Catherine Creek vicinity (Trips 9 and 10) are more than you have the time or energy to tackle, then consider the two easier loops described here. Except for high viewpoints, these trails include everything that the longer hikes have to offer and, for extra credit, they throw in a small waterfall and (for the daring) a chance to walk on top of a rock arch. With excellent scenery, relatively easy trails, and acres of wildflowers, it's not surprising that these trails are popular. On spring weekends the parking lot fills rapidly. Try to visit early in the day or on a weekday.

DIRECTIONS Take Exit 64 off Interstate 84 at Hood River, turn north, and cross the toll bridge over the Columbia River ($.75 per vehicle as of 2007). Turn east (right) on State Highway 14, and drive 5.9 miles to a junction with Old Highway 8. Turn left, proceed 1.5 miles, and then park in an unmarked gravel lot on the north side of the road.

Two equally attractive and worthwhile loop trips are possible. The easier option is a paved, wheelchair-accessible, figure-eight nature trail that starts from the south side of the road and travels a few dozen yards to a junction at the start of the loop. Either direction is equally attractive, but most hikers turn left (clockwise) and wind around on a beautiful flower-spangled tableland for 0.2 mile to a viewing area above Catherine Creek's rocky gorge. Below you to the northeast is small but lovely Catherine Creek Falls. Scramble routes lead down to the falls, but to protect the sensitive vegetation, hikers are discouraged from going beyond the overlook.

The paved loop trail continues south and west from the overlook winding gradually downhill past ephemeral ponds, twisted oak trees, scattered serviceberry and other bushes, and countless types of wildflowers. Signs identify some of the more common and unusual species, but you will be sorry if you forgot to bring a good wildflower guide. At 0.4 mile is a junction with a shortcut return trail. For the longer loop, go straight, still on a paved trail, and pass some nice viewpoints looking south over the Columbia River. Eventually the trail loops back to the east, goes left at a second junction with the shortcut trail, and makes a couple of gentle switchbacks back to the close of the loop and your car.

For the longer and more rugged northern loop, go through the gate on the north side of the road and head right (northeast) on a wide gravel path signed "020." This trail goes across a grassy, wildflower-covered tableland and then drops into the basalt-lined canyon of Catherine Creek to a junction at 0.3 mile. You veer right, almost immediately cross the creek

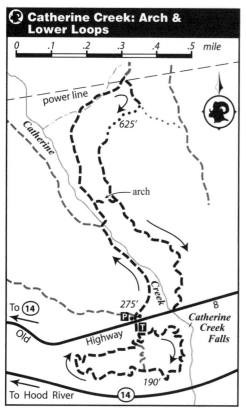

Catherine Creek: Arch & Lower Loops

0   .1   .2   .3   .4   .5 mile

power line

Catherine

625'

arch

Creek

To (14)

275'

8

Catherine
Creek
Falls

Old

Highway

P

T

190'

To Hood River   (14)

Past the old corral the trail goes more steeply uphill and then curves to the right, paralleling a power line through a wide break in the rimrock. Just after you cross under the power line you turn right on an unsigned but obvious trail. This path climbs to an open oak-dotted tableland and then branches off in a confusion of sketchy use paths. Head southwest over a low hill, and you will soon pick up a more recognizable trail.

Once found, the trail goes downhill, always staying close to the top of the rim on the east side of Catherine Creek's canyon. There are nice views into the canyon and south to the Columbia River and its surrounding ridges. About 0.4 mile from the junction near the power lines, a small side path leads to the top of Catherine Creek's arch. From above it is difficult to pick out the arch from among the other ledges and pinnacles along this basalt cliff, so you have to look carefully. Those afraid of heights should probably skip the steep and narrow side trail that travels along the top of the arch, but it makes for a fun diversion for more daring hikers. To close the loop, continue winding downhill for 0.5 mile to a junction with the road just east of where it crosses Catherine Creek. It is an easy 0.1-mile walk along the road shoulder back to the trailhead.

on a plank bridge, and then walk 250 yards up an old road/trail to the broken-down remains of a wooden corral and barn. On the basalt cliff-face just east of the corral is the large rock arch you will visit later in the trip.

Rock arch above Catherine Creek

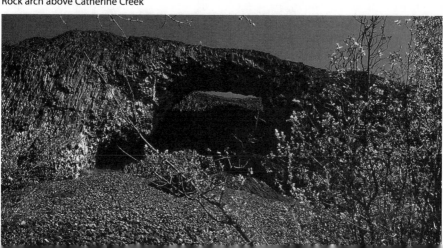

TRIP 12 Herman Creek Pinnacles

Distance	6.0 miles, Out-and-back
Elevation Gain	950 feet
Hiking Time	3 hours
Optional Map	Green Trails *Bonneville Dam*
Usually Open	All year (except during winter storms)
Best Time	Mid-March to June
Trail Use	Dogs OK, horseback riding
Agency	Columbia River Gorge National Scenic Area
Difficulty	Moderate
Note	Good in cloudy weather

HIGHLIGHTS This is the easiest of several possible destinations radiating from the Herman Creek Trailhead. Happily, it may also be the most interesting option, combining rich greenery with visits to lovely Herman Creek, a wispy waterfall, and a pair of fascinating rock spires. Add the good possibility of solitude, and this hike qualifies as one of the author's favorites.

DIRECTIONS Leave Interstate 84 at Cascade Locks Exit 44, and drive the main road (Wa Na Pa Street) through town. At the east end of town turn left on Forest Lane, following signs for the airport. Drive this road 2.0 miles to an overpass over the freeway. Turn left after the overpass, and, 0.3 mile later, turn right at a sign for Herman Creek Campground. This narrow paved road climbs a short distance to a junction with the marked spur road to the trailhead on the right.

The path starts out in a shady forest of stately Douglas fir and bigleaf maple, whose limbs and trunks sprout the usual growth of moss and licorice fern. The lazy route switchbacks uphill to cross a power line access road, curves into the canyon of Herman Creek, and makes two more switchbacks, before coming to a trail fork. The main Herman Creek Trail goes left, but you bear right for this trip and make a pleasant descent on a semi-open hillside to a metal bridge spanning Herman Creek.

From the rushing creek, the path climbs a hillside with a nice mix of forest and talus slopes, where you may hear or see pikas. This charming species, which looks like a diminutive small-eared rabbit, normally prefers the rocky slopes of the high mountains, but it also finds surprisingly good habitat at low elevations throughout the Columbia River Gorge.

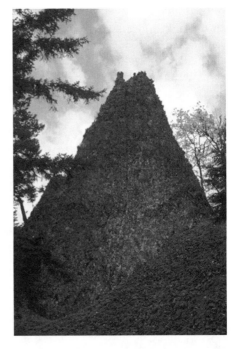
Pinnacle on Pacific Crest Trail near Herman Creek

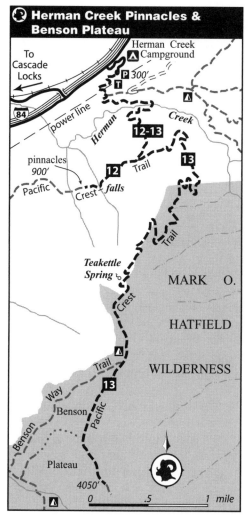

About 0.9 mile from Herman Creek, you meet the Pacific Crest Trail and bear right on this famous path, which goes initially through woods and then across two large rocky areas. You splash through a small creek at the base of a wispy waterfall and, about 250 yards later, come to a pair of crumbly rock spires on your right.

A short side trail takes you to the base of these free-standing landmarks, but photographers will be frustrated by the pinnacles because they are difficult to capture on film. One reason is that, for most of the year, their location beneath the north-facing cliffs of the Gorge ensures that they receive virtually no sunshine. Those who want some additional exercise can continue hiking west on the PCT for about 1.3 miles to Dry Creek and then make the short side trip upstream to spectacular Dry Creek Falls.

TRIP 13 Benson Plateau via the Pacific Crest Trail

see map on p.279

Distance	14.0 miles, Out-and-back
Elevation Gain	4000 feet
Hiking Time	7 to 9 hours
Optional Map	Green Trails *Bonneville Dam*
Usually Open	May to October
Best Time	June
Trail Use	Dogs OK, backpacking option, horseback riding
Agency	Columbia River Gorge National Scenic Area
Difficulty	Strenuous

HIGHLIGHTS No matter how you get there, Benson Plateau is a worthwhile goal. The flowers, especially beargrass, are abundant, the views are superb, and there are nice camps for backpackers to make this an overnight adventure. Unfortunately, there is no easy route to the top. Among the many difficult routes to choose from, the well-graded Pacific Crest Trail is probably the least demanding. It is also the least scenic, however, so you have to make a choice between exhaustion and exhilaration.

DIRECTIONS Leave Interstate 84 at Cascade Locks Exit 44, and drive the main road (Wa Na Pa Street) through town. At the east end of town turn left on Forest Lane, following signs for the airport. Drive this road 2.0 miles to an overpass over the freeway. Turn left after the overpass, and, 0.3 mile later, turn right at a sign for Herman Creek Campground. This narrow paved road climbs a short distance to a junction with the marked spur road to the trailhead on the right.

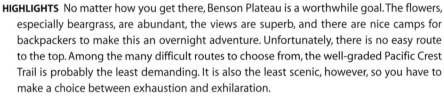

The path starts in a shady forest of stately Douglas fir and bigleaf maple, whose limbs and trunks sprout the usual growth of moss and licorice fern. The lazy route switchbacks uphill to cross a power line access road, curves into the canyon of Herman Creek, and makes two more switchbacks, before coming to a trail fork. The main Herman Creek Trail goes left, but you bear right for this trip and make a pleasant descent of a semi-open hillside, to a metal bridge spanning Herman Creek. Once across the bridge, the path climbs a hillside with a nice mix of forest and talus slopes for 0.9 mile to a junction with the Pacific Crest Trail (PCT).

Turn left and travel southbound on the PCT as it gently traverses a scree slope where pikas scurry about and squeak at passing hikers. Then you enter forests of Douglas fir and western hemlock, which will block the view almost all the way to

the top of Benson Plateau. Between here and there, however, are dozens of irregularly spaced switchbacks and traverses that take you back and forth across a ridgeline, on a steady, moderate, uphill grade. Although never especially steep, it is still an awfully long way up, so take plenty of rest stops as you climb. There is no water available, so carry an extra quart or two, especially on hot days.

About 3 miles up the ridge, you reach a decent viewpoint at a small helicopter landing spot, where you can rest and enjoy views of Herman Creek Canyon, Nick Eaton Ridge, and the area around Cascade Locks. It is also near this point that the vegetation changes, from low-elevation Douglas fir and western hemlock, to high-elevation Pacific silver and noble fir and western white pine. You will also see plenty of beargrass, always a good sign in the Gorge that you are nearing the top of your climb. In June of favorable years, the 3-foot-tall stalks of beargrass, with its clustered white flowers, put on a terrific show. After two more long switchbacks, look for a short, usually unsigned, side path to Teakettle Spring on your right. This little seepage is your only source of water after Herman Creek.

Several more switchbacks take you up to the edge of Benson Plateau, where the climb becomes much easier, and the scenery improves. You walk past a waterless camp and along a wide forested crest that extends northeast from the main Benson Plateau, to reach a junction with the Benson Way Trail. For the best views, stay left on the PCT as it travels along the eastern edge of the plateau, past several small meadows carpeted with wildflowers. Here, you will have outstanding views of the rugged Columbia River Gorge and distant Mt. Hood.

About 1.2 miles past the Benson Way junction is a junction with the Ruckel Creek Trail. The best view in the area is 100 yards straight ahead on the PCT. From this grandstand, you can look southeast to Woolly Horn Ridge, bald-topped Tomlike Mountain, pointed Chinidere Mountain, and distant Mt. Hood. Backpackers should know that the best camp on the plateau is about 0.3 mile west on the Ruckel Creek Trail, although it is popular with equestrians, so you may be sharing the camp with horses.

In the wildly contorted, up-and-down landscape of the Columbia River Gorge, the flatness of Benson Plateau is something of an oddity. This surface is the top layer of the ancient lava flows that buried the entire area between 10 and 17 million years ago. Since then, the Columbia River and its many tributaries have eroded the hard basalt rock by almost 4000 feet. So this flat remnant gives you some perspective both on the extent of the original lava flows and on the almost unbelievable amount of erosion that has diminished them over time.

TRIP 14 Herman Creek Trail

Distance	4.8 to 15.0 miles, Out-and-back
Elevation Gain	900 to 2700 feet
Hiking Time	2 to 8 hours
Optional Map	Green Trails *Bonneville Dam*
Usually Open	March to November
Best Time	Late March to June
Trail Use	Dogs OK, backpacking option, horseback riding
Agency	Columbia River Gorge National Scenic Area
Difficulty	Moderate to Difficult
Note	Good in cloudy weather

HIGHLIGHTS Herman Creek is one of the major streams of the Columbia River Gorge, and the trail up its canyon is an important artery for longer trips into the backcountry. However, the trail is also fine for shorter outings to more modest destinations. Unlike the trail up better-known Eagle Creek, the Herman Creek Trail stays above the stream on woodsy hillsides, where the only evidence of the creek is the sound of its cascading water. That's not to say that the trail is dull. Quite the contrary, there may be no major waterfalls to enjoy

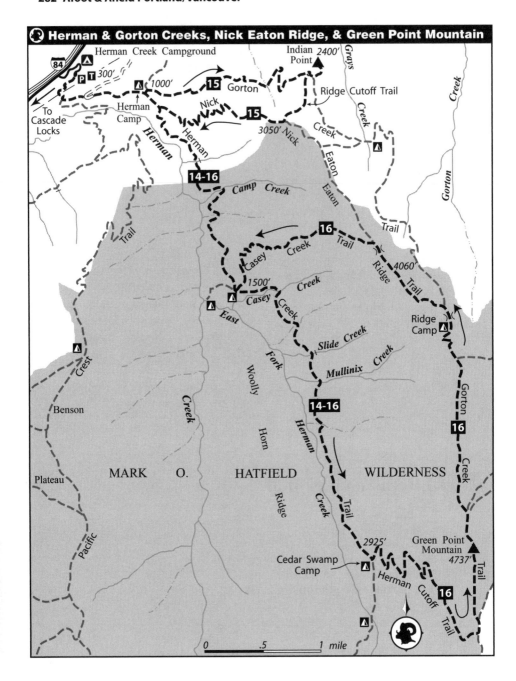

Herman & Gorton Creeks, Nick Eaton Ridge, & Green Point Mountain

Herman Creek Campground

84

300'

To Cascade Locks

Herman Camp

1000'

Gorton

15

Nick

15

Herman

Herman

Indian Point 2400'

Ridge Cutoff Trail

Grays

Creek

3050' Nick

Creek

Eaton

Gorton

14-16

Camp Creek

Eaton

16 Trail

Ridge

Trail

4060'

Casey Creek

Crest

Trail

1500'

Casey Creek

East

Slide Creek

Mullinix Creek

Ridge Camp

Creek

Fork

Woolly

16

Gorton

Benson

Creek

Horn

Herman

Plateau

MARK O. HATFIELD WILDERNESS

Ridge

Creek

Trail

Creek

Pacific

2925'

Green Point Mountain 4737'

Trail

Cedar Swamp Camp

Herman Cutoff Trail

16

0   .5   1 mile

on the main creek, but there are plenty of delicate, wispy falls on side creeks. In addition, the forests here are some of the loveliest in the Gorge. And finally, unlike the extremely popular trail up Eagle Creek, on this trail it is possible to stop and enjoy the scenery, without the fear of being trampled by armies of fellow hikers.

DIRECTIONS Leave Interstate 84 at Cascade Locks Exit 44, and drive the main road (Wa Na Pa Street) through town. At the east end of town turn left on Forest Lane, following signs for the airport. Drive this road 2.0 miles to an overpass over the freeway. Turn left after the overpass, and, 0.3 mile later, turn right at a sign for Herman Creek Campground. This narrow paved road climbs a short distance to a junction with the marked spur road to the trailhead on the right.

The trail begins by winding uphill through a forest of stately bigleaf maple and Douglas fir. Were it not for all the traffic sounds from Interstate 84, the forest would be quiet, but that adjective certainly doesn't apply now. The wide path ascends, passes under a set of power lines, and then continues gradually uphill through attractive, open forests, with lots of spring and early summer wildflowers, such as twisted stalk, inside-out flower, and tiger lily. The traffic sounds fade away as you turn the corner of a minor ridge and enter the canyon of Herman Creek. Two uphill switchbacks take you up to a fork in the trail, where you go left (uphill), staying on the Herman Creek Trail.

In a few hundred yards you arrive at a potentially confusing junction with a closed jeep road. Go straight—ignoring the unsigned routes that head downhill to the right and sharply back to the left—and walk 50 feet to a switchback, where you bear right (uphill) and climb slowly up the west side of a slope. Once at the top of the ridge, you walk on the level about 0.2 mile to long-abandoned Herman Camp, where several trail junctions are found. Go straight on the old road, now just a wide trail, and walk another 250 yards to a junction with the Nick Eaton Trail, where you go straight again and amble lazily along, mostly on the level or slightly downhill, until the old road ends and the route becomes an actual foot trail.

A little less than 1 mile from Herman Camp, you come to a tall, lacy waterfall, just above the trail on an unnamed side creek. After this, you climb a little to an opening in the forest where picturesque oak trees frame good views of Herman Creek Canyon and heavily forested Woolly Horn Ridge. This is a good turn-around point, if you want an easy hike.

Shortly after the viewpoint, you enter the Mark O. Hatfield Wilderness Area and then make a mostly level detour into and out of the side canyon holding Camp Creek, which has an easy rock-hop crossing. Still wandering along at a gentle grade and carefully watching your step to

Falls along lower Herman Creek Trail

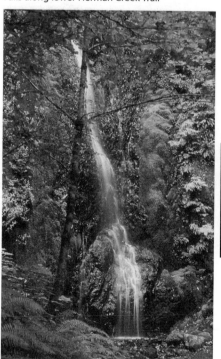

avoid the trailside poison oak, you make some minor ups and downs for the next 1.5 miles to a good campsite beside a junction with the Casey Creek Trail. For an interesting side trip, turn right, walk through the camp, and veer right on a sometimes steep 0.3-mile trail that drops to the confluence of Herman Creek and East Fork Herman Creek. There is an inviting campsite here, or you can simply eat your lunch, enjoying the cascading stream, mossy rocks, cavorting dippers, and dense, overhanging vegetation.

This spot is another good turnaround point, but if you're still going strong, get back on the Herman Creek Trail and begin a long, gradual climb for the next 3.3 miles. Along the way, you cross a half dozen or more splashing side creeks, not all of which have names or flow all year. The second one, Slide Creek, feeds a tall, wispy waterfall that drops over a scenic cliff just above the trail.

None of the creeks has a bridge, but only Mullinix Creek cannot be easily crossed with dry feet. Here, you can either make a simple ford or scramble a few yards upstream to carefully cross on a log. All of this water provides habitat for dense riparian vegetation, dominated by devil's club, with its enormous, foot-wide leaves that hide rows of nasty thorns underneath.

The long climb eventually takes you to a junction with the Herman Cutoff Trail, which goes off to the left just before a tiny creek near Cedar Swamp Camp. The trail shelter that used to stand here is gone, but it is still a pleasant place to spend the night or eat your lunch beneath big, old-growth western hemlocks and western red cedars. For dayhikers this is the last logical turnaround point, unless you are really athletic and plan to make a long loop via Green Point Mountain (See Trip 16).

TRIP 15 Gorton Creek & Nick Eaton Ridge Loop

Distance	8.0 miles, Loop
Elevation Gain	2600 feet
Hiking Time	4½ hours
Optional Map	Green Trails *Bonneville Dam*
Usually Open	April to early November
Best Time	May
Trail Use	Dogs OK, backpacking option, horseback riding
Agency	Columbia River Gorge National Scenic Area
Difficulty	Difficult

see map on p.282

HIGHLIGHTS This excellent loop trip provides a nice sampling of what makes ridge walks in the Columbia River Gorge so nice. In most hiking areas, hikers are satisfied if the trail includes a single major highlight, such as a mountain lake, a high viewpoint, or a flower-covered meadow. But Gorge hikes always manage to come up with several highlights in the same package. On this trip, for example, you can enjoy lush forests, a spectacular rocky overlook, and brightly colored wildflower meadows—all in one compact trip. The only typical Gorge feature lacking is a waterfall, but let's not be greedy.

DIRECTIONS Leave Interstate 84 at Cascade Locks Exit 44, and drive the main road (Wa Na Pa Street) through town. At the east end of town turn left on Forest Lane, following signs for the airport. Drive this road 2.0 miles to an overpass over the freeway. Turn left after the overpass and, 0.3 mile later, turn right at a sign for Herman Creek Campground. This narrow paved road climbs a short distance to a junction with the marked spur road to the trailhead on the right.

The trail begins by winding uphill through a forest of bigleaf maple and Douglas fir with lots of ferns and poison oak crowding the tread. The path passes under a set of power lines and then continues gradually uphill through attractive woods. You round a small ridge to enter the canyon of Herman Creek and then follow two uphill switchbacks to a fork in the trail, where you bear left (uphill).

In a few hundred yards, you arrive at a potentially confusing junction with a closed jeep road. Go straight—ignoring unsigned routes that head downhill to the right and sharply back to the left—and walk 50 feet to a road switchback, where you bear right (uphill) and climb slowly on a road up the west side of a slope.

The dense forest canopy here provides lots of shade, and it keeps the forest floor remarkably free of ground-cover plants. Shortly after the route levels off, you arrive at long-abandoned Herman Camp and a confusing set of junctions.

The main jeep track goes straight, but you turn left to enter the old camp area and pick up the Gorton Creek Trail at a small sign to the southeast. Follow this hiker-only trail as it ascends a lovely open forest, without a hint of the claustrophobic feeling often associated with trails in the Gorge. In early May, white-blooming forest wildflowers brighten the forest floor—baneberry, vanilla leaf, star-flowered smilacina, false Solomon's seal, twisted stalk, valerian, and white anemone. You may hear the occasional train whistle, but freeway sounds are only a distant murmur. Wind in the trees and bird songs are a pleasure for your ears.

You continue at a moderate uphill grade for 2.6 miles, including six short switchbacks, to a junction with the Ridge Cutoff Trail. So far, there have been only occasional small breaks in the tree cover, limited to partially obstructed views. Now, you can satisfy your hankering for broader vistas by making a superb side trip to nearby Indian Point. To reach it, go straight at the junction and walk about 50 yards, and then turn left on an unsigned side trail that goes steeply downhill. In about 0.1 mile, this trail leads to the dramatic views from Indian Point, a rocky outcropping on the side of a cliff. Adventurous hikers can scramble over the rocks to the top of the point, where they can spot Mounts Adams and St. Helens, and enjoy fine views up and down the Columbia River.

To complete the main loop, return to the junction with the Ridge Cutoff Trail and turn south. The trail climbs steeply at first, levels off, and then comes to an area with an abundance of May wildflowers. Look for red-flowering currant, blue anemone, red paintbrush, yellow wood violet, and thick patches of yellow glacier

Indian Point

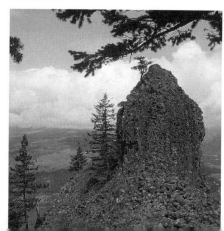

lilies. The almost constant Gorge winds whistle pleasantly through the trees and help to cool off sweaty hikers.

The path tops out at a junction with the Nick Eaton Trail, where you turn right and descend in forest 0.4 mile, before enjoying the trip's next highlight, a series of open meadows with some of the best flower gardens in the Columbia River Gorge. There are plenty of lomatium, prairie star, strawberry, larkspur, ballhead waterleaf, paintbrush, stonecrop, serviceberry, and enough other species to blanket the hillside with a rainbow of colors. The views are also good, especially of the gaping canyon of Herman Creek, Woolly Horn Ridge, and Benson Plateau, with fine vistas to the west, down the Colum-

bia River. The dozens of steep downhill switchbacks that wind through the meadows can be tough on your knees, but amid such scenery, who can complain? The meadows are frequently broken by forested sections that add shade and variety to the hike.

Sadly, the meadows are with you for only about 0.5 mile before you reenter forest and drop through several dozen more switchbacks. The trees get larger as you descend, eventually including really grand old specimens of Douglas fir and western hemlock. The woodsy path bottoms out at a junction with the wide Herman Creek Trail. To close the loop, simply turn right and, in about 200 yards, reach the trail junction at Herman Camp.

TRIP 16 Green Point Mountain Loop

Distance	19.6 miles, Semiloop
Elevation Gain	4300 feet
Hiking Time	9 to 12 hours
Optional Map	Green Trails *Bonneville Dam*
Usually Open	Late May to early November
Best Time	June
Trail Use	Dogs OK, backpacking option, horseback riding
Agency	Columbia River Gorge National Scenic Area
Difficulty	Strenuous

see map on p.282

HIGHLIGHTS This book includes dayhikes of all lengths and difficulty levels, so hikers of all abilities have a range of options to meet their needs. Near the high end of the difficulty range is this loop over Green Point Mountain. At nearly 20 miles, this hike is a major challenge, but for those ready for that challenge, it is well worth the effort. The view from atop Green Point Mountain is the equal of any in the Portland/Vancouver region, and before you even get there, you'll pass waterfalls along the Herman Creek Trail and travel through miles of some of the finest forests in the Columbia River Gorge. Backpackers can make this into a pleasant weekend trip, with a night at Cedar Swamp Camp.

DIRECTIONS Leave Interstate 84 at Cascade Locks Exit 44, and drive the main road (Wa Na Pa Street) through town. At the east end of town turn left on Forest Lane, following signs for the airport. Drive this road 2 miles to an overpass over the freeway. Turn left after the overpass, and 0.3 mile later turn right at a sign for Herman Creek Campground. This narrow paved road climbs a short distance to a junction with the marked spur road to the trailhead on the right.

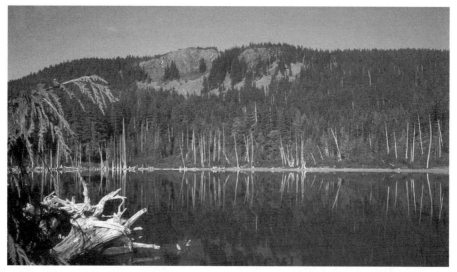

Green Point Mountain over Rainy Lake

The trail begins by winding uphill through a forest of bigleaf maple and Douglas fir and then passes under a set of power lines. From there, you continue gradually uphill around a small ridge and make two uphill switchbacks to a fork in the trail. Bear left (uphill) and, in a few hundred yards you arrive at a potentially confusing junction with a closed jeep road. Go straight—ignoring unsigned routes that head downhill to the right and sharply back to the left—and walk 50 feet to a road switchback, where you bear right (uphill) and climb slowly on the road up the west side of a wooded slope. Once at the top of the ridge, you walk on the level for about 0.2 mile to long-abandoned Herman Camp, where several trail junctions are found.

Go straight on the old road, now just a wide trail, and walk another 250 yards to a junction with the Nick Eaton Trail. You go straight again to continue on the gently graded Herman Creek Trail for 1 mile to a tall waterfall on an unnamed side creek. Then you pass a good viewpoint and move in and out of side canyons to a campsite next to a junction with the

Casey Creek Trail. This is the beginning of the loop trip.

After this campsite, the formerly gentle Herman Creek Trail steepens, continuing south, and steadily gains elevation for the next 3.3 miles. Along the way, you cross a half dozen splashing side creeks, skirt another tall waterfall, and move through dense forests. The long climb eventually takes you to a junction with the Herman Cutoff Trail, which goes to the left, just before Cedar Swamp Camp. If you are enjoying this as a two-day backpacking trip, this comfortable site is the most logical place to spend the night.

To reach Green Point Mountain, turn east on the Herman Cutoff Trail, cross a sluggish little creek, and begin a steady climb. In the next 2.3 miles, you make nine long switchbacks up a heavily wooded hillside. The switchbacks keep the grade from becoming overly steep, but the trail is still tiring. Finally, you come to a small abandoned building at a junction with an old jeep road.

Turn left here and almost immediately leave the road in favor of the Gorton Creek Trail, which runs uphill along a ridgeline. In a little less than 1 mile, you come to the open summit of Green Point Mountain, where you can sit down and enjoy the view. From here, you can see all the major volcanic snow peaks in the region, as well as most of the recognizable high points in the Columbia River Gorge, all the way west to Larch Mountain. The most impressive sights, however, are looking east down to Rainy Lake, and northeast to the bald, rocky summit of Mt. Defiance.

Reshoulder your pack and drop down the trail on the north side of Green Point Mountain to a junction. Bear left here and make a very gradual descent in open forests for 1.5 miles to the next junction, where you bear left again and descend a series of short, rather steep, switchbacks. At the bottom of these switchbacks is a saddle and a sign identifying Ridge Camp. A smaller sign directs you to the

nearest water, at the end of a 0.2-mile spur trail to the east.

To close the loop, you contour across open slopes on the east side of Nick Eaton Ridge for a short distance and then come to a junction with the Nick Eaton Trail. Bear left and walk near the crest of the ridge, savoring some excellent views from several openings along the way. At the next saddle, you come to another junction, where you turn left on the Casey Creek Trail on which you will lose all of the elevation you gained before. The trail is rather narrow and quite steep as it loses 2500 feet in 2.1 miles, which explains why you don't want to make this loop in the opposite direction. As compensation for jammed toes, you are treated to some good views and abundant wildflowers in a steep meadow about halfway down. Eventually, you get back to the junction near the campsite on the Herman Creek Trail, turn right, and return to your car.

TRIP 17 Gorge Trail: Herman Creek to Wyeth Campground

Distance	5.3 miles, Point-to-point
Elevation Gain	800 feet
Hiking Time	2½ hours
Optional Map	USFS *Trails of the Columbia Gorge*
Usually Open	All year
Best Times	April to May and late October
Trail Use	Dogs OK
Agency	Columbia River Gorge National Scenic Area
Difficulty	Moderate
Note	Good in cloudy weather

HIGHLIGHTS This rarely traveled trail was constructed in the late 1990s as a section of the low-elevation Gorge Trail. Most hikers are unaware of its existence, as no other guidebooks include this trip. Those who discover this route find it to be a welcome link in the interconnected trail system of the central Gorge because it makes some excellent loop trips possible. Backpackers and sturdy dayhikers looking to visit Herman Creek and North Lake can use this trail to visit both areas, without having to retrace their steps.

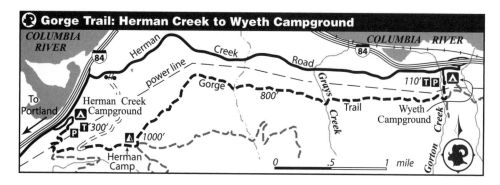

Gorge Trail: Herman Creek to Wyeth Campground

The leisurely route is also a pleasant dayhike in its own right, providing a quiet stroll through forests and over talus slopes, with nice views of the Columbia River and surrounding cliffs. The route is open all year (except during winter storms) and is easy enough for hikers of virtually any ability level, especially when it is done as a point-to-point trip with a short car shuttle. As on most low-elevation routes in the Gorge, poison oak is common here. Learn to recognize and avoid it. The hike is described from west to east.

DIRECTIONS Leave Interstate 84 at Cascade Locks Exit 44, and drive the main road (Wa Na Pa Street) through town. At the east end of town turn left on Forest Lane, following signs for the airport. Drive this road 2 miles to an overpass over the freeway. Turn left after the overpass and, 0.3 mile later, turn right at a sign for Herman Creek Campground. This narrow paved road climbs a short distance to a junction with the marked spur road to the trailhead on the right.

To leave a second car at the Wyeth Trailhead, go east on Interstate 84 to Wyeth Exit 51. Turn right at the end of the exit road, and almost immediately turn right again on Herman Creek Road. After 0.1 mile, turn left into Wyeth Campground, and drive through this comfortable and attractive area, keeping right at all intersections, to the signed trailhead parking lot.

The trail begins by winding uphill through a stately forest of bigleaf maple and Douglas fir, with lots of ferns and poison oak crowding the tread. The path passes under a set of power lines and then continues gradually uphill through attractive woods. You round a small ridge to enter the canyon of Herman Creek and then follow two uphill switchbacks to a fork in the trail, where you veer left (uphill). In a few hundred yards you arrive at a potentially confusing junction with a closed jeep road.

Go straight—ignoring unsigned routes that head downhill to the right and sharply back to the left—and walk 50 feet to a road switchback. Bear right (uphill) and slowly climb up the west side of a wooded slope. Shortly after the route levels off, you arrive at long-abandoned Herman Camp and a confusing set of junctions. The poorly signed Gorge Trail begins at the northeast corner of the camp area on your left.

The path sets a leisurely course through the dappled sunshine of an open forest, with lots of vine maple and bracken fern forming an understory. The eastbound trail goes along at a level or very slight downhill grade, in and out of little canyons, most of which have no water. The scenery doesn't change much as you hike, but it's never dull, because of the mixed forests and lush greenery. An abundance of vine maple make this quiet hike enjoyable in late October, although by then almost no sunshine reaches these north-facing slopes.

About 1 mile from Herman Camp, you cross a steep, narrow skid road and continue your nearly level traverse. As you continue east, you pass the base of some moss-covered scree slopes, where you can catch glimpses of the towering cliffs of Nick Eaton Ridge on your right. Three types of ferns, as well as Oregon grape and thimbleberry, compete for dominance on the forest floor, while Douglas fir, western red cedar, and western hemlock vie with deciduous species, such as Pacific dogwood and bigleaf maple, for dominance above.

The trail comes close to and briefly follows a parallel set of power lines and then crosses a large rocky slope with good views of the Columbia River. Conveniently, busy Interstate 84 is hidden from view by trees, making for more attractive photographs. On this rocky slope, listen for the peeping sounds of pikas, cute little guinea-pig-like creatures, who find good habitat among the rockslides in the Gorge. The next landmark is the easy crossing of two branches of splashing Grays Creek, followed by another scree slope with disappointing river views but excellent looks up to the cliffs and rocky pinnacles to the south. This nicely varied mix of forest and occasional scree slopes continues as you slowly descend, gradually approaching the power lines and freeway on your left. The path bottoms out as it detours briefly inland to a wooden bridge over rushing Gorton Creek and then immediately hits a junction with the Wyeth Trail. To close your hike, turn left and soon arrive at the Wyeth Campground and Trailhead.

TRIP 18 Wyeth Trail to North Lake

Distance	11.4 miles, Out-and-back
Elevation Gain	3800 feet
Hiking Time	6 to 7 hours
Optional Map	Green Trails *Bonneville Dam*
Usually Open	Mid-May to November
Best Time	June
Trail Use	Dogs OK, backpacking option, fishing
Agency	Columbia River Gorge National Scenic Area
Difficulty	Strenuous

HIGHLIGHTS Like many other Gorge hikes, the Wyeth Trail will provide you with a really good workout. It's a long way up from the Columbia River, near sea level, to North Lake at the top. In fact, mountain climbers often use this path as a conditioning hike in the spring. Fortunately, the climb is well shaded by trees, and the woods are always attractive, so there are compensations for all the sweat.

DIRECTIONS Take Exit 51 off Interstate 84 east of Cascade Locks, and turn right at the end of the exit road. You immediately turn right again on Herman Creek Road and, after 0.1 mile, turn left into Wyeth Campground. Keep right at all intersections in this comfortable and attractive campground to reach the signed trailhead parking lot.

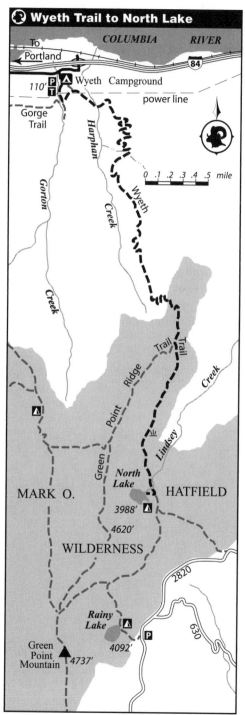

Wyeth Trail to North Lake

COLUMBIA RIVER

To Portland

84

110' Wyeth Campground

power line

Gorge Trail

Harphan

Gorton

Creek

Wyeth

Creek

0 .1 .2 .3 .4 .5 mile

Trail

Trail

Ridge

Point

Green

Lindsey

Creek

North Lake

MARK O.

3988'

4620'

HATFIELD

WILDERNESS

2820

Rainy Lake

4092'

630

Green Point Mountain

4737'

The wide trail follows an old road for about 150 yards to a signed junction. To the right, the Gorge Trail heads west to Herman Creek, while straight ahead is an old trail that is no longer used. You turn left and cross a hillside above the parking lot, before coming to an unsigned junction with a spur trail that heads sharply left, back to the campground. You go straight, cross an open area under a set of power lines, and then go back into the trees.

Next, you hop across the clear waters of 6-foot-wide Harphan Creek and turn uphill. Up to this point, you have done only some modest ups and downs, from here on, however, the downgrades disappear, and steady uphill is all you get.

Very quickly, the trees make a transition from mostly bigleaf maple to mostly Douglas fir, while sword fern and Oregon grape cover the forest floor. Before long, you reach the first of what will be many switchbacks. The first 10 are rather long and well graded, following a recently realigned route. At the end of these, you cross a tiny but reliable creek, where you can splash your head with water and take a short rest.

Above this, you make a series of much shorter and somewhat steeper switchbacks, before you break out of the woods and reach a small but welcome rocky clearing, above the steep slopes of Harphan Creek Canyon. There is a nice variety of wildflowers here, and fine vistas to the Carson area in Washington. Both make good excuses to stop climbing for a while and take another needed rest stop.

For the next mile, you alternate between trees and open rocky areas, affording you a pleasant variety of scenery. The uphill grade is sometimes steep, sometimes only moderate, but it never ceases.

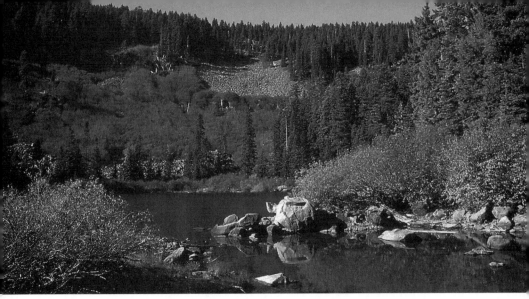

North Lake

Finally, after the last open clearing, you make eight more switchbacks and come to a junction with the Green Point Ridge Trail, a possible loop option for athletic hikers. More important, you have now completed virtually all of the uphill.

To reach North Lake, bear left at the junction, and travel through a higher-elevation forest of Pacific silver fir and western white pine. The trail now loses a little elevation, as you cross a marshy area and an open slope with nice views east to distinctive Mt. Defiance, the highest landmark on the Oregon side of the Columbia River Gorge. Cross a couple of tiny creeks, and then make a final uphill push to North Lake, which you reach by taking a short side trail to the right.

After all that effort you might be a little disappointed with North Lake. It is formed by an earthen dam and has lots of dead snags around its shores, so it's not the most aesthetically pleasing pool in the Portland/Vancouver region. It does, however, boast several decent campsites on its south shore and a good view of the talus slopes of Green Point Mountain, to the southwest.

If you have enough energy to visit a somewhat prettier pool and to make a loop with great views, bear left around North Lake and soon come to a junction. You bear right here and walk very gradually uphill in forest to a second junction. If you want to visit Rainy Lake, go left and come to this attractive mountain lake in about 0.3 mile. Like North Lake, Rainy Lake has some snags, but it also has a first-rate view of Green Point Mountain and very nice camps for backpackers. This lake is also accessible by a very short trail that connects with a nearby logging road, so you should expect some company.

If you want to make the loop, turn right at the junction before Rainy Lake and climb a mix of woodsy slopes and open rocky areas for 0.6 mile to a four-way junction on top of a ridge. To return to the Wyeth Trail, go north at this junction and follow the Green Point Ridge Trail, which closely follows the edge of the ridge above North Lake. After 1.5 miles, you bear right at a junction and continue downhill another 1.2 miles, back to the junction with the Wyeth Trail mentioned earlier. This optional loop adds a total of 2.3 miles and 800 feet of elevation gain to your hike.

TRIP 19 Shellrock Mountain

Distance	2.8 miles, Out-and-back
Elevation Gain	1300 feet
Hiking Time	2½ hours
Optional Map	Green Trails *Hood River* (trail not shown)
Usually Open	All year (except during winter storms)
Best Time	All year
Trail Use	Dogs OK
Agency	Columbia River Gorge National Scenic Area
Difficulty	Moderate

HIGHLIGHTS Not maintained by any land agency and not shown on any map, the trail partway up Shellrock Mountain joins a long list of such overlooked routes lacing the isolated parts of the Columbia River Gorge. Built to access a U.S. Geological Survey station, this little-known and rarely traveled path features very convenient access, excellent views, and some interesting history. The route is a real gem, but it is not good for hikers with children due to some exposed sections and a rather steep grade. Although not necessary on every trail, high-topped boots are essential on this hike because the very uneven and rocky trail seems designed to give you a sprained ankle, especially when the rocks are wet, and you are traveling downhill. Since the trail is not maintained, please do your part to keep it up by removing any deadfall and helping to rebuild obliterated sections.

DIRECTIONS Drive Interstate 84 east from Portland to a spot 0.7 mile beyond Milepost 52, and pull off the freeway into a small unmarked gravel area just off the right shoulder. There is a guardrail here with a small white sign stating PROPERTY OF DEPT. OF TRANSPORTATION—HIGHWAY DIVISION. In order to return to Portland after your hike, you will have to get back on the eastbound lanes of Interstate 84, and drive to Exit 56 at Viento State Park, where you can turn back west. Be very careful when you get back on the freeway as there is no merge lane.

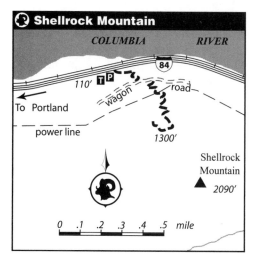

Shellrock Mountain

COLUMBIA RIVER

To Portland

110' wagon road

power line

1300'

Shellrock Mountain ▲ 2090'

0 .1 .2 .3 .4 .5 mile

Hop over the guardrail and walk east on a section of the old scenic highway, through a tunnel of trees. Traffic zips by on the busy freeway just a few yards to your left, and poison oak crowds the route, but the hiking is easy and the forest is attractive. After less than 100 yards, look for a small path on the right and turn onto it.

This well-graded trail ascends a slope of moss-covered rocks in five evenly spaced switchbacks to a junction with a section of a historic 1872 wagon road. Much of the stonework used to build this old route is still visible and interesting to explore. Also visible are increasingly good

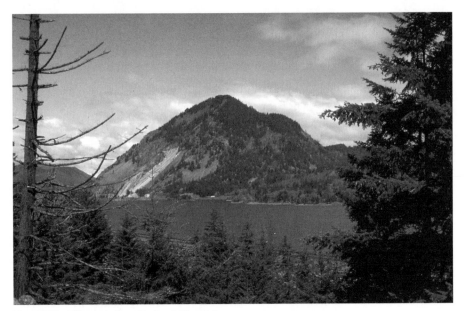

View of Wind Mountain from Shellrock Mountain

views across the Columbia River to Wind and Dog mountains.

Bear left (uphill) on the old wagon road, and follow it for about 80 yards to where the road starts to curve into the trees. Turn sharply right here on an obvious trail, and resume switchbacking up the rocky slope. Even though you never quite escape the sounds of big rigs barreling along Interstate 84, the trail is otherwise remarkably wild and attractive. It climbs steadily and rather steeply in 10 switchbacks all the way to the top of the rocky slope. The view from here is especially good looking east down the Gorge to Mitchell Point and north to Dog and Augspurger mountains.

You may want to call it quits here, as the trail beyond this point becomes less distinct and much more rugged and overgrown. There is also a lot more poison oak to deal with, so you must be careful where you step. If you decide to trudge on, follow the sketchy up-and-down route into the trees and make a series of five switchbacks and short but difficult traverses, before you eventually emerge from the trees at an old wooden overlook and survey site. From here, you can enjoy a quiet lunch while taking in the nice view.

There is no trail beyond this point to the actual summit of Shellrock Mountain, about 1 mile away and 800 feet higher. The bushwhack to the top is extremely difficult, and the view is almost entirely blocked by trees, so it's not worth the effort.

TRIP 20 Mount Defiance Trail

Distance	11.9 miles, Out-and-back or Loop
Elevation Gain	4800 feet
Hiking Time	8 to 12 hours
Optional Map	Green Trails *Hood River*
Usually Open	Late May to October
Best Time	June
Trail Use	Dogs OK
Agency	Columbia River Gorge National Scenic Area
Difficulty	Strenuous

HIGHLIGHTS At 4960 feet, Mt. Defiance is the highest point directly overlooking the Columbia River Gorge. The loftiness of this spot ensures that visitors enjoy an exceptional view, extending from the familiar Cascade snow peaks, to the agricultural Hood River Valley, to the mighty river far below. The height also ensures that since the hike starts at near sea level, it will be a difficult challenge. The elevation gain is truly daunting, so this hike should be left solely to the fittest athletes. Serious mountain climbers looking for a conditioning hike love this outing, but all others should think twice.

DIRECTIONS Drive east on Interstate 84 to Starvation Creek Exit 54, and park in the small lot for Starvation Creek State Park. This exit is accessible only to eastbound traffic, so on your return you have to continue east to Exit 56 at Viento State Park to get back on the westbound lanes.

The signed path begins from the west end of the lot and follows the highway shoulder, separated from the noisy traffic by a concrete barrier. The perfectly level trail slowly works away from the freeway, although the sounds of cars and trucks remain dominant as you wander through the woods. Much of the route follows the historic Old Columbia River Highway, which ensures an easy grade, but you'll need to watch your step to avoid poison oak, a very common plant in the eastern Gorge.

Just 0.3 mile from the trailhead, a tiny sign marks the steep Starvation Cutoff Trail, which goes up the slope on your left. Go straight and catch a glimpse of Cabin Creek Falls as you continue walking west to a much better view of Hole-in-the-Wall Falls on Warren Creek. This 100-foot falls isn't exactly human-made; it has always existed. But in 1938 highway engineers diverted the flow into a tunnel so drivers on the old highway could avoid a shower.

A little past the bridge over Warren Creek is a junction with Starvation Ridge Trail, going back to the left. The Mount Defiance Trail goes straight and passes beside the rather short but lovely Lancaster Falls, a 20-foot-high spreading cascade of water.

Up to this point the trail has remained almost level, but since you know the hike gains 4800 feet, logic dictates that the uphill must begin soon, and it does. A little less than 0.5 mile from Lancaster Falls, the path cuts to the left and launches into the expected ascent, with two dozen short switchbacks. The grade isn't excessively steep, but it's consistently uphill, so your calves and Achilles tendons better be prepared. The ascent is also bone dry, so

Eastern Columbia River Gorge

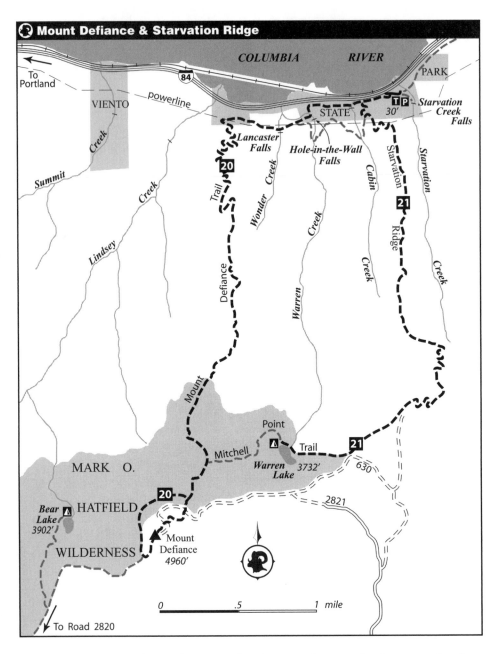

Mount Defiance & Starvation Ridge

carry an extra quart of water in your pack for hydration.

The first switchbacks climb the east side of the heavily wooded ridge, while the later ones (and there are lots of later ones) cut back and forth near the crest of the ridge. While most of the route is in deep woods, a couple of grassy and rocky openings provide decent views of Lindsey Creek Canyon to the west and welcome excuses for rest stops.

The climbing doesn't end when the switchbacks do, because after an all-too-brief level stretch, you resume charging up the ridge. At about the 3200-foot level are the first beargrass plants. This is usually a welcome sign in the Gorge, indicating that your climb is almost over, but that disappointingly isn't the case here. Compensation comes in the form of views from openings in the trees near the edge of some rocky talus slopes.

You turn right at the junction with the Mitchell Point Trail, which goes east to Warren Lake, and resume climbing. About 0.2 mile later, look for a possibly unsigned trail to the right, and turn onto this route as it gradually ascends a view-packed talus slope on the west side of Mt. Defiance's summit. On the south side of the peak you reach a junction, where you turn left and make the short final push to the top.

Even though you share the open summit with a jeep road and a microwave station, these only briefly detract from the view. There is a lot to look at in every direction, so allow some time to take it all in. Below you to the west is sparkling Bear Lake, and spreading out from there are various recognizable high points like Tanner Butte, Tomlike Mountain, and Indian Mountain. To the northwest are Table Mountain, Silver Star Mountain, and decapitated Mt. St. Helens. Rising prominently to the north is snowy Mt. Adams. To the east are the Columbia River, Hood River Mountain, and the distant wheat fields of the Columbia Plateau. Most striking is the view south to horn-shaped Mt. Hood. Hikers familiar with the region can spend hours picking out familiar places. Before spending those hours, however, keep in mind that you still face a long hike back down before the day ends, and while going down may sound easy, countless hikers who have suffered from bad knees and jammed toes after completing the descent would beg to differ.

For variety on the return trip, you can take a shorter but less scenic trail from the top that switchbacks down through woods and crosses the closed jeep road twice before getting back to a junction with the Mount Defiance Trail. Another return loop option is the long, steep Starvation Ridge Trail (see Trip 21), although this path serves better as the uphill leg of a loop returning via the Mount Defiance Trail.

Hikers who want to visit the summit of Mt. Defiance but who can't handle the rigors of the Mount Defiance Trail, have the option of taking a much easier route from Forest Road 2820 to the south that gains only 1500 feet in 2 miles. Although easier on the body, this trail is less scenic and requires an extra hour or more of driving on bumpy gravel roads.

TRIP 21 Starvation Ridge to Warren Lake

see map on p.296

Distance	8.6 miles, Out-and-back or Loop
Elevation Gain	3800 feet
Hiking Time	5 to 7 hours
Optional Map	Green Trails *Hood River*
Usually Open	May to October
Best Time	June
Trail Use	Dogs OK (but the trail can very difficult for them), backpacking option, fishing
Agency	Columbia River Gorge National Scenic Area
Difficulty	Strenuous

HIGHLIGHTS So you've looked at the distance and elevation gain totals for the Mount Defiance Trail (Trip 20) and decided that, even though you're in good shape, that trip is beyond your abilities. Before you give up on getting to the top of Mt. Defiance, consider the two other options that reach the same goal. The first is a relatively easy backdoor approach, from a logging road to the south. Although pleasant, this trail requires a drive of almost two hours, so it is beyond the range of this book.

Another option is to do the trip as a two-day backpacking loop. For this approach, hike up the Starvation Ridge Trail, spend the night at scenic Warren Lake, and then return on the Mount Defiance Trail. It won't be much fun hauling your gear up to Warren Lake, but you'll have all day to do it, and you can cool off at day's end with an invigorating dip in a lovely mountain lake. The trip is also worth taking separately as a dayhike to Warren Lake, which is the trip described here.

DIRECTIONS Drive east on Interstate 84 to Starvation Creek Exit 54, and park in the small lot for Starvation Creek State Park. This exit is accessible only to eastbound traffic, so on your return you have to continue east to Exit 56 at Viento State Park to get back on the westbound lanes.

The signed path begins from the west end of the lot and follows the highway shoulder, separated from the noisy traffic by a concrete barrier. After 0.2 mile, you turn left on the sketchy Starvation Cutoff Trail and switchback steeply up through attractive Douglas-fir and bigleaf-maple forests for 0.5 mile to a junction with the Starvation Ridge Trail. You turn left here and make a series of 10 uphill switchbacks to a good viewpoint beneath a power line tower.

From here, the trail turns right and ascends rather steeply up a narrow ridge, mostly under a canopy of big trees. You keep this up for 2 exhausting miles, never straying far from the ridge crest, despite a few short switchbacks. There is one good viewpoint along the way but little else to break up the steady climb. A break does come eventually, when the grade of the climb lessens a little so that you can cross a small rocky area and then contour across a brushy slope with decent views of distant Mt. Adams.

The trail then goes up a series of short switchbacks, crosses a scree slope, and comes to the edge of an old clear-cut. This landmark may not be aesthetically pleasing, but it does provide you with the opportunity to congratulate yourself on completing most of the uphill.

The trail curves to the right, away from the logging scar and works gradually uphill in deep woods of smaller, high-elevation trees, like Pacific silver fir. Beargrass blossoms brighten the way in June. At the top of a couple shorter switchbacks, you hit the end of another road and logged area. You skirt this spot and soon reenter deep woods, now traveling on a basically level trail. You pass a mediocre viewpoint, and 0.3 mile later reach an unsigned junction with the Mitchell Point Trail.

The path to the left goes 50 yards to a closed logging road, but you turn right and descend slightly for 0.4 mile to Warren Lake. This lovely pool is backed by a scenic rockslide and provides good swimming for tired hikers. The shore has a fair amount of brush, but there are a couple of good campsites at either end of the lake. Mosquitoes can be bothersome in June and early July.

If you are continuing to Mt. Defiance, keep hiking on the Mitchell Point Trail as it rounds the northwest side of Warren Lake and climbs a scenic, mostly open slope with good views. The trail reenters woods and, 0.8 mile from Warren Lake, comes to a junction with the Mount Defiance Trail. To reach the summit, turn left and follow the trail uphill, as described in Trip 20. If you are doing this trip as a loop, it is marginally easier on the knees to go up the Starvation Ridge Trail and down the slightly better graded Mount Defiance Trail.

TRIP 22 Starvation Creek Explorations

Distance	0.1 to 9.2 miles, Loops
Elevation Gain	50 to 2200 feet
Hiking Time	30 minutes to 5 hours
Optional Map	Green Trails *Hood River* (some trails not shown)
Usually Open	All year (except during winter storms)
Best Time	April
Trail Use	No dogs (too dangerous for them), partly wheelchair accessible
Agency	Columbia River Gorge National Scenic Area
Difficulty	Moderate

HIGHLIGHTS Most hikers who come to Starvation Creek are looking to tackle the long, rugged climbs of Mt. Defiance (Trip 20) or Starvation Ridge (Trip 21), but these trips have two big drawbacks. The first and most obvious is their difficulty, well beyond the ability level of most dayhikers. The second problem is that they climb to elevations that are snowbound several months of the year. Both of these problems can be avoided by spending your time on the lower trails around Starvation Creek. These scenic paths provide enough exercise for a decent workout, without making you feel like you just survived army basic training. They also remain open all year, so on a sunny early spring day you can check out some lovely country without having to strap on snowshoes.

DIRECTIONS Drive east on Interstate 84 to Starvation Creek Exit 54, and park in the small lot for Starvation Creek State Park. This exit is accessible only to eastbound traffic, so on your return you have to continue east to Exit 56 at Viento State Park to get back on the westbound lanes.

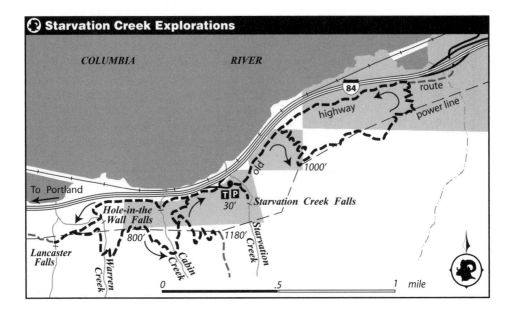

Starvation Creek Explorations

COLUMBIA   RIVER

route
84
highway
power line
1000'
To Portland
30'   Starvation Creek Falls
Hole-in-the
Wall Falls
800'   1180'
Lancaster
Falls
Cabin Creek
Warren Creek
Starvation Creek
0   .5   1   mile

Start your explorations by walking the paved, 150-yard trail up to 186-foot-high Starvation Creek Falls. In recent years, this trail has been blocked off well back from the towering falls, so the view is no longer as good as old timers remember, but you will still want to spend some time gazing up in awe at the portion of the falls you can see.

If you're in the mood for history rather than wilderness, then your next exploration should be the wide trail going east toward Viento State Park. This gently graded, 1.1-mile segment of the historic Old Columbia River Highway has a paved surface and visits several good viewpoints just above Interstate 84. The trail stays near the busy and noisy freeway the entire way, so it's not terribly wild, but it is interesting, especially if you take the time to read the interpretive signs near the trailhead, which inform you of the history of this road.

A rugged option for hikers who aren't allergic to poison oak is to follow the old highway west for about 250 yards, then turn right on an unsigned and hard-to-find path that steeply climbs several irregular and overgrown switchbacks to the base of a power line tower. From here, you turn left (east) and follow another rough use path for 1 mile past several more viewpoints and power line towers. When you reach the top of a rocky slope, turn left on a path covered with loose rocks and descend this rough trail back down to the old highway. Although there are good views on this hike, the thickets of poison oak along this loop route are virtually impossible to avoid. Only experienced route-finders should try this trail, and then only in winter and early spring before the poison oak gets too frisky and its poisonous toxin isn't as virulent.

Probably the best of the options lead from the Mount Defiance Trail west of the parking lot. This path initially follows the freeway shoulder, with a concrete barrier separating you from the traffic, and then veers away from the freeway onto segments of the old highway.

The woodsy path goes below wispy Cabin Creek Falls, which is hard to see from the trail, and then past Hole-in-

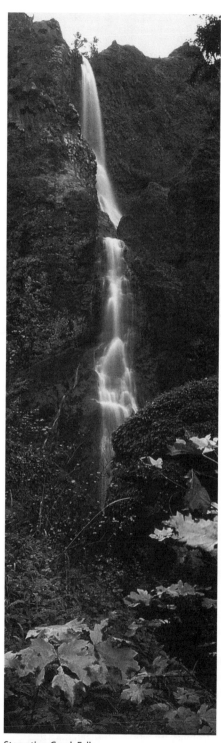

Starvation Creek Falls

the-Wall Falls, whose natural flow was diverted in 1938 by highway workers but is still impressive. After crossing Warren Creek on a bridge, the trail continues to a junction with the Starvation Ridge Trail. Before turning left on this path, take 15 minutes to go straight on the Mount Defiance Trail for 0.2 mile to visit 20-foot-high Lancaster Falls. After returning to the junction, turn onto the Starvation Ridge Trail, climb to a crossing of Warren Creek in the woods above Hole-in-the-Wall Falls, and then ascend a grassy wildflower meadow to a dramatic clifftop overlook. From here, you can see the entire Starvation Creek area, as well as hulking Dog Mountain across the river in Washington.

The trail then switchbacks downhill, crosses Cabin Creek, and comes to a junction with the Starvation Cutoff Trail. Before taking this return leg of the loop, consider going straight on a worthwhile side trip up 10 short switchbacks under a set of power lines to a final good viewpoint at the base of a power line tower. To close this dramatic loop, return to the junction with the Starvation Cutoff Trail, and descend this steep route for 0.5 mile back to the Mount Defiance Trail.

Eastern Columbia
River Gorge

TRIP 23 Wygant Trail Loop

Distance	8.5 miles, Semiloop
Elevation Gain	2100 feet
Hiking Time	4 to 5 hours
Optional Map	Green Trails *Hood River* (part of trail not shown)
Usually Open	March to early December
Best Time	Late March through mid-May
Trail Use	Dogs OK (but beware of poison oak)
Agency	Oregon State Parks, Columbia River Gorge region
Difficulty	Difficult

HIGHLIGHTS This little-known route offers hikers a lot of variety in a relatively small package. It starts with a treat for history buffs by following a short section of the historic old Columbia River Highway and then visits a quiet creek canyon and a string of spectacular viewpoints that provide unusual perspectives of the eastern Columbia River Gorge. Before setting out on this adventure, however, be warned that poison oak is extremely abundant in this area. This leafy menace is probably more of a hazard along this trail than on any other hike described in this book. Hikers must watch their step, wear long pants, and wash all of their clothes immediately upon their return.

DIRECTIONS Drive Interstate 84 to Mitchell Point Overlook Exit 58, and take the short exit road to a parking lot. Since Exit 58 has access only to and from the eastbound lanes of Interstate 84, in order to return to Portland you will have to continue east to Hood River Exit 62, and then turn around to get on the westbound lanes.

The signed Wygant Trail follows a closed road that goes west from the lower (southwest) end of the parking lot. Walk about 250 yards, and then as the road turns left, take a signed footpath that veers right and into the trees. This trail takes you to a log bridge over small Mitchell Creek and then descends slightly to join a section of the Old Columbia River Highway.

After 0.3 mile, you leave this old road, which is being invaded by mosses and poison oak, and walk up a little gully through open Douglas-fir forests. About 1 mile from the trailhead is a junction with the Chetwoot Trail, which is the return route of the recommended loop. You go straight and, a few yards later, pass a side trail to a viewpoint on your right. Only hikers who aren't allergic to poison oak should take this overgrown route, as the stuff is unavoidable.

You turn south, pass under a set of power lines, cross Perham Creek on a log bridge, and turn north again, crossing back under the same power lines. The next highlight is a spectacular little viewpoint in an open area just on your right. Almost 200 feet directly below this overlook is busy Interstate 84, but your attention will be drawn much more to the outstanding views of Mitchell Point to the east and Dog Mountain to the northwest. In April, a whole array of delicate wildflowers bloom on this open slope, providing colorful foregrounds for photographs.

This viewpoint makes a good turnaround point for hikers who don't want to do a lot of climbing. If you are up for a bit more exercise, however, follow the trail as it turns sharply south into the Douglas-fir woods and begins climbing. You cross under the power lines yet again

⊕ Wygant Trail & Mitchell Point

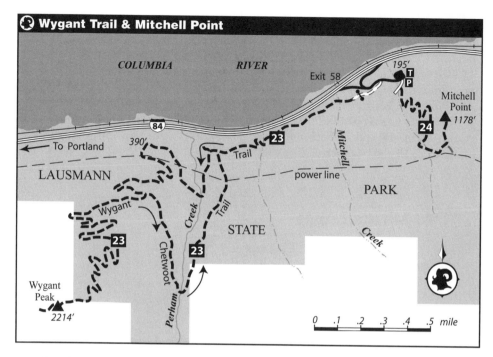

COLUMBIA   RIVER

Exit 58

195'

Mitchell Point
1178'

84

To Portland   390'

Trail

23

LAUSMANN

power line

PARK

Wygant

STATE

Creek

Trail

23

Creek

Chetwoot

23

Wygant
Peak

2214'

Perham

0   .1   .2   .3   .4   .5 mile

and make a series of short switchbacks, followed by a long traverse and one more switchback, to a junction with the Chetwoot Trail. If you want to visit higher viewpoints, turn right and make first a traverse, then a series of long switchbacks for 0.5 mile to an excellent higher viewpoint at a clifftop break in the trees on a ridge. From here, you can even look over the hills on the Washington side of the Gorge to see a small part of Mt. Adams.

The trail above this point is not maintained very well, but experienced hikers can follow the narrow route as it ascends a series of 15 short switchbacks for the next 1.2 miles, mostly in dense forest, to the top of Wygant Peak. The view here is rather disappointing, but if you continue downhill through the trees to the northeast for about 200 yards, you will emerge at a nice, private meadow with excellent views to the west.

Mitchell Point from the Wygant Trail

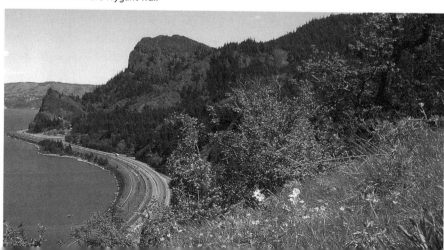

To resume the recommended loop, go back down the trail 1.7 miles to the Chetwoot Trail junction and hike that gently graded and irregularly maintained path as it makes a long downhill traverse into the canyon of Perham Creek. You make a bridgeless crossing of that little stream, then turn north and traverse the oak-studded slopes east of the creek. The oaks here are mostly of the harmless Oregon white oak variety, but not-so-harmless poison oak is also common. You intersect the power lines a final time and come to the rough power line access road. Jog to the right along this road for about 50 feet to reacquire the trail and then quickly return to the junction with the Wygant Trail.

TRIP 24 Mitchell Point

Distance	2.4 miles, Out-and-back
Elevation Gain	1200 feet
Hiking Time	1½ hours
Optional Map	Unnecessary
Usually Open	All year (except during winter storms)
Best Time	Late March through April
Trail Use	Dogs OK (but dangerous at the top)
Agency	Oregon State Parks, Columbia River Gorge region
Difficulty	Difficult

HIGHLIGHTS Although thousands of motorists drive past prominent Mitchell Point every day, few bother to stop at small Lausmann State Park at its base. Fewer still take the hike to the top of this rugged monolith to enjoy the terrific views and flowers there. One reason is that very few people even know that it is possible to hike to the summit. Even so-called "comprehensive" guidebooks on trails in the Columbia River Gorge overlook this fine route, despite easy highway access and big rewards at the end of a good trail. Here is your opportunity to correct this oversight.

DIRECTIONS Drive Interstate 84 to Mitchell Point Overlook Exit 58, and take the short exit road to a parking lot. Since Exit 58 has access only to and from the eastbound lanes of Interstate 84, in order to return to Portland you will have to continue east to Hood River Exit 62 and then turn around to get on the westbound lanes.

The unsigned Mitchell Point Trail leaves from the upper (southeast) corner of the parking lot. The route follows a paved path heading toward the restroom building, but after about 75 feet you bear left onto an obvious, but unsigned, old gravel road. The gravel route loops to the right for about 100 yards, then you veer left on an obvious foot trail into the trees. This trail climbs moderately steeply in lush woods of Douglas fir and bigleaf maple, above a trickling seasonal creek on your right, then it switchbacks to the left, away from the creek, and climbs steeply on a rocky path. The forest here is broken by open, rocky areas that are rimmed by twisted specimens of Oregon white oak, as well as the less welcome, shiny-leafed poison oak crowding the trail. You'll hear plenty of traffic sounds from the freeway below, but you'll also enjoy many spring wildflowers, such as lomatium, Oregon grape, larkspur, and prairie star.

Two more switchbacks take you up to and across a scree slope directly below the sheer cliffs of Mitchell Point. From this open, rocky area, you'll get your first good views across the Columbia River, to Dog and Wind mountains and large Drano Lake, which are cut off from the river by a bend in Washington State Highway 14. You briefly leave the scree in favor of woods and then switchback and recross the rocks at a higher elevation with even wider vistas. Leaving the rocks a second and final time, the trail's grade gets less severe, as you continue through Douglas-fir forests, with lots of vine maple forming an understory, and common plants like vanilla leaf, Oregon grape, and various mosses on the forest floor.

As the freeway sounds fade, you emerge from the trees in a brushy saddle south of Mitchell Point and then enter an open swath beneath a set of power lines. The somewhat overgrown but easy-to-follow path now climbs a little more to a trail junction. The trail to the right goes a short distance to a power line access road, but your route turns left and follows the open spine of a ridge. Abundant late April wildflowers here include arrowleaf balsamroot, lupine, onion, and fringecup. Twisted oak trees frame good pictures of the rocky summit of Mitchell Point directly ahead. Views up and down the Gorge are superb, and they improve with every step as you ascend to the usually windy summit.

The exposed top isn't recommended for acrophobics, but it allows you to look east to small farms near Hood River, north to a tiny bit of the top of Mt. Adams, northwest to Dog and Wind mountains, and west to such landmarks as Mt. Defiance and Table Mountain. At

the base of the towering cliffs on the west side of Mitchell Point, you can see the freeway exit and the entire route of this hike. The jagged spine of Mitchell Point continues a short distance north from the high point, but the rocks are far too dangerous for exploration on foot.

Looking north along the jagged spine of Mitchell Point and to the Columbia River

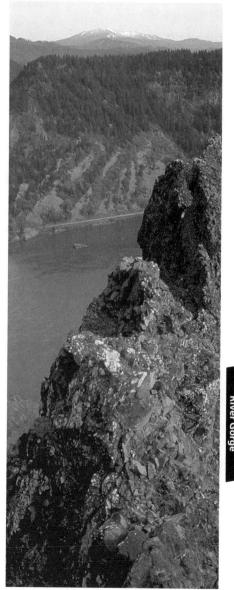

TRIP 25 Hood River Mountain

Distance	1.8 to 2.9 miles, Loop
Elevation Gain	600 feet
Hiking Time	1 to 3 hours
Optional Map	None
Usually Open	March to November
Best Time	Late April to mid-May
Trail Use	Good for kids, dogs OK, mountain biking, horseback riding
Agency	Private property (SDS Lumber Company)
Difficulty	Easy

HIGHLIGHTS You won't find this leg-stretcher in any other guidebook—there isn't even a sign at the trailhead, but this lack of publicity is no reflection on the trail's worth. The stunning view from the trail's end extends from a flower-covered hillside down to the orchards of the Hood River Valley, and up to the horn-shaped spire of Mt. Hood. Few trails provide so much reward for so little effort. If you time your visit for late April or early May, the flower show alone is worth the trip.

This property is owned by the SDS Lumber Company in Bingen, Washington. The company prohibits motorized travel, but it is kind enough to allow public access for all other users. It is important that visitors not abuse this privilege to ensure that respectful hikers and mountain bikers can continue to enjoy this area.

DIRECTIONS Take Hood River Exit 64 off Interstate 84, and drive south on State Highway 35. After 0.4 mile, turn left on East Side Road, and follow it 1.5 miles to the turnoff for Panorama Point County Park. Keep straight on East Side Road, and 0.4 mile after the park turnoff turn left on Old Dalles Road. Drive east on this paved route for 2.1 miles to a saddle beneath a set of power lines. Park on the side of the road, but be sure not to block access to the gated road going north from the pass.

The hike begins by going over a low berm on the south side of the road and following a wide mountain biking trail. The path is easy to follow as it goes through open woods of second-growth Douglas fir, ponderosa pine, and Oregon white oak. In early May the trail is lined with numerous flowering shrubs, the most prominent of which are white-blooming serviceberry and red-flowering current. After about 0.5 mile, the path briefly levels out and then intermittently climbs for another 0.4 mile, before you rather suddenly emerge from the brush at the open, grassy summit of Hood River Mountain.

Sit back and enjoy! Gentle breezes blow over the summit, carrying butterflies to pollinate the many flowers that carpet the open slopes. The most abundant of those wildflowers are yellow balsamroot and lomatium, red paintbrush, and blue lupine and larkspur. Views are superb, with Mt. Adams and part of Mt. Rainier visible to the north, and a snippet of Mt. St. Helens to the northwest. Most spectacular of all, though, is the view of horn-shaped Mt. Hood over the orchards and farms of the Hood River Valley. Convenient flat-topped rocks provide nice "chairs" on which to sit and enjoy the view without trampling the flowers. For

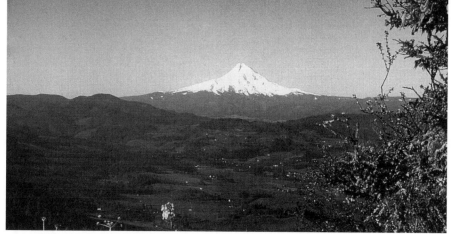

Mt. Hood from Hood River Mountain

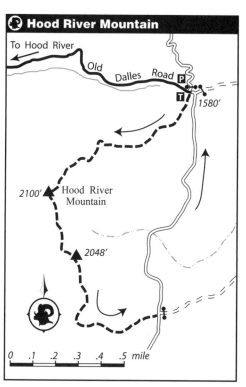

Hood River Mountain

To Hood River

Old Dalles Road

1580'

2100' Hood River Mountain

2048'

0   .1   .2   .3   .4   .5 mile

maximum enjoyment, bring a wildflower identification guide, a good friend, and a picnic lunch.

You could simply return the way you came, but for more exercise, consider making a loop out of this trip by continuing south along the summit ridge. The wildly scenic up-and-down path follows along the edge of a flower-covered meadow that provides great views as you hike. About 0.6 mile from the top, the route curves to the left, away from the summit ridge. You then drop through more meadows to another unsigned trailhead on a gravel road. To complete the loop, simply turn left and walk this little-traveled road 1.1 miles back to your car.

Eastern Columbia
River Gorge

Chapter 6
Mount Hood Area

At 11,237 feet, glacier-clad Mount Hood towers over the forested peaks and ridges of its namesake national forest, serving as the undisputed king of the Portland skyline. The majestic peak also acts as a magnet for outdoor lovers, attracting skiers, anglers, photographers, out-of-state visitors, and pretty much everybody else to its slopes throughout the year. Since a significant percentage of those visitors are hikers, many of the

hundreds of miles of trails here are (justifiably) crowded. With a little effort, however, solitude-seeking pedestrians should have no trouble finding quiet paths to enjoy their favorite pastime.

The mountain offers every sort of terrain and never disappoints. Here you will find our region's best alpine landscapes, its finest wildflower displays, the only glaciers, some of the deepest canyons, and just about anything else in the way

Atop Mt. Hood

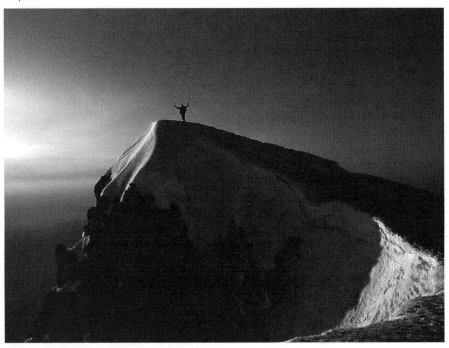

Mount Hood Area

of scenery a hiker could want. With the higher elevations, the hiking season is considerably shorter than in the Columbia River Gorge, Coast Range, or Willamette Valley. So although a few paths along the lower Salmon River are open all year, most trails do not open until at least June, and the highest trails won't be snow free until about mid-July.

Access to the west side of the mountain, the only part of the peak reachable by a one-hour drive from Portland, is from U.S. Highway 26. For most residents, the quickest way to reach this road is to drive east on Interstate 84, leaving that freeway at Wood Village Exit 16. From there you drive south on 242nd Avenue for about 3.5 miles, and then turn left (east) on Burnside Street, which soon merges with Powell Boulevard/Highway 26 on its way to Sandy, Zigzag, and the countless scenic hiking opportunities beyond.

TRIP 1 Douglas Trail to McIntyre Ridge & Wildcat Mountain

Distance	3.0 miles to McIntyre Ridge, Out-and-back;
	3.2 miles to Wildcat Mountain, Out-and-back
Elevation Gain	700 feet to McIntyre Ridge, 950 feet to Wildcat Mountain
Hiking Time	2 to 3 hours
Optional Map	Green Trails Cherryville & Government Camp (with many shorter options)
Usually Open	June to October
Best Time	Late June to mid-July
Trail Use	Good for kids, dogs OK
Agency	Zigzag Ranger District, Mt. Hood National Forest
Difficulty	Moderate

HIGHLIGHTS Although this hike starts in a human-made eyesore, it soon becomes a very pleasant up-and-down ridge walk in the western part of the Salmon-Huckleberry Wilderness. Using this higher-elevation "backdoor" trailhead allows you to let your car tackle most of the uphill, avoiding the long climbs required for other viewpoint trails in this wilderness. In addition, with the closure of the road to the old McIntyre Ridge Trailhead (Trip 2) the Douglas Trail now provides the easiest access to the spectacular meadows of McIntyre Ridge. Visitors are attracted, not only to the easier trail and fine views, but also to the flowers because in early July of favorable years the open woods here come alive with the blossoms of pink rhododendrons and white beargrass.

DIRECTIONS Drive U.S. Highway 26 for 2 miles east of Sandy, and then turn south (right) on S.E. Firwood Road, where the highway makes a sweeping curve to the east. Drive this road 3.4 miles, through two intersections, to a four-way junction. Turn left here on S.E. Wildcat Mountain Drive, and climb this paved road for 9.5 miles to where it enters National Forest land and becomes a one-lane paved road. Just 0.6 mile later, turn right on an unsigned paved route, and continue another 0.8 mile to a junction. You bear right and, 0.2 mile later, park at the far end of an ugly and much abused old rock quarry, now the local playground for all-terrain vehicle enthusiasts and illegal target shooters. To locate the unsigned trailhead, walk about 150 feet east to an upper gravel lot and pick up the obvious trail going east into the trees.

The Douglas Trail, as this foot-and-horse path is called, immediately enters a mountain-hemlock and Douglas-fir forest, with lots of bracken fern, beargrass, and rhododendrons in the understory. Only 250 yards from the quarry, you reach the first highlight, a fine clifftop view looking south to Old Baldy and the heavily forested Eagle Creek drainage. Pinemat manzanita and ground-hugging juniper add to the scenery from this open viewpoint, as do scattered wildflowers like stonecrop.

The trail soon reenters the woods and climbs, sometimes near a generally unseen logging road on your left, to a junction with the McIntyre Ridge Trail. The signpost here is often vandalized by target shooters and may not be standing, but the junction is obvious.

To reach the open meadows atop McIntyre Ridge, turn left at the junction and go gradually up and down through

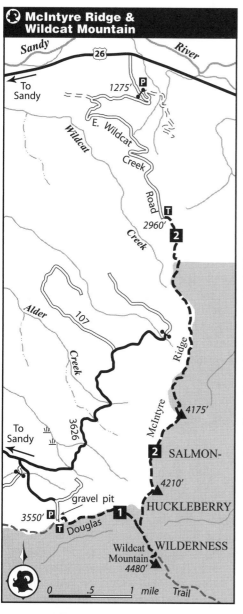

**McIntyre Ridge &
Wildcat Mountain**

Sandy

River

26

To
Sandy

1275'

P

E. Wildcat

Wildcat

Creek

Road

T

2960'

2

Creek

Alder

107

Creek

3626

McIntyre

Ridge

4175'

To
Sandy

2

SALMON-

4210'

gravel pit

3550'

P

HUCKLEBERRY

T

Douglas

1

Wildcat

WILDERNESS

Mountain

4480'

0   .5   1   mile   Trail

forests and thickets of huckleberries. After about 0.6 mile you enter a large ridgetop meadow with a small bench and a knockout view to the east of Mt. Hood. In early summer of favorable years the meadow is alive with wildflowers, especially beargrass, but also a variety of smaller flowers. Look for lupine, cliff penstemon, yarrow, and lomatium, among others. The trail continues to the north passing more viewpoints and pretty meadows, but the first meadow has the best views.

To reach Wildcat Mountain, go straight at the McIntyre Ridge junction and climb steadily for 0.5 mile to a possibly unsigned junction. Turn right and walk 100 yards uphill to the top of the peak. The summit has decent views, although brush and small trees often get in the way.

For athletic types, it is possible to follow the Douglas Trail east for another 6 miles, with access to trails that connect to Huckleberry Mountain (Trips 4 & 5) and Salmon Mountain (Chapter 7, Trip 8).

If you can arrange a car shuttle, another fun option is to leave a car at the Wildwood Recreation Site and hike down off Huckleberry Mountain along the Boulder Ridge Trail (Trip 4). This way the hike is almost all downhill.

Atop McIntyre Ridge

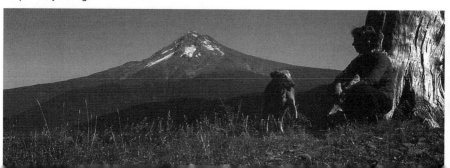

TRIP 2 McIntyre Ridge

see map on p.311

Distance	15.0 miles with road walk, Out-and-back
Elevation Gain	3100 feet
Hiking Time	7 hours
Optional Map	Green Trails *Cherryville*
Usually Open	May to early November
Best Time	Mid-June to mid-July
Trail Use	Dogs OK, horseback riding
Agency	Zigzag Ranger District, Mt. Hood National Forest
Difficulty	Difficult

HIGHLIGHTS Once the best and the easiest ridge walk in the Salmon-Huckleberry Wilderness, the McIntyre Ridge Trail recently became a much longer hike. To combat the extensive damage done by all-terrain vehicles (ATVs), the Bureau of Land Management recently closed the access road, adding 6.4 miles and 1700 feet of elevation gain to the round-trip hike. A shorter approach to the ridge is described in Trip 1, but lovers of the old trail still prefer the longer route for the added exercise, the better forests, and the string of meadows before you reach the end. Hike them both and make your own choice.

DIRECTIONS Take U.S. Highway 26 east from Sandy about 11 miles to Milepost 36, and turn right (south) on E. Wildcat Creek Road. If it helps to have a landmark, this turnoff is right next to a large brown-and-white sign that says MT. HOOD RECREATIONAL AREA—WELCOME. Climb this narrow gravel road 0.7 mile, and park where the road is gated closed.

The hike begins with a 3.4-mile walk up gravel E. Wildcat Creek Road. It is uphill virtually the entire way and rather dull, but never steep. Stick with the main road at all intersections and you will end up at a large clear-cut where several recovering ATV trails obscure the trailhead. To find the hiking trail, follow the motorcycle tracks to the southeast corner of the old clear-cut, where you will see a sign for the McIntyre Ridge Trail in the uncut trees just beyond the clearing.

The gently graded trail does go up and down quite a bit but manages to slowly gain elevation, staying mostly in the forests. At 1.5 miles from the old trailhead, you ascend consistently for about 0.5 mile to reach the first of McIntyre Ridge's fine meadow viewpoints. The most memorable vista, as always, is looking east to Mt. Hood.

Although it is a worthwhile spot for a rest stop, don't turn around at this first viewpoint—better rewards lie ahead. The trail moves inland a little and climbs steadily, in a half dozen small switchbacks, to the edge of a much larger meadow, which is filled with the tough, grassy leaves and tall white blossoms of beargrass. Not every year is graced with good beargrass displays—because the individual plants bloom in two- and three-year cycles—but in off years, other flowers take up the slack, especially lavender cliff penstemon, yellow lomatium and stonecrop, and blue lupine and larkspur.

This meadow, which in addition to flowers has a first-rate view of Mt. Hood, is a worthwhile destination all by itself, but it's hard to stop here. To see more, your first challenge is to find the right trail. The meadow has a couple of confusing unsigned junctions that have obviously led many hikers astray. The proper route goes to the right on what is initially a rather faint path. Soon it gets more distinct and climbs through the trees to a final meadow that is the largest of all, complete with a bench for hikers to sit and rest. Beargrass is even more abundant here, and the views are truly superb, featuring not just Mt. Hood, looming impressively over Huckleberry Mountain to the east, but also west to Portland and the farm country of the Willamette Valley. Bring a sack lunch to enjoy this spot in style.

TRIP 3 Wildwood Recreation Site Trails

Distance	0.8 to 4.0 miles, Loops
Elevation Gain	0 to 100 feet
Hiking Time	1 to 3 hours
Optional Map	Trailhead brochure
Usually Open	All year
Best Time	All year
Trail Use	Good for kids, dogs OK (on leash), wheelchair accessible
Agency	Bureau of Land Management Salem District
Difficulty	Easy
Note	Good in cloudy weather

HIGHLIGHTS In the foothills of the Cascade Mountains near Zigzag, the Wildwood Recreation Site is a wonderful day-use facility complete with picnic areas, interesting interpretive material, and several easy but excellent hiking trails. The site has become justifiably popular with families looking for a quick nature outing and school groups on field trips (weekdays in May are often crowded with schoolchildren). Hikers are also beginning to discover the park, which features a convenient network of gentle trails, nice forest and stream scenery, and access to longer trails into the Salmon-Huckleberry Wilderness (see Trip 4).

DIRECTIONS Drive U.S. Highway 26 east to just past Milepost 39, and then turn right (south) at a sign for the Wildwood Recreation Site. Pay your day-use fee at the entrance station ($3 per vehicle as of 2007), proceed 0.4 mile, and then turn left into the large trailhead parking lot.

There is plenty of exploring to do here and it is all worthwhile. Start with the 0.8-mile wheelchair-accessible Wetland Trail Loop. To find it, take the trail that leaves from the east side of the parking lot just left of the restrooms and soon cross an arcing bridge over the beautiful Salmon River. At 0.1 mile is a signed junction at the start of the loop. Turn sharply left and soon begin walking on a long boardwalk. The trail passes numerous signs informing visitors about the diverse plants and animals that inhabit this area's forest, ponds, and wetlands. Quiet hikers stand a good chance of seeing some of that wildlife, including salamanders and newts, great blue herons, various ducks, red-winged blackbirds, fish, and maybe even a beaver. At four places along the boardwalk dead-end side trails go left to viewing areas over the water. At the southwest end of the loop is a junction.

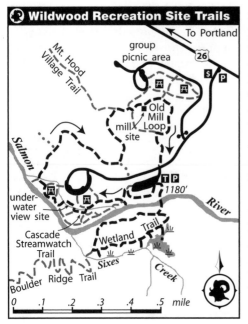

Wildwood Recreation Site Trails

To Portland

group picnic_area

26

Mt. Hood Village Trail

Old Mill Loop

mill site

Salmon

under-water view site

Cascade Streamwatch Trail

Wetland Trail

Sixes

Boulder Ridge Trail

River

Creek

1180'

0   .1   .2   .3   .4   .5   mile

following signs that keep you on the main paved path at several junctions over the next 0.2 mile. Along the way you twice cross a small side channel of the Salmon River before coming to an underwater viewing window that allows you a unique perspective of a forest stream. Here you are likely to see small trout and salmon, snails, mud skipper fish, and other underwater inhabitants usually missed by hikers.

You cross the side channel a third time and then come to a junction. The return portion of the Cascade Streamwatch Trail goes left, but for the longer loop turn right, still on paved trail, and loop around the outside of a dispersed picnic area with some lovely sites right along the river. This is a good place to enjoy lunch under the shade of moss-draped vine maples and towering western red cedars and western hemlocks. You may also be entertained by watching dippers feeding in the Salmon River. In the autumn watch for migrating Chinook salmon.

At the western end of the picnic area loop, turn left at a junction, following signs to the group picnic area. This gravel path winds through gorgeous forest with lush greenery and small forest wildflowers. In April and May look for such flowers as trillium, wood violet, false lily-of-the-valley, bleeding heart, and candyflower. After 120 yards a dead-end side trail goes left on its way to a quiet spot on the Salmon River.

The main trail goes right at the junction, immediately crosses a final bridge over the side channel, and continues its almost level meandering in dense forest. After passing a junction with a closed trail, the now-dirt path goes uphill briefly and then turns right. Another 0.2 mile and you make a 90-degree left turn at a junction with a second closed trail. Several more minor ups and downs take you

The Boulder Ridge Trail goes left on its way to Huckleberry Mountain (Trip 4). To return to your car, turn right and walk along a packed gravel trail that stays fairly close to the clear Salmon River back to the bridge and parking lot.

With more time and energy a longer loop should be next on your agenda. Start at the trailhead information kiosk and go southwest on the paved Cascade Streamwatch Trail. Stylistic blue and white signs identify this trail for its entire length. The first 150 yards travel through the forest between the parking lot and the Salmon River with some nice overlooks of that lovely stream. You then follow a boardwalk downhill to a junction, turn sharply left, and soon come to a four-way junction. For a quick side trip, turn left, hike a few yards down a spur trail to an interpretive display about watersheds, and then walk down to the river to obtain a partial view of Mt. Hood.

Return to the four-way junction, and go straight (northwest) on the inland loop of the Cascade Streamwatch Trail, to a junction with the trail to Mt. Hood Village. Go straight and, just 50 yards later, come to another junction. You turn right this time, walk 25 yards, and reach a junction with the gravel Old Mill Loop Trail. It is slightly shorter to return to the car by turning right here, but it is more interesting to turn left on the loop and soon reach the moss-covered stone remains of an old sawmill. Continue 0.35 mile clockwise around the loop, ignoring a side trail to the group picnic area, to a junction at the south end of the loop. Turn left at a sign directing you back to the Cascade Streamwatch Trail, walk 0.2 mile, and come to a crossing of the paved access road directly across from the turn-off to the trailhead parking lot.

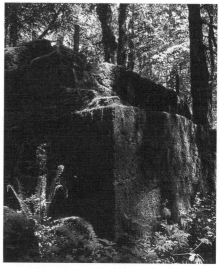

Ruins of an old sawmill

TRIP 4 Huckleberry Mountain via Boulder Ridge

Distance	10.5 miles, Out-and-back
Elevation Gain	3100 feet
Hiking Time	5 to 7 hours
Optional Map	Green Trails *Government Camp*
Usually Open	Late May to October
Best Time	Mid-June to mid-July
Trail Use	Dogs OK
Agency	Zigzag Ranger District, Mt. Hood National Forest
Difficulty	Difficult

HIGHLIGHTS Like most of the ridge walks in the Salmon-Huckleberry Wilderness, the long trail up Huckleberry Mountain provides both good exercise and fine views from the summit. From the small, rocky meadows at the top, you can take in a vista that includes, not only snow-covered peaks like Mounts Jefferson, St. Helens, and nearby Hood, but also the rapidly growing developments around the towns of Wemme and Zigzag, and a whole array of ridges and lower summits spread out in every direction. Tiny wildflowers at your feet are a perfect small-scale complement to the large-scale views.

DIRECTIONS Drive U.S. Highway 26 east to just past Milepost 39, and then turn right (south) at a sign for the Wildwood Recreation Site. Pay your day-use fee at the entrance station ($3 per vehicle as of 2007), proceed 0.4 mile, and then turn left into the large trailhead parking lot.

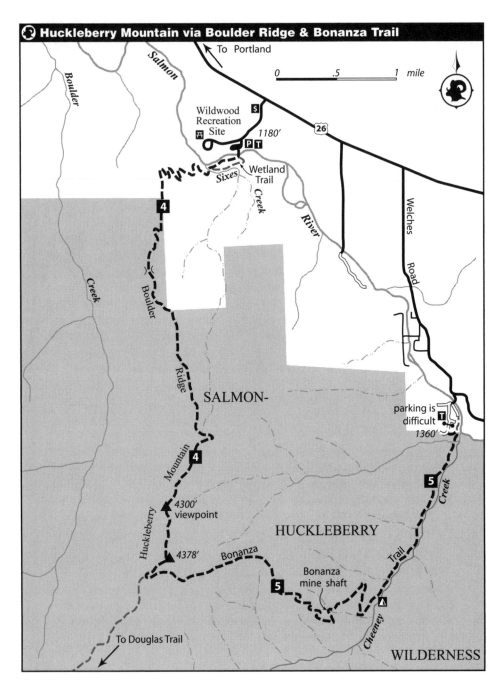

The trail begins from the eastern edge of the parking lot just left of the restrooms and soon crosses an arcing bridge over the Salmon River. At 0.1 mile is a fork with a Wetland Nature Trail Loop, where you go straight and follow the river downstream. The gravel path wanders on the level through a shady forest of red alder and Douglas fir, passes a junction with the upper portion of the nature trail loop, crosses small Sixes Creek on a bridge, and begins to climb.

The first part of the climb is a series of switchbacks and traverses that combine to lead you steadily, but not overly steeply, up a forested hillside. The route levels off a little after about 1.7 miles, where you briefly follow a long-abandoned logging road. Near the start of this section, you are treated to a good view of Mt. Hood and Hunchback Mountain. In June the forests host lots of Pacific rhododendron covered with pink blossoms. In early July, the open areas come alive with foxglove, daisy, beargrass, iris, and other wildflowers.

You enter the wilderness at the 2-mile point in your hike, shortly after which you make two quick switchbacks and climb to a ridge-crest saddle. A short side trail leads to a second good view that extends over the same scene as before, but it is improved by the added elevation. Now you work southeast, ascending along a narrow ridge. At one point you gain an excellent perspective to the west of Wildcat Mountain, McIntyre Ridge, and trailless Boulder Creek Valley.

After more climbing, you leave the ridgetop and cross a north-facing slope with a small, trickling creek, before coming to a ridgeline where the trail makes a sharp right. From here the trail climbs a ridge overgrown with beargrass for a final 1 mile to a fine viewpoint in some rocky meadows on the high ridge of Huckleberry Mountain. The mountain's highest point lies 0.3 mile to the south, but the views are much better here.

TRIP 5 Huckleberry Mountain via Bonanza Trail

Distance	11.4 miles (plus any road walking), Out-and-back
Elevation Gain	3250 feet
Hiking Time	5 hours
Optional Map	Green Trails *Cherryville, Government Camp*
Usually Open	Mid-May to November
Best Times	Late May and June
Trail Use	Dogs OK
Agency	Zigzag Ranger District, Mt. Hood National Forest
Difficulty	Difficult

HIGHLIGHTS The Bonanza Trail provides a less crowded alternative to the Boulder Ridge route up Huckleberry Mountain (Trip 4), but solitude isn't the only good reason to take this trail. The first 1.6 miles follow Cheeney Creek, a delightful wilderness stream with lots of gentle riffles, small pools, chutes, and short waterfalls. The path also passes the old Bonanza Mine, an interesting rocky tunnel that is well worth a look. On the downside, this narrow, sloping path receives only irregular maintenance, so you may have to deal with blowdown and some brush along the route. The biggest problem, however, is with parking. There is no reasonable parking near the trailhead, and local landowners have aggressively discouraged hikers from trying to access the trail (sometimes even towing away cars parked at the trailhead). You can try to park along Welches Road about 0.2 mile away, although parking there is also very limited. The best plan is to either be dropped off at the trailhead, or to park at a distant location and bike to the starting point.

DIRECTIONS Drive U.S. 26 east from Portland to a traffic light in Welches near Milepost 40.5. Turn right (south) on Welches Road, and proceed 2 miles to the junction with E. Bridge Street. If you are looking to park your car, try to find some room on the very narrow road shoulder somewhere in this area. To find the trailhead, drive or walk Bridge Street for 0.1 mile, and then turn left on Grove Lane (the second left after a bridge over the Salmon River). Follow this narrow gravel road past isolated homes and cabins for 0.1 mile to where the road makes a 90-degree left turn. Look here for a possibly unsigned jeep road going straight (uphill) that is blocked by a chain.

Follow the closed jeep road uphill for 0.1 mile, and then veer left (downhill) on a possibly unsigned trail. In 0.2 mile this path makes one rounded switchback and descends to an unsigned junction on the flats near Cheeney Creek. You go sharply right (upstream) and walk 100 yards to another unsigned junction. The trail to the left simply dead-ends at a pool in the creek. You go straight and soon come to a fairly easy rock-hop crossing of an unnamed tributary creek.

The trail's next section is a nearly level ramble through small meadows and beneath a thin canopy of red alders, bigleaf maples, and a few western hemlocks. The hiking is delightful and easy, and you can usually hear, if not see, the rippling water of Cheeney Creek off to the left. At 1.1 miles the trail becomes a little more rugged as it goes up and down just above the lovely creek passing through a moss-draped forest of western red cedars. In May look for thick stands of pink Scouler's corydalis blooming beside the trail. Shortly after a possible campsite at 1.6 miles, the trail begins climbing away from the creek. In two long switchbacks you ascend to the long-abandoned shaft of Bonanza mine.

From here, the narrow and sometimes brushy trail becomes progressively steeper, first in a lengthy uphill traverse and then in 10 irregularly spaced switchbacks. The final mile is gentler, gradually ascending a wooded hillside to a junction atop the long ridge of Huckleberry Mountain.

There is no view here, so to get a better payoff for your efforts, turn sharply right and climb 0.3 mile to the high point of Huckleberry Mountain where there is a small opening with decent views. For even better views, descend along the trail to the north another 0.3 mile to a large opening. Here you will enjoy the hike's best view of Mt. Hood, as well as several nearby creek valleys and forested ridges.

TRIP 6 Hunchback Mountain

Distance	4.0 to 9.0 miles, Out-and-back
Elevation Gain	1600 to 2900 feet
Hiking Time	2 to 6 hours
Optional Map	Green Trails *Government Camp*
Usually Open	Mid-May to October
Best Time	June
Trail Use	Dogs OK
Agency	Zigzag Ranger District, Mt. Hood National Forest
Difficulty	Difficult

HIGHLIGHTS Forested Hunchback Mountain rises sharply from the lowlands around Zigzag and extends to the southeast like a 6-mile-long green finger. Along the way, several knuckles and warts rise up, providing high viewpoints for hikers on the Hunchback Trail. The long, generally lonesome trail has very easy road access and follows the entire length of this prominent ridge, providing hikers with both exercise and good views.

DIRECTIONS Drive U.S. Highway 26 to the east end of Zigzag, and turn right into the Zigzag Ranger Station, almost exactly opposite the intersection with E. Lolo Pass Road. Park in the portion of the large lot just east of the ranger station that is specifically marked for trail users.

The trail starts in the lush Douglas-fir, western-red-cedar, and western-hemlock forests that are so typical of the Portland/Vancouver region. The forest floor is dominated by five different species of fern: ground-hugging deer fern, the delicate fronds of maidenhair and lady fern, and 3- and 4-foot-tall bracken and sword fern. Almost immediately the trail begins climbing up to the first switchback, next to a rock wall that holds back the flow of an insignificant trickle of cool water. Beyond this rocky cistern, three more switchbacks take you to a short downhill section. You will need the respite this provides, as the next 14 switchbacks become increasingly steep.

During the first part of this climb, you hear traffic speeding by on Highway 26. By the time you near the top of the ridge, however, these sounds are only a memory, and bird song and breezes are all that you hear. The thinning soils and harsher environment gradually cause the forests to become more open. Rhododen-

dron, beargrass, and salal are the dominant cover species. After finally topping the ridge and walking around the right side of a little knob, look for a side trail that heads left, back to a viewpoint atop the knob. This view of the Zigzag Valley and a tiny part of the top of Mt. Hood is enough for many hikers, who turn back here, fully satisfied.

To continue to higher viewpoints, stick with the Hunchback Trail as it becomes much more rugged, with lots of steep uphill sections and some downhill sections, always staying at or near the jagged, rocky ridge crest. About 0.5 mile from the knob, you pass another possible turnaround point, at an excellent viewpoint on the spine of the ridge. This view features an unusually good perspective of the many ridges and high points in the Salmon-Huckleberry Wilderness to the south and west. Most notable are Huckleberry Mountain, the Cheeney Creek Valley, Salmon Butte, and Salmon Mountain. Colorful cliff penstemon, stonecrop,

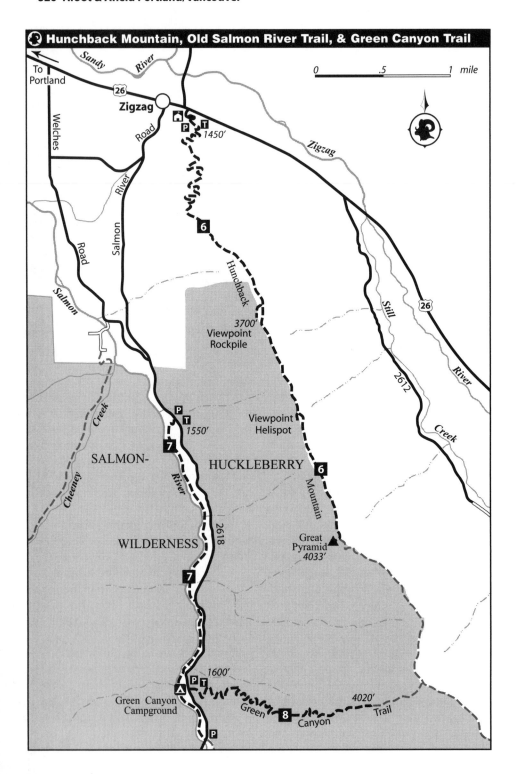

Hunchback Mountain, Old Salmon River Trail, & Green Canyon Trail

To Portland

Sandy River

Welches

26

Zigzag

Road

Salmon River Road

Salmon

Salmon

Cheeney Creek

0   .5   1 mile

Zigzag

Still

26

2612

River

Creek

1450'

6

Hunchback

3700'
Viewpoint
Rockpile

P
T
1550'

7

SALMON-

HUCKLEBERRY

Viewpoint
Helispot

6

Mountain

River

2618

7

WILDERNESS

Great
Pyramid
4033'

1600'
P **T**

Green Canyon
Campground

Green

8

Canyon

Trail

4020'

P

saxifrage, yarrow, and paintbrush grow amid the rocks.

Those who want still more views and exercise should push on, climbing steeply in forests to a signed 100-yard spur trail that goes to Viewpoint Rockpile. The name itself is an adequate description, although it is also worth mentioning that this particular pile of large rocks supports a population of pikas and provides the best views of Mt. Hood on this hike. Back on the main Hunchback Trail, you make a final short climb and then begin a long stretch of gentle hiking. For the next mile, the trail either stays level or makes a gentle ascent, passing through a dense forest with little or no ground cover. Views are blocked by trees, but the hiking is easy and pleasant. As the ridge begins to narrow again, you come to another signed, but sketchy, spur trail to VIEWPOINT HELISPOT 260. The views here are partly blocked by growing trees, but they are worth a look.

After this viewpoint junction, both the ridge and the trail get much narrower and rougher, with many short, steep ups and downs. The path stays mostly on the east side of the ridge, but for one extended stretch it follows a 2-foot-wide rocky catwalk right along the spine. After a final steep climb, you reach a viewless high point and the trail turns right. If you go downhill on the main trail another 150 yards, you reach a final viewpoint spur trail, this one to Great Pyramid. This rocky viewpoint has trees blocking most directions, but it provides good vistas southeast to Devils Peak.

With a car shuttle you can make a long one-way adventure out of this hike. Just continue north over the steep ups and downs along Hunchback Ridge, and then take either the Green Canyon Trail (Trip 8) or the Cool Creek Trail down from Devils Peak (Trip 11).

TRIP 7 Old Salmon River Trail

Distance	5.2 miles, Out-and-back
Elevation Gain	150 feet
Hiking Time	2½ hours
Optional Map	Green Trails *Government Camp*
Usually Open	All year
Best Time	April to November
Trail Use	Good for kids, dogs OK, fishing, backpacking option
Agency	Zigzag Ranger District, Mt. Hood National Forest
Difficulty	Easy
Note	Good in cloudy weather

HIGHLIGHTS Stately old-growth forests and a beautiful clear river are the highlights of this easy hike, which is suitable for children and usually open all year. Another nice feature is that there is no bad season for this stroll, as the scenery changes little from month to month. Anglers should note that this portion of the Salmon River is managed as a catch-and-release trout stream, and fishing for salmon or steelhead is prohibited.

DIRECTIONS Take U.S. Highway 26 to the town of Zigzag, and turn south onto E. Salmon River Road, just west of the junction with E. Lolo Pass Road. Follow this paved route for 2.7 miles to the marked lower trailhead for the Old Salmon River Trail, at a pullout on the right.

The trail wastes no time in plunging down through old-growth western-hemlock and western-red-cedar forests. The dense forests provide plenty of shade, making this a pleasantly cool trip even on the hottest summer day. The canopy of magnificent old trees helps to make rainy winter days more comfortable as you hike beneath a natural umbrella.

In the darkness below the trees, the forest floor is covered with oxalis and sword fern, while mosses drape from every tree limb. As you travel upstream, the trail sometimes approaches the road, so you may see or hear cars, but the murmuring "river music" and the calls of dippers dominate throughout the hike. The gentle path never does much up or down, and it uses quaint little plank bridges to cross tiny tributary creeks.

You drop down to the banks of the rushing Salmon River, and then turn south and begin the gentle upstream walk. Along the way, the trail passes several short side trails to the river that are all worth taking and often lead to excellent riverside campsites. Several short spur routes also go left up to the road if you want to shorten the hike. The forest and river scenery doesn't change much as you hike, but it is so pleasant you wouldn't really want it to. At the 1.5-mile point the trail intersects and follows the road shoulder for 200 yards before returning to the riverside forests in a stand of bigleaf maple and red alder. Above this you enjoy more of the same river-and-forest scenery for the next 0.5 mile, until you come to Green Canyon Campground. Staying near the river, you skirt around the campground and then go 0.4 mile farther to a reunion with the road, just below the large parking lot for the Salmon River Trail.

TRIP 8 Green Canyon Trail

Distance	5.6 miles to highest viewpoint, Out-and-back
Elevation Gain	2450 feet
Hiking Time	3 hours
Optional Map	Green Trails *Government Camp*
Usually Open	Mid-May to October
Best Time	June
Trail Use	Dogs OK
Agency	Zigzag Ranger District, Mt. Hood National Forest
Difficulty	Difficult
Note	Good in cloudy weather

see map on p.320

HIGHLIGHTS Starting from the green depths of the Salmon River Canyon, the Green Canyon Trail climbs a woodsy hillside all the way up to the ridge between Hunchback Mountain and Devils Peak. The U.S. Forest Service reopened this old route in the mid-1980s to give hikers access to long loop options on the Hunchback and Salmon River trails, but the path is worth hiking all by itself. The forests are just as enjoyable in cloudy weather as in the sun, but blue skies are preferable near the top, if you want to enjoy the fine view from there.

DIRECTIONS Take U.S. Highway 26 to the town of Zigzag, and turn south onto E. Salmon River Road, just west of the junction with E. Lolo Pass Road. Follow this paved route about 4.7

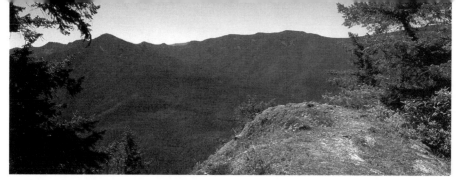

Overlook near the top of Green Canyon Trail

miles to Green Canyon Campground. Directly opposite the campground entrance road, look for a small brown sign for the Green Canyon Trail. Turn into the campground, and immediately park in a small lot on the left side of the entrance road.

The trail starts by crossing a low-lying area of dense shrubbery, under a canopy of old-growth bigleaf maple, western red cedar, and western hemlock, with mosses hanging from nearly every limb. Relatively few birds live in the darkness of this dense forest. Two lively singers who do seem to thrive in this habitat are the winter wren and the chestnut-backed chickadee, which both fill the green depths with their rollicking songs.

The path gradually leaves the rain forest by curving off to the right, switchbacking to the left, and making a long traverse up the hillside. Douglas firs are added to the mix of trees as you climb, and the ground cover is now mostly vanilla leaf, sword fern, Oregon grape, and oxalis with its shamrock-shaped leaves.

The trail makes a series of 15 uphill switchbacks, mostly in forest, but with a couple of small, steep meadows that are home to flowers and some twisted oak trees. Because the uphill is fairly steep and the tread quite narrow, it is not open to horses.

After this first set of switchbacks, you turn left, follow the top of a minor ridge, and then traverse the steep left side of the ridge. When you come to a second ridge, there is a small opening with a nice view up to Devils Peak. From this viewpoint, you go up and down along the spine of

this little ridge and then move to its left side and begin switchbacking again.

At the last of eight switchbacks that take you nearly to the top of the final ridge, there is a junction with an unsigned use path that goes straight for 50 yards to a small, rocky overlook. From this dramatic viewpoint, you can see Salmon Butte and other nearby forested ridges, but the best view is down into the green depths of the Salmon River Canyon, more than 2000 feet below. The impressive scene is enhanced by the many flowers that live here, including lots of larkspur, paintbrush, and a particularly beautiful pink penstemon.

This viewpoint is the recommended stopping point because it is a long way to the next highlight along this route. However, if you are interested in a long, rugged dayhike or backpacking loop, you can continue through open forest along a ridge for 0.6 mile to a junction with the Hunchback Trail. Turn right here, wander up and down (mostly up) for 2.4 miles to Devils Peak, and then continue 1.6 miles to the isolated car campground at tiny Kinzel Lake. From here, you descend a rather steep, switchbacking trail, down to the Salmon River Trail, where you turn right and walk back on this popular path to the road just 0.3 mile from the Green Canyon Trailhead.

Mount Hood Area

TRIP 9 Salmon River Canyon

Distance	7.2 miles to canyon viewpoint, Out-and-back
Elevation Gain	900 feet
Hiking Time	3 to 4 hours
Optional Map	Green Trails *Government Camp, High Rock*
Usually Open	March to December
Best Time	May
Trail Use	Good for kids, dogs OK, backpacking option, fishing
Agency	Zigzag Ranger District, Mt. Hood National Forest
Difficulty	Moderate
Note	Good in cloudy weather

HIGHLIGHTS The Salmon River Canyon is the scenic highlight of the Salmon-Huckleberry Wilderness and has been a popular hiking destination for decades. The first couple miles of this trail travel through one of the best old-growth forests in Portland/Vancouver region, staying close to the banks of the river. After this, the trail traverses steep, forested slopes well above a string of spectacular waterfalls inaccessible to all but the most daring adventurers equipped with ropes and, frankly, not much common sense. But, you don't have to be a risk taker to enjoy this hike—even the main trail provides outstanding scenery, including sloping meadows that allow hikers plenty of great views and a memorable outdoor adventure.

DIRECTIONS Take U.S. Highway 26 to the town of Zigzag, and turn south onto E. Salmon River Road, just west of the junction with E. Lolo Pass Road. Follow this paved route for 5 miles to a large gravel parking area on the left, just before a bridge over the Salmon River.

The trail begins beside a prominent sign on the east side of the road and then works its way upstream on the Douglas-fir-covered slopes above the water. After curving down to a viewpoint above a large, deep pool in the river, you wander lazily through an exceptionally impressive old-growth forest of massive Douglas fir, western red cedar, and western hemlock. Moss hangs from the limbs and covers the trunks of these old giants, while ferns and new young trees grow up out of nurse logs, where some of the trees have succumbed to time and blown down onto the forest floor.

The forest continues to inspire awe as you keep working upstream, passing many glassy pools, small rapids, and quiet riffles in the clear waters of the river. After about 2 miles, you come to Rolling Riffle Camp, below the trail on the right, which is a popular spot for families on summer weekends. Please camp only in the designated sites, to avoid damaging the land.

Shortly after this camp, the trail pulls away from the water and climbs at a gentle but steady grade up the hillside north of the river. You cross several small tributary creeks along the way, allowing you to douse your head if the weather gets too hot for comfort. The trees are smaller now, as these slopes are less protected than the river-level flats, and are subject to periodic wind and fire.

Shortly after climbing out of a good-sized side canyon, the trail splits and a short, pebble-strewn loop path bears to the right, out to an open, meadowy slope

Salmon River Canyon

with outstanding views up the canyon. Almost 600 feet below, the river cascades in the depths of the cliff-walled chasm. This is a rewarding turnaround spot that provides hikers with the best canyon view on the trip.

If you are continuing up the canyon, return to the main trail, and look for several short scramble paths dropping to the right in the next few tenths of a mile. These routes lead to stunning overlooks of towering Final and Frustration falls on the main stem of the river, but the paths are extremely steep. The small rocks on the tread make the route slippery and much too dangerous for anyone who isn't quite experienced and sure-footed. *People have fallen off and died in accidents* *from these cliffs, so take these warnings seriously!*

Most dayhikers turn around here, but really athletic types, and those making this into a backpacking adventure, can continue up the canyon. You traverse, generally on the level to a camp at Goat Creek and then gradually ascend to a junction with the Kinzel Lake Trail. Here you have a choice. You can stick with the Salmon River Trail, which climbs gradually up this lovely, forested canyon all the way to the upper trailhead south of Trillium Lake, or you can turn left on the Kinzel Lake Trail.

The latter path climbs steeply for 2 miles to the primitive car campground at tiny Kinzel Lake, where you meet the

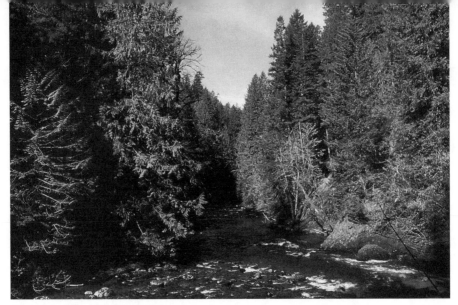

Salmon River near Rolling Riffle Camp

Hunchback Trail. Turn west on this path and follow it past Devils Peak and down to a saddle where you meet the Green Canyon Trail. You can then descend on this trail to the E. Salmon River Road just 0.3 mile north of your car. The total length of this difficult loop trip is 15.7 miles.

TRIP 10 Salmon Butte

Distance	8.6 miles, Out-and-back
Elevation Gain	2800 feet
Hiking Time	4 to 5 hours
Optional Map	Green Trails *Government Camp, High Rock*
Usually Open	June to late October
Best Time	Mid- to late June
Trail Use	Dogs OK
Agency	Zigzag Ranger District, Mt. Hood National Forest
Difficulty	Difficult

HIGHLIGHTS There are two types of hikes in the Salmon-Huckleberry Wilderness: canyon routes that follow cascading streams and viewpoint excursions that start in deep woods and climb to ridgetop vistas. The Salmon Butte Trail is among the best of the latter type. This hike has one big advantage over other viewpoint options; the trail is never steep, and it follows an even, gentle grade throughout. That said, it's still a 2800-foot climb, so be prepared for some exercise.

DIRECTIONS Take U.S. Highway 26 to the town of Zigzag, and turn south onto E. Salmon River Road just west of the junction with E. Lolo Pass Road. Follow this paved route 5 miles to a bridge over the Salmon River, and then continue straight on a gravel road 1.7 miles to a small pullout on the left and an easily overlooked brown sign pointing to the Salmon Butte Trail.

Start by hiking 0.1 mile on an old road that is rapidly being encroached upon by young cedar, Douglas fir, western hemlock, and vine maple. This road ends at an old parking area where the Salmon Butte Trail veers to the left and becomes a true footpath. The trail climbs through an old clear-cut, now so overgrown it's hard to tell it ever was one, except for the universally young age of the trees. You'll know

when you leave the old clear-cut because the trees get taller and the canopy thicker. The deep shade of this old-growth forest leaves the ground largely devoid of undergrowth, but there are lots of old downed trees that require you to take a winding route to avoid them.

The climb remains gradual as you go up a woodsy hillside. You round a ridge at a small rocky meadow with decent views of the forested ridge of Salmon Mountain to the west. The undergrowth becomes thicker as you ascend another hillside that boasts a particular abundance of rhododendrons, which are covered with showy pink blossoms in mid- to late June, the ideal time for this hike. A series of six moderately graded, but irregularly spaced, switchbacks takes you to a tantalizing ridgetop view, where you can see the top half of Mt. Hood.

Now you follow the ascending ridge through a tunnel of conifers, with beargrass lining the trail as you climb. Five more switchbacks take you to a junction with a long-abandoned jeep road. Turn right here, and follow this rocky track another 0.3 mile to the open summit of Salmon Butte, a former lookout site that still sports the fine views typical of such locations. Mt. Hood, of course, dominates the skyline to the north-northeast, but you can also spot Mt. Adams in Washington, and look south to Olallie Butte and Mt. Jefferson. On very clear days you can even see the Three Sisters in the distance to the south.

Mt. Hood from atop Salmon Butte

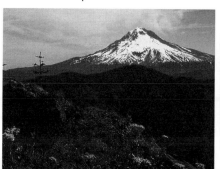

TRIP 11 Devils Peak

Distance	8.0 miles, Out-and-back
Elevation Gain	3200 feet
Hiking Time	4½ to 6 hours
Optional Map	Green Trails *Government Camp*
Usually Open	June to October
Best Time	June
Trail Use	Dogs OK, backpacking option
Agency	Zigzag Ranger District, Mt. Hood National Forest
Difficulty	Difficult

HIGHLIGHTS The logic behind place names is sometimes hard to understand. Consider the Cool Creek Trail to the top of Devils Peak. Far from being evil, beautiful Devils Peak is the perfect sort of place to eat your lunch and marvel at God's handiwork. The Cool Creek Trail is another example. The long climb is anything but cool, and you never even get close to a creek. But, putting aside confusing names, this is a highly enjoyable hike, if you are up for the challenge of a substantial elevation gain.

DIRECTIONS Drive 1.4 miles east of Zigzag on U.S. Highway 26, and then turn right on paved Still Creek Road. After 0.1 mile, you bear right at a confusing fork. Follow the single-lane paved road another 2.8 miles to the end of pavement. Almost 0.5 mile later, look carefully in the trees on the right for a small brown sign for the Cool Creek Trail. Park in a small pullout on the left, about 50 yards west of the trailhead.

The trail starts in a dense low-elevation forest of old-growth western hemlock and western red cedar, with lots of lush moss, deer fern, oxalis, delicate lady fern, and other ground-level species covering the forest floor. It is all very attractive but a little daunting since you know that before the day is done you must climb from this low-elevation forest all the way up to a high-elevation environment. The path wastes no time in accomplishing this feat, foregoing a gentle warm-up in favor of an immediately steep ascent.

Not far from the trailhead, you pass through dense thickets of salal, which, surprisingly, is mixed with beargrass. Normally you don't encounter beargrass until much higher elevations, but on this shady, north-facing slope the plant survives at elevations below 2000 feet.

After briefly following the spine of a minor ridge, you make an uphill traverse to the left and climb a series of short switchbacks to an opening in the forest. The sloping, open hillside looks like it has been selectively logged, which, in a way, it has. In this case, however, the selecting was done not by humans but by natural avalanches and windstorms that toppled many of the trees. The result is a hillside with sparse forests, lots of June-blooming rhododendrons, and your first good views on the hike. From this slope, you can look north to the low, forested ridge of Flag Mountain, farther north to higher Zigzag Mountain, and above them both to glacier-clad Mt. Hood.

After switchbacking up this slope, you traverse to the right and cross a seasonal trickle, which is your only chance to cool off by dousing your head. Continuing uphill, the grade eases off somewhat as you enter a quiet, mid-elevation forest, with lots of 100-foot-high hemlocks,

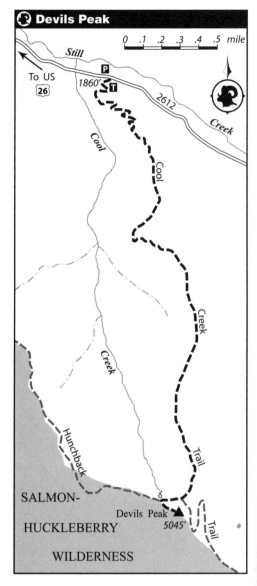

an abandoned section of trail. Here you turn right and resume the gradual climb.

The trees get smaller as you get higher. The dominant species are now mountain hemlock and Pacific silver and noble fir. The final 0.5 mile is up a slowly narrowing rocky ridge, with some excellent views of Mt. Hood. In addition to views, the rocky meadows support a good variety of wildflowers, including wallflower, paintbrush, lomatium, larkspur, phlox, and purple penstemon.

The climb ends at a junction with the Hunchback Trail, where you turn right. Walk about 100 yards on this trail, turn left at a junction, and walk a short spur trail to the top of Devils Peak.

The weather-beaten fire-lookout building at the summit is no longer used for fire detection, but it is kept open as a historic structure and a shelter for backpackers. Views are pretty good from the lookout building, but growing trees now obstruct many of the best vistas. Views of Mt. Hood are actually better from the ridge below. Perhaps the best views from the top are looking south to rounded Olallie Butte and pointy Mt. Jefferson.

Lookout atop Devils Peak

8-foot-high rhododendrons, 3-foot-high huckleberries, and 6-inch-high bunchberries filling all the levels of this ecosystem.

The trail steadily but no longer very steeply ascends through these peaceful woods for about 0.5 mile and then climbs a few steep switchbacks. At the top of these switchbacks are a tiny cairn and an unsigned junction with

TRIP 12 Flag Mountain

Distance	4.4 miles, Out-and-back
Elevation Gain	1200 feet
Hiking Time	2 hours
Optional Map	Green Trails *Government Camp*
Usually Open	Mid-March to November
Best Time	Mid-March to June
Trail Use	Good for kids, dogs OK
Agency	Zigzag Ranger District, Mt. Hood National Forest
Difficulty	Moderate
Note	Good in cloudy weather

HIGHLIGHTS Although mostly a forest walk, the rarely traveled Flag Mountain Trail includes at least one good viewpoint that is an ideal lunch spot. Another benefit of this trip is that the stiff climb in the first mile ensures that you'll get a good workout, despite this hike's short distance.

DIRECTIONS Drive U.S. Highway 26 east from Zigzag for 2 miles to the east end of the tiny town of Rhododendron. Turn right on poorly signed Road 20, a narrow paved route that begins in a tunnel of large trees. Stay on this road for 1.7 miles, past several driveways to summer homes, and then turn left on gravel Road 20-E. About 50 yards later, look on your right for a small sign for the Flag Mountain Trail. There is room to park about three cars on the left side of the road.

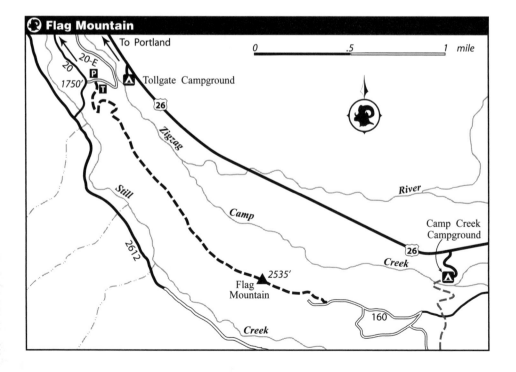

This quiet path starts in a typical, low-elevation forest of western hemlock and western red cedar, with an abundance of sword fern, salal, and Oregon grape on the forest floor. You immediately pass two summer homes and then steeply ascend a woodsy hillside in four switchbacks. You'll hear the sounds of traffic on Highway 26 as you climb, but the cars are out of sight and not overly intrusive. When you top the ridge for the first time, solid forest breaks briefly at a tiny rock outcropping, providing decent views of Hunchback Mountain to the southwest.

Despite never escaping the sounds of Highway 26, the character of this trail remains very wild as you make an often steep climb along the mountain's camel-back ridge. The steep sections are mixed with welcome level bits, until you reach the top, at a fine viewpoint. Here, you get a good perspective of the deep-green Zigzag Valley, Enola Hill, West Zigzag Mountain, and snowy Mt. Hood, which towers over the green ridges. The shrubbery near the summit includes not only the salal and sword ferns from below, but a smattering of such mid-elevation favorites as manzanita and Pacific rhododendron.

This view is the highlight of the hike, but for more exercise you can continue east on the trail as it makes some gently graded ups and downs along the viewless ridge. The last 0.6 mile is nearly all downhill, and you lose about 300 feet in a straightforward descent to a trailhead on isolated gravel Road 160.

TRIP 13 Still Creek Trail

Distance	3.2 miles, Out-and-back
Elevation Gain	300 feet
Hiking Time	2 hours
Optional Map	Green Trails *Government Camp*
Usually Open	March to December
Best Time	April
Trail Use	Good for kids, dogs OK
Agency	Zigzag Ranger District, Mt. Hood National Forest
Difficulty	Easy
Note	Good in cloudy weather

HIGHLIGHTS There is something very soothing about walking through an old-growth forest, and the Still Creek Trail amply demonstrates why. This classic and easy ramble takes you through a quiet cathedral forest with all the lush greenery, deep shade, and impressively large trees that make hiking in our area so good. This is a perfect choice for hikers who want an easy leg-stretcher on a day when the skies are gloomy or the higher Mt. Hood trails are still covered with snow.

DIRECTIONS Drive U.S. Highway 26 about 4.8 miles east of Zigzag, and turn right into the Camp Creek Campground. After 0.1 mile, you turn right on the campground road and drive to the turnaround at the west end. There is room for two cars, directly across from a large pedestrian bridge over the creek.

You begin the hike by crossing the bridge and immediately turning left on the Still Creek Trail. From here, you wander upstream beside the clear water of rollicking Camp Creek, where you can look and listen for gray-colored dippers zipping above the water, and even diving into it, to feed on insect larvae and other prey. The creek's banks are overgrown with a beautiful mix of western hemlock, Douglas fir, western red cedar, and Pacific yew, with long strands of moss hanging from every limb.

The path switchbacks away from the creek and takes you through more old-growth woods, whose shady canopy provides nice cool temperatures even on hot summer days. In April, the forest floor is brightened by the white blossoms of trillium. You cross an unobtrusive one-lane paved road and then wander at an uneven but mostly level grade through a forest of big old trees to a crossing of a more primitive dirt road.

From here, you travel through denser woods and then slowly leave the big trees. You then cross a steeper hillside, where you will hear the splashing of Still Creek, below you on the right. The open forest here is home to perky chestnut-backed chickadees, which break the quiet with their raspy calls. One or two partial openings in the forest allow you to glimpse heavily wooded Hunchback Ridge to the southwest, but this remains basically a forest ramble. The last 0.2 mile drops about 150 feet to a poorly signed trailhead on gravelly Still Creek Road. For a good lunch spot, cross the road and drop to an unofficial car campsite beside lovely Still Creek. Return the way you came.

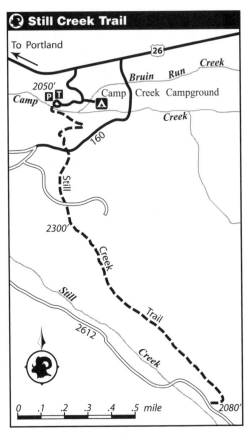

The author on the Still Creek Trail near Zigzag

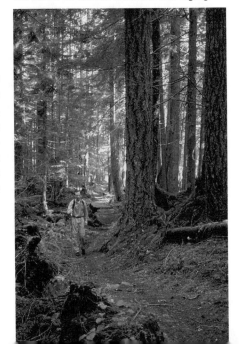

TRIP 14 Buck Peak

Distance	16.0 miles, Out-and-back
Elevation Gain	2600 feet
Hiking Time	7 to 9 hours
Optional Map	Green Trails *Government Camp*
Usually Open	June to October
Best Times	Mid-June to mid-July and mid-August to September
Trail Use	Dogs OK, horseback riding, backpacking option
Agency	Zigzag Ranger District, Mt. Hood National Forest
Difficulty	Strenuous

HIGHLIGHTS The Pacific Crest Trail (PCT) runs 2650 miles from Mexico to Canada through the mountains of California, Oregon, and Washington, but you can tackle short segments close to home. One such segment is the route going north from Lolo Pass. Although the scenery doesn't compare to other trails higher on Mt. Hood, it is still very pleasant, and the view from Buck Peak provides ample compensation for your efforts. Additional compensation comes in the form of delicious huckleberries that ripen in late August.

DIRECTIONS Follow U.S. Highway 26 to Zigzag, and turn north on E. Lolo Pass Road. Climb this good paved road 10.6 miles to Lolo Pass, where the pavement ends and the PCT crosses the road. The best parking is 100 feet down gravel Road 1810, which turns right from the pass.

Pick up the northbound PCT, and walk a short distance through a brushy area to a clearing beneath a set of power lines. While far from natural, this opening provides good views of Mt. Hood, and plenty of sunshine for the abundant Pacific rhododendrons, which bloom from mid-June to mid-July. After the power lines, you reenter a forest of lodgepole pine, Douglas fir, Pacific silver fir, and mountain hemlock. Although there are only a few wildflowers on this slope, in late August and September the huckleberry bushes lining the trail provide an even better treat, or at least a tastier one.

The trail generally stays on the Hood River side of the watershed divide, but occasionally it passes onto the west side of the ridge and travels briefly in the Bull Run Watershed. This large basin provides the City of Portland with its famously clean drinking water. To protect this water quality, hikers are not allowed to travel off-trail, and camping is strictly prohibited. Keeping these restrictions in mind, you make a long, generally uphill traverse of the east side of a forested divide and then round a ridge on the northeast shoulder of Sentinel Peak.

From here, the trail curves left (west) and goes downhill briefly, before leveling off in a long wooded saddle. You then pass two more low, unnamed summits and come to a junction with trail 617, heading down to Lost Lake.

Go straight on the PCT, which travels uphill for about 250 yards and then passes a short side trail leading to a nice campsite beside Salvation Spring. Four uphill switchbacks now take you through an indistinct saddle between two minor high points titled Preacher's Peak and Devils Pulpit.

Continuing north, you stay in the forest on the huckleberry-lined trail as

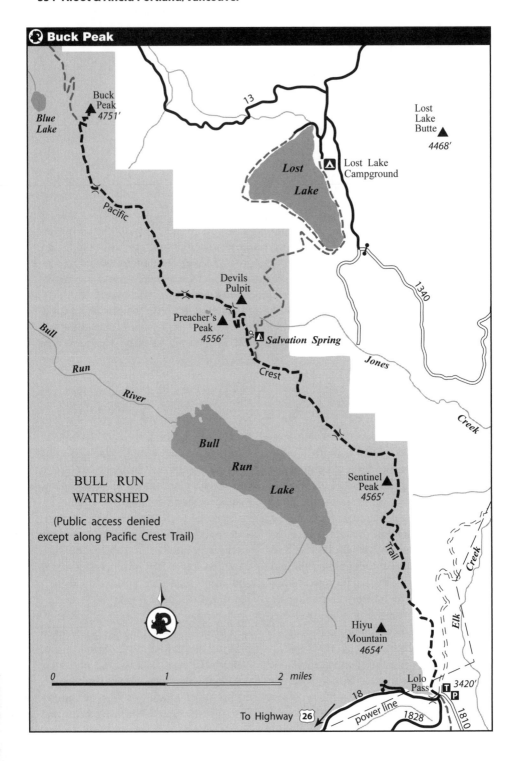

Blue
Lake

Buck
Peak
4751'

Lost
Lake
Butte
4468'

Lost
Lake

Lost Lake
Campground

13

1340

Pacific

Devils
Pulpit

Preacher's
Peak
4556'

Salvation Spring

Crest

Jones

Bull

Run

River

Creek

Bull

Run

Lake

BULL RUN
WATERSHED

(Public access denied
except along Pacific Crest Trail)

Sentinel
Peak
4565'

Trail

Hiyu
Mountain
4654'

0   1   2 miles

Lolo
Pass
3420'
P

Elk

Creek

18

power line

1828

1810

To Highway 26

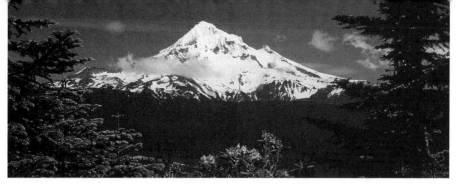
Mt. Hood from the Pacific Crest Trail near Lolo Pass

it drops to yet another saddle, northwest of Preacher's Peak, and regains the lost altitude by going over a rounded knoll. Going downhill once again, you drop to another pass and then climb to a junction.

To reach Buck Peak, turn right at this junction and ascend rather steeply for 0.4 mile to the summit. Views from the top are very good, although not of the 360-degree variety as trees block several angles. Mt. Hood is the star attraction, but you will also enjoy looking east toward triangle-shaped Lost Lake and smooth-sided Lost Lake Butte.

Since you are now 8 miles from the trailhead, you've probably gotten enough exercise. If you want more exercise, however, just go back down to the PCT and keep walking north. You'll hit Canada eventually.

TRIP 15 McNeil Point via McGee Creek

Distance	8.9 miles, Out-and-back or Semiloop
Elevation Gain	2700 feet
Hiking Time	4½ hours
Optional Map	Green Trails *Government Camp, Mount Hood*
Usually Open	Mid-July to mid-October
Best Times	Late July to mid-August and early October
Trail Use	Backpacking option, dogs are allowed (the trail is too rough and difficult for most)
Agency	Hood River Ranger District, Mt. Hood National Forest
Difficulty	Difficult

HIGHLIGHTS For great scenery, you really can't go wrong on any trip near timberline on Mt. Hood. This wonderful outing doesn't disappoint, so bring plenty of film and a sense of awe—both are mandatory for maximum enjoyment. Another good item to bring along is an alpine wildflower guide. The number and variety of wildflowers here rival or surpass any other hike in this book. If you can visit on a weekday, you'll enjoy the views and wildflowers in relative solitude.

DIRECTIONS Follow U.S. Highway 26 to Zigzag, and turn north on E. Lolo Pass Road. Climb this good paved road for 10.6 miles to Lolo Pass, where the pavement ends and the Pacific Crest Trail crosses the road. Take the second right turn, onto gravel Forest Road 1810, and drive 1.5 miles. Then turn sharply right at a small brown sign for the McGee Creek Trail. In just 0.2 mile, this narrow gravel road comes to the trailhead, at a pullout on the right.

Mount Hood Area

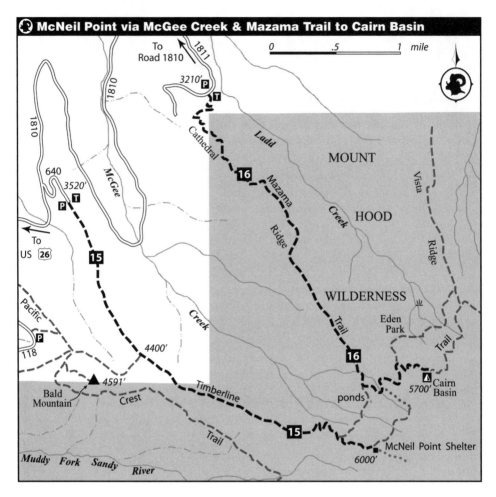

The trail, which is only intermittently maintained, follows a rocky old roadbed for 0.1 mile and then becomes a true footpath in a pretty forest of mountain hemlock, Douglas fir, and Pacific silver fir. The first few miles of trail are lined with wild berries, especially blueberries, which ripen in mid- to late August. The uphill grade is moderately steep for the first 1.3 viewless miles. It leads to a junction with the Timberline Trail and a wilderness permit sign-in station.

You turn left at the junction and continue making a moderate ascent as the trees gradually get smaller at the higher altitudes. Finally, the uphill abates, and the path breaks out of the forest in two large ridgetop meadows with terrific views of Muddy Fork Canyon and Yocum Ridge to the south, as well as Sandy Glacier, on the slopes of Mt. Hood, to the east. Lots of showy wildflowers in July and early August, especially beargrass and lupine, add to the scene. After some small ups and downs, the trail leaves the meadows, reenters forest, and makes four short, uphill switchbacks. Just after the last of these is an unsigned, but obvious, fork in the trail, at a small clearing choked with early August wildflowers.

For the direct route to McNeil Point, you turn right, onto an extremely steep and rugged trail. Please walk carefully, to avoid injuring yourself or tumbling rocks onto others below. It is also important that you stay on the trail to avoid damaging the flowers and trees, which have a hard enough time living in this harsh alpine environment.

The unofficial trail charges up a steep slope initially through a wildflower meadow that sports thousands of "old-man-of-the-mountains" (the midsummer incarnation of western pasqueflower), paintbrush, lupine, bistort, valerian, aster, and groundsel, among other showy blossoms. After the meadow, you scramble uphill, sometimes having to use your hands to crawl over boulders and exposed roots. After 0.5 mile of this lung- and thigh-busting experience, you are rewarded with rather sudden relief at McNeil Point Shelter. This old rock structure sits right at timberline, with only a few wind-whipped whitebark pines and mountain hemlocks in its vicinity. Camping here is discouraged, both to protect the fragile vegetation and to avoid the sometimes severe winds to which McNeil Point is exposed. It does make a magnificent lunch stop, however, and for that purpose, it is highly recommended. You can spend hours soaking in the view of Mt. Hood, the Portland area (all too often hidden under the haze of pollution), and

three distant volcanoes in Washington state—Mounts Rainier, Adams, and St. Helens.

For a gentler return route and a chance to enjoy even more of this magnificent scenery, turn east from the shelter and follow a gently contouring footpath that crosses meadowy slopes and lingering snowfields. After about 0.6 mile, turn left and follow another boot path downhill, through a wide gully with lots of wildflowers. One especially abundant flower is spiraea, whose clusters of pink blossoms saturate the mountain air with a lovely perfume.

Where the use path hits the Timberline Trail, you turn left and quickly pass a junction with the newly reopened Mazama Trail, which goes to the right, down Cathedral Ridge (Trip 16). After this junction, you cross several small creeklets and then go up and down through wildflower meadows. Along the way, you pass two very photogenic snowmelt ponds, before getting back to the junction with the path up to McNeil Point Shelter. From here, you simply return to your car the way you came.

A slightly shorter and *much* more crowded approach to this magnificent area is from the Top Spur trailhead (see Trip 17), but by starting from McGee Creek, you avoid most of the crowds.

Mt. Hood from McNeil Point

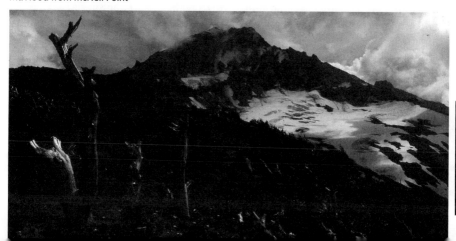

TRIP *16* Mazama Trail to Cairn Basin

Distance	7.2 miles, Out-and-back or Semiloop
Elevation Gain	2400 feet
Hiking Time	3 to 4 hours
Optional Map	Green Trails *Government Camp, Mount Hood*
Usually Open	Mid-July to October
Best Time	Late July to mid-August
Trail Use	Dogs OK, backpacking option
Agency	Hood River Ranger District, Mt. Hood National Forest
Difficulty	Difficult

see map on p.336

HIGHLIGHTS The old trail up Cathedral Ridge was abandoned by the U.S. Forest Service in the 1980s after heavy blowdown made reopening and maintaining this scenic route too expensive. Taking matters into their own hands, members of the Mazamas, a Portland-based climbing and hiking club, used lots of hard work by volunteers to cut through logs and reroute the trail to allow hikers to once again enjoy this scenic path.

The new trail was dedicated in 1994 to commemorate the club's 100th anniversary, and it was officially renamed by the Forest Service in honor of the Mazamas. Local pedestrians owe a debt to the group, as the trail is very scenic and now provides the best-graded option of the several feeder trails on the mountain. Once you reach the famous Timberline Trail, there are all kinds of options for exploring an alpine wonderland that is the match of anything in the American West.

DIRECTIONS Follow U.S. Highway 26 to Zigzag, and turn north on E. Lolo Pass Road. Climb this good paved road for 10.6 miles to Lolo Pass, where the pavement ends and the Pacific Crest Trail crosses the road. Take the second right turn, onto gravel Forest Road 1810, drive for 5.6 miles, and then turn right on Forest Road 1811. Follow this narrow gravel route for 2.5 miles to the signed trailhead parking area on the left.

Start hiking in a recovering clear-cut on a little ridge above loudly cascading Ladd Creek. When the clear-cut ends, you enter forest and come to a wilderness permit and registration box, where you can obtain a free permit. Keep winding steadily uphill on this very well-built path, through a predominantly mountain-hemlock forest with a ground cover of almost solid bunchberry, a plant that features perky little four-petaled flowers in early summer and orange berries in late summer.

The trail switchbacks three times up a large talus slope and then enters a shady hemlock forest with lots of head-high Pacific rhododendron blooming in late June. The trail then makes 14 short switchbacks up to the top of Cathedral Ridge, where a sign marks your entry into the Mount Hood Wilderness. From here, you climb more gradually, generally staying on the ridge's forested west side. As the snow melts in July, these forests come alive with thousands of beautiful white avalanche lilies.

At the top of an extended steeper section, the forest cover breaks, and you enter a gorgeous little ridgetop glade with lots of pink heather blooming in July. Above this, you traverse a heavily forested hillside and then climb beside a small rockslide, through meadows, and past a shallow seasonal tarn. There are great views across this tarn directly ahead to Mt. Hood's rugged north face. Shortly after this is the signed junction with the Timberline Trail.

The possibilities for exploring are numerous and outstanding. The easiest choice is to turn left (east) and go about 0.5 mile over a low ridge and across several small creeks to Cairn Basin, which has excellent camps, lots of flowers, and partially obstructed views of Mt. Hood. From there, you can drop to the wildflower bonanza of Eden Park or just keep going east on the Timberline Trail to Elk Cove, Cloud Cap, and beyond. Another option is to follow unofficial trails up to the McNeil Point Shelter (Trip 15). The most challenging option is to make the tough cross-country scramble up Barrett

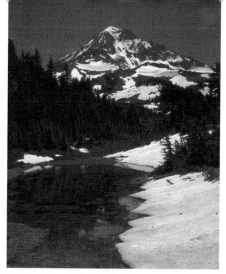

Mt. Hood from Mazama Trail

Spur to where you can look down on either side to the deep crevasses of Ladd and Coe glaciers. No matter what you choose, it's all great, so enjoy!

TRIP 17 Bald Mountain from Top Spur

Distance	1.6 to 10.6 miles, Out-and-back
Elevation Gain	500 to 1900 feet
Hiking Time	1 to 4 hours
Optional Map	Green Trails *Government Camp, Mount Hood*
Usually Open	Mid-June to October
Best Time	Mid-June to mid-July
Trail Use	Good for kids (short option), dogs OK, backpacking option
Agency	Zigzag Ranger District, Mt. Hood National Forest
Difficulty	Easy to moderate

HIGHLIGHTS It's almost sinfully easy to reach the great views of Mt. Hood from Bald Mountain. After a ridiculously short 0.8-mile amble, you hardly feel worthy of being able to sit back amid acres of wildflowers, looking up at a drop-dead-gorgeous view of Oregon's highest mountain. This is an ideal location to show out-of-shape visiting relatives why you rave so much about the beauties of the Pacific Northwest. Locals who feel guilty about how easy it all is or who just want to get more exercise can extend this hike past more great mountain scenery, either up to the alpine country around McNeil Point or on a long loop trip that explores the canyon of Muddy Fork Sandy River.

DIRECTIONS Drive U.S. Highway 26 to Zigzag, and turn north on E. Lolo Pass Road. After 4.3 miles, turn right on paved Forest Road 1825. In 0.7 mile, go straight on Forest Road 1828, and climb this narrow paved route for about 5.5 miles to a junction with gravel Forest Road 118. You bear right here, following signs to Top Spur Trailhead and then continue another 1.7 miles to the trailhead. Parking can be tight here on summer weekends.

Bald Mountain Loop

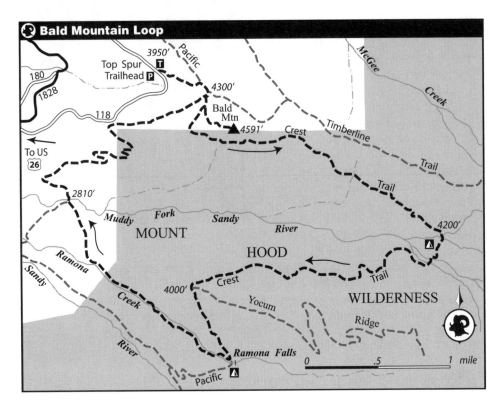

The trail climbs away from the road in a shady, mid-elevation forest of Douglas fir and western hemlock. In season, hikers in this forest can enjoy blooming bunchberries (June) or pick huckleberries (late August). Before you've even had a chance to break a sweat, you come to a junction with the Pacific Crest Trail (PCT), where you turn right. Just 50 yards later you find a confusing junction and a choice of trails.

To visit the summit of Bald Mountain, simply turn slightly to the right, walk south on the PCT for about 150 yards, and then bear left on an unsigned trail. This path climbs for 0.2 mile to the summit, with its up-close-and-personal look at the west face of Mt. Hood. This scene will satisfy most people, but for an equally good view with much better flowers, return to the PCT and walk south, looping around to the south side

of Bald Mountain. The trail breaks out of the trees and crosses steeply sloping meadows with lots of flowers in June and July and even better views of Mt. Hood than you had at the summit.

Hikers who want more exercise and are considering taking the long loop into Muddy Fork Canyon need to take into account that that route requires that they ford the Muddy Fork Sandy River. This ford can be a little tricky in early summer, which is unfortunate, because that is when the flowers on Bald Mountain are at their best. The crossing can also be a problem on hot afternoons when meltwater from the snow and ice on Sandy Glacier swell the stream. If this doesn't deter you, follow the PCT gradually downhill, first across the open hillside and then back into the trees where you lose the view of Mt. Hood. This well-graded path crosses several small creeklets, before coming to a campsite and the ford of Muddy Fork Sandy River. This glacial stream changes its course from time to time, but it usually has two or three main branches spread out over about 0.4 mile. In the morning, you can probably hop across with dry feet, but wading and a sturdy walking stick as a third leg may be required in the afternoon.

Once across the flow, you pass more campsites and begin the winding traverse of the north side of Yocum Ridge. The route has some ups and downs and crosses several small tributary creeks, but it isn't terribly strenuous. The trail is, however, subject to frequent washouts, which require expensive reconstruction efforts and closure of the route from time to time. Before you leave, call ahead to make sure the trail is open.

As usual on a north-facing slope, the cool, wet conditions support dense vegetation of thimbleberry, devil's club, bracken fern, monkeyflower, and other greenery that overhangs the trail, which soak you to the bone when the plants are covered with either morning dew or water from a recent rain. The traverse ends by descending a little before you get to the ridge crest, where you meet the Yocum Ridge Trail.

Go straight at this junction, staying on the PCT, and descend a drier south-facing hillside to a junction just before you reach Ramona Falls. You can get to this extremely popular spot by a much shorter trail (see Trip 19), but the crowds only slightly diminish your enjoyment of this classic cascade, which tumbles veil-like over a basalt cliff face. Backpackers must camp a minimum of 500 feet from the falls, preferably in the designated camping area south of the falls.

For the loop trip, you leave the PCT and travel west down the forested valley of Ramona Creek. Cross and then parallel this beautiful, clear creek for about 1 mile. Cross the creek again and bear to the right, away from the water. Turn right at a junction and almost immediately cross the rushing Muddy Fork Sandy River, this time, fortunately, on a bridge.

The most strenuous part of the trip now takes you up seven long and irregularly spaced switchbacks on a forested hillside. The route is totally dry, so be sure to save enough water to quench your thirst on this final climb. You top out on a ridge and then climb at a more gentle pace back to the junction with the PCT near Bald Mountain.

If you don't want to deal with the ford of the Muddy Fork, a second alternative for a longer hike follows the Timberline Trail east from Bald Mountain. This path goes up along a wildly scenic ridge with lots of views and flowers, all the way to Cairn Basin and McNeil Point. For a complete description of this route, see Trip 15.

TRIP 18 Bald Mountain from Lolo Pass

Distance	6.8 miles, Out-and-back
Elevation Gain	1600 feet
Hiking Time	3 to 4 hours
Optional Map	Green Trails *Government Camp*
Usually Open	June to October
Best Time	Mid-June to mid-July
Trail Use	Dogs OK, horseback riding
Agency	Zigzag Ranger District, Mt. Hood National Forest
Difficulty	Moderate

HIGHLIGHTS The classic view of Mt. Hood from the meadowy slopes of Bald Mountain can be reached by a very short and easy stroll from the Top Spur Trailhead (Trip 17). In some unexplainable way, however, the same view is better when you feel like you've "earned" it by taking a longer approach. One such longer route follows the Pacific Crest Trail (PCT) south from Lolo Pass. In addition to sharing the same famous view, this route has other attributes that you won't find on the shorter alternative.

First, you'll get more exercise, which is, after all, one of the reasons to go hiking. Second, the hike takes you through some very attractive woods that might be worth a visit all by themselves. Finally, even though the destination will probably be fairly crowded, you can at least approach it in relative solitude while you hike.

DIRECTIONS Follow U.S. Highway 26 to Zigzag, and turn north on E. Lolo Pass Road. Climb this good paved road 10.6 miles to Lolo Pass, where the pavement ends and the PCT crosses the road. The best parking is 100 feet down gravel Road 1810, which turns right from the pass.

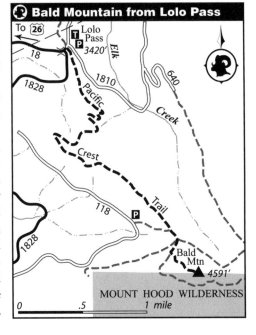

Start on the southbound PCT in an old clear-cut next to the parking area. Trees are now up to 20 feet high here, but the old clear-cut still has an open feeling with lots of beargrass and Pacific rhododendron. In late June and early July, the display of color from these two species is a special treat.

After leaving the clear-cut, the trail enters a hemlock-and-fir forest and climbs at a moderate grade. A dozen switchbacks lead you up a relatively dry hillside, before you switchback again and cross a wetter, more open slope above a small puddle (calling it a "pond" would be an overstatement). Shrubs like thimbleberry, rhododendron, devil's club, and gooseberry have taken advantage of the extra sunshine here to grow in profusion.

After crossing the slope, you reenter forest and hit the top of a ridge where you get a nice view north down the valley of West Fork Hood River. From here, you turn up the ridge and contour around the south side of a forested knoll before returning to the ridge crest. You then gradually lose elevation for about 0.4 mile to a junction with the shortcut from Top Spur. Go straight, and 50 yards later come to a confusing junction.

For the best views bear right, staying on the PCT, and walk about 150 yards to an unsigned junction. To go to the top of Bald Mountain, bear left and walk this use path 0.2 mile to the summit. The view east to Mt. Hood is very good but that's about all you can see because trees block the vistas in all other directions.

For a more photogenic scene, go back to the PCT and loop around in the trees to the south side of Bald Mountain. Here, you enter the huge, steeply sloping meadows that gave Bald Mountain its name. These meadows sport lots of wildflowers and have terrific views of the Muddy Fork Valley and Mt. Hood to the east and Yocum Ridge to the south. Photographs—you'll kick yourself if you forgot to bring a camera—are best in the late afternoon when the lighting is most dramatic.

TRIP 19 Ramona Falls Loop

Distance	6.9 miles, Semiloop
Elevation Gain	1000 feet
Hiking Time	3 to 4 hours
Optional Map	Green Trails *Government Camp*
Usually Open	Late April to November
Best Time	Mid-May to July
Trail Use	Good for kids, dogs OK, backpacking option
Agency	Zigzag Ranger District, Mt. Hood National Forest
Difficulty	Moderate
Note	Good in cloudy weather

HIGHLIGHTS The Ramona Falls Loop has long been the most popular dayhike on the west side of Mt. Hood—hardly surprising since the 120-foot falls is a masterwork of nature, cascading beautifully over a moss-covered basalt cliff in a perfect fan shape. In addition to the falls, the hike allows you to enjoy some decent views of Mt. Hood, as well as a gorgeous walk along a quiet creek in a cool forest. Until recently, this fairly easy hike was even easier because a rough dirt road took you to a trailhead 1.2 miles closer to the falls. The road, however, was miserable to drive, and it forced people to choose between hiking an additional round-trip distance of 2.4 miles and putting their cars through the torture. Flood damage in 1996 closed the road.

DIRECTIONS Drive U.S. Highway 26 to Zigzag, and turn north on E. Lolo Pass Road. After 4.3 miles, turn right onto paved Forest Road 1825, which you follow for 1.2 miles, over a bridge, and then go left at a fork, staying on Road 1825. About 1.5 miles later, you bear left at a junction and quickly arrive at the large parking area for the Ramona Falls Trail.

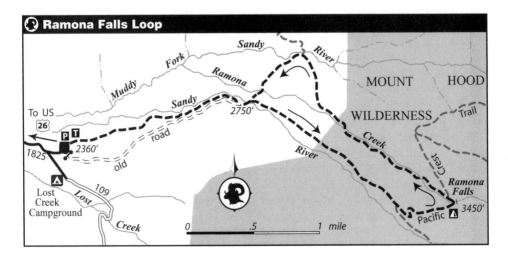

Ramona Falls Loop

The trail leaves from the northeast end of the parking lot and travels up the wide valley of the Sandy River. The trail is sandy and rocky for much of the way, but it does go in and out of some lodgepole pines and hemlocks, providing at least some shade. After about 0.6 mile, the trail meets the closed road and parallels it all the way to the upper trailhead.

Once you reach the old trailhead, you cross the Sandy River on a metal bridge from which you can look up the canyon to Mt. Hood. About 100 yards later is a trail junction amid the short trees and brushy willows of this glacial floodplain. Since this is the start of the loop, either fork will work, but you'll have a slightly shorter trip to the falls if you turn right.

This up-and-down path gradually works up the wide glacial valley of the Sandy River, sometimes near the unstable banks of the muddy stream and sometimes in open forests struggling to survive this inhospitable environment. The area appears rather desolate and is completely dry, so it is better to hike this section in the cool of the morning not the heat of the afternoon.

After 1.5 miles, you reach a junction with the Pacific Crest Trail, where you bear left onto it. You make two quick switchbacks and wander through increasingly interesting and attractive woods for 0.5 mile to a designated camping area. Backpackers should use *this* camp, as wilderness rules require that you camp at least 500 feet from the falls. The falls is a short distance ahead, and it immediately demonstrates why it was worth the hike. The area near the base of this classic falls

Ramona Falls

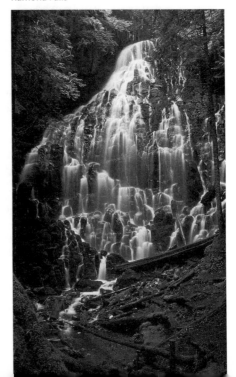

has been beaten to death by admirers, so what vegetation used to exist has been replaced by rocks and dirt, but the falls itself remains as charming as ever.

You cross a bridge at the base of the falls, bear left at a junction, and walk down a lush valley beside strikingly beautiful Ramona Creek. This clear stream tumbles over mossy rocks and flows beside water-loving plants as it makes its way down the gently sloping terrain. The contrast between the shady, green environment beside this stream and the virtual wasteland along the glacial flow of the Sandy River is striking. After the second crossing of the creek, veer right, away from the water.

At a junction near the Muddy Fork Sandy River, turn left (south) and walk a mostly level but very rocky and sandy trail over a low ridge. After crossing a bridge over Ramona Creek, the trail returns to the junction just before the bridge over the Sandy River.

TRIP 20 Yocum Ridge

Distance	17.4 miles, Out-and-back
Elevation Gain	3800 feet
Hiking Time	8 to 11 hours
Optional Map	Green Trails *Government Camp, Mount Hood*
Usually Open	Mid-July to September
Best Times	Late July and August
Trail Use	Dogs OK (but it's difficult for them in places), backpacking option
Agency	Zigzag Ranger District, Mt. Hood National Forest
Difficulty	Strenuous

HIGHLIGHTS Beyond the crowds at Ramona Falls, adventurous hikers can ascend a long ridge on the western spur of Mt. Hood to one of the most dramatic places in Oregon. The flowers, views, and close-up looks at the towering rocks and jagged glacial ice of Oregon's highest mountain are truly memorable.

The name Yocum Ridge honors an important man in the history of this part of Oregon. Oliver C. Yocum was only a boy when he emigrated to Oregon with his family in 1847. He made his mark on the state decades later as the developer of the Government Camp hotel and resort, still the most popular tourist area on Mt. Hood. As a long-time resident and climber, he probably guided more people to the top of Mt. Hood than any other person has. There is no better place to absorb the scenery and admire this early resident's exploits than atop the alpine ridge bearing his name.

DIRECTIONS Drive U.S. Highway 26 to Zigzag, and turn north on E. Lolo Pass Road. After 4.3 miles, turn right onto paved Forest Road 1825, which you follow for 1.2 miles, over a bridge, and then go left at a fork, staying on Road 1825. About 1.5 miles later, you bear left at a junction and quickly arrive at the large parking area for the Ramona Falls Trail.

The sandy trail leaves from the northeast end of the parking lot and travels up the wide valley of the Sandy River. After about 0.6 mile, the trail meets a closed road and parallels it all the way to an old, upper trailhead. Now you cross the Sandy River on a metal bridge and, about 100 yards later, turn right at a

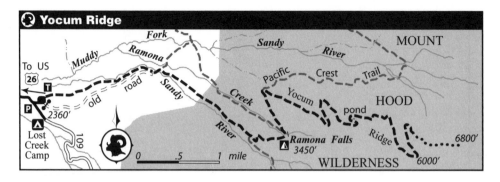

junction. From here you walk an up-and-down path up the wide and rather desolate glacial valley of the Sandy River.

After 1.5 miles, you reach a junction with the Pacific Crest Trail (PCT), where you bear left onto it, make two quick switchbacks, and go 0.5 mile to Ramona Falls. You cross a bridge below this lovely cascade, then turn right onto the PCT at a junction, and go gradually up a hillside past dripping, moss- and fern-covered cliffs. At the top of the ridge, you meet the Yocum Ridge Trail and turn right.

This path goes up the south side of the wooded ridge, often traveling through jungles of Pacific rhododendron, where spiders put up thousands of webs for the first hiker of the day to break through. You pass a rocky slope and then switchback up to the wide summit of the ridge. Another long switchback with occasional steep sections takes you up to a tiny shallow pond. Beyond the pond, the forest

gradually becomes more open and the meadows more attractive as you continue gaining elevation. In early summer, these openings come alive with masses of yellow glacier lilies and white avalanche lilies.

All around you now is some of the most beautiful country in Oregon. The trail passes through gorgeous sloping meadows with scattered subalpine fir and mountain hemlock adding scenic contrast. Flowers abound, including bistort, columbine, beargrass, lupine, paintbrush, wallflower, larkspur, and so many others that it would take pages to list them all. The most awe-inspiring scenery starts when you arrive at a stunning overlook above steep-walled Sandy River Canyon, where you can look up to the craggy ice sheet of Reid Glacier. An adjective like "dramatic" hardly seems adequate.

The main trail switchbacks to the left from this viewpoint, going up the ridge

Mt. Hood from Yocum Ridge

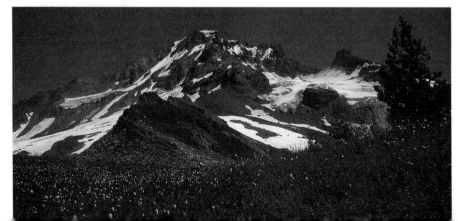

beneath some towering rock formations. When you top out on the ridge crest, the trail turns to the right and climbs up the spine of the ridge. You soon climb above treeline and wander through alpine terrain that features unrestricted views, ranging from Mt. Rainier in the north to Mt. Jefferson to the south.

Finally, the diminishing trail comes to a rocky cliff, which athletic hikers can scale by steep, but not overly dangerous, routes up snowfields to a glorious alpine plateau. Follow this high ridge as far as you like; it leads all the way to the base of Sandy and Reid glaciers. Just sitting back and enjoying the incredible views is more than enough for most hikers. On hot afternoons, hikers are often startled by loud cracking sounds coming from the moving ice of the glaciers.

Backpackers can haul their sleeping bags up to this paradise to enjoy gorgeous sunsets and the nighttime lights of the city of Portland. If you want to enjoy this experience, however, keep in mind that the area is extremely fragile and that the only available water is obtained from the semipermanent snowfields. If you are not backpacking, be sure to leave enough time to make the long walk back to your car.

TRIP 21 Cast Lake & Ridge

Distance	11.2 miles, Out-and-back or Loop
Elevation Gain	2500 feet
Hiking Time	5½ to 6 hours
Optional Map	Green Trails *Government Camp*
Usually Open	Mid-June to October
Best Times	Mid-July and mid- to late August
Trail Use	Dogs OK, backpacking option, fishing, horseback riding
Agency	Zigzag Ranger District, Mt. Hood National Forest
Difficulty	Difficult

HIGHLIGHTS There are three big attractions in the Zigzag Mountain area: acres of blooming beargrass, fields of scrumptious huckleberries, and lots of outstanding views of Mt. Hood and beyond. Any one of these features would be more than enough to recommend a hike here.

The trail up Cast Ridge includes all three attractions, making for something close to hiking perfection. If you've come to see the beargrass in mid-July, keep in mind that beargrass plants bloom in two- and three-year cycles. As a result, in some years almost none bloom, but every six years, when the two- and three-year cycles coincide, the displays of tall white blossoms are breathtaking. Huckleberries are more consistent than beargrass. In the latter part of August these open ridges produce a tasty feast for both hikers and black bears. Most consistent of all, of course, is the view. On any clear day, Mt. Hood's snowy massif rises impressively to the northeast.

DIRECTIONS Follow U.S. Highway 26 to Zigzag, and turn north on E. Lolo Pass Road. After 4.3 miles, turn right onto paved Forest Road 1825, and drive 1.2 miles, over a bridge and to a junction. Turn right on Road 380, following signs to the Horseshoe Ridge Trail, and go 0.5 mile, passing Riley Horse Camp, to a small sign for the Cast Creek Trail on your left. Just past the trailhead is a small parking pullout on the right.

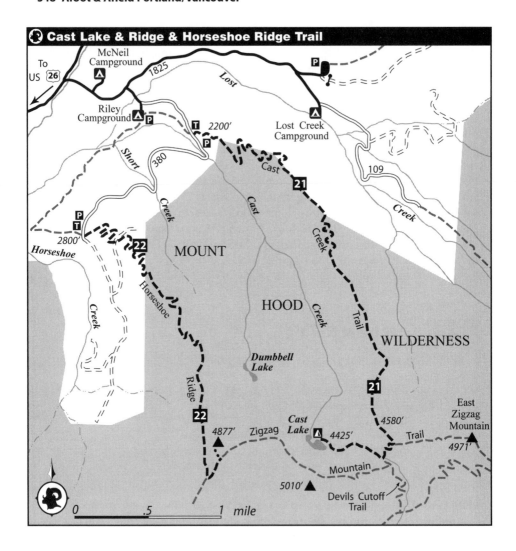

Cast Lake & Ridge & Horseshoe Ridge Trail

The dusty, horse-pounded route makes long, moderately steep traverses and switchbacks in a cool forest of western hemlock, Douglas fir, and western red cedar. This trail used to be a rather steep footpath, until the U.S. Forest Service, largely for the benefit of equestrians, rerouted the trail and added several new switchbacks. The uphill grade is much gentler now, but the trail is also 1.5 miles longer.

At the 13th switchback, you come to an obvious but viewless ridgeline. Here, the undergrowth abruptly changes to a distinctive mid-elevation mix of rhododendron, manzanita, and beargrass. From here, you stay level—even lose some elevation—as you travel east along the ridgetop for the next 0.5 mile. After the climbing resumes, 10 gradual switchbacks lead to some breaks in the trees, providing partial views of snowy Mt. Hood. By this time, the trees are smaller specimens, mostly western white pine and lodgepole pine. In July, it is also near here that you start to encounter more wildflowers and the first of the soon-to-be-abundant huckleberry bushes. The last 0.3 mile of the trail follows a view-packed, mostly open ridge.

At the junction with the Zigzag Mountain Trail, you have a choice of destinations. To the left, the best high viewpoint in the area, East Zigzag Mountain, is only 0.5 mile away. If you prefer a swim, turn right and go downhill a few hundred yards to the Cast Lake Trail. You turn right here and hike 0.4 mile to this pleasant lake with its fair to good camps and fine swimming opportunities. Unfortunately, there is no good view of Mt. Hood from the lake, and the shore is brushy in spots. Nevertheless, this is the only reliable water in the area.

Backpackers spending the night at Cast Lake, or fit dayhikers making the loop connection to the Horseshoe Ridge Trail (Trip 22) can explore beyond the Cast Lake turnoff. To do so, stick with the trail toward West Zigzag Mountain as it passes through a pretty little meadow with lots of pink spiraea in July and early August. Shortly after this meadow, you turn right at the junction with the Devils Cutoff Trail and climb, sometimes steeply, to some of the finest beargrass and huckleberry meadows in the state of Oregon. If you are continuing on to the Horseshoe Ridge Trail, you pass through many lovely meadows before reaching the trail junction, which is about 0.1 mile past an obvious high point in the ridge.

TRIP 22 Horseshoe Ridge Trail

Distance	6.3 miles, Out-and-back or Loop
Elevation Gain	2100 feet
Hiking Time	6 hours
Optional Map	Green Trails *Government Camp*
Usually Open	Mid-June to October
Best Times	Mid-July and mid- to late August
Trail Use	Dogs OK, horseback riding
Agency	Zigzag Ranger District, Mt. Hood National Forest
Difficulty	Difficult

see map on p.348

HIGHLIGHTS This pleasant hike has all the attractions of the neighboring Cast Creek Trail (Trip 21)—huckleberries, views, and beargrass, but it also has at least one big advantage over the other trail. It gets a lot less horse traffic and so is less dusty and more pleasant for the hiker.

DIRECTIONS Follow U.S. Highway 26 to Zigzag, and turn north on E. Lolo Pass Road. After 4.3 miles, turn right onto paved Forest Road 1825, and drive 1.2 miles, over a bridge and to a junction. Turn right on Road 380, following signs for the Horseshoe Ridge Trail, and go 2.1 miles to a small sign for the trail on your left. There is room for a few cars at a pullout near the trailhead.

The path is uphill all the way, and it wastes no time on preliminaries. You begin with six quick switchbacks in dense forests and then make a diagonal crossing of a closed road. Beyond the road, the trail continues uphill at a steady, sometimes tiring pace through a viewless forest of Douglas fir, western hemlock, and western red cedar.

This terrain is made for switchbacks, and the trail succumbs to this necessity with 16 sharp turns and several rounded curves that amount to long switchbacks. As you near the upper reaches of the ascent, the ground cover becomes a thick green mat dominated by oxalis the vanilla leaf, star-flowered smilacina, and other plants that provide variety.

After finally leaving the trees, you contour across the open southwest side of the ridge through a meadow covered with huckleberries and various wildflowers. Look for beargrass, goldenrod, paintbrush, lupine, and fireweed. Plan on spending plenty of extra time enjoying the flowers or picking huckleberries.

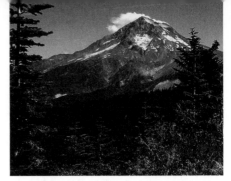

Mt. Hood from the Zigzag Mountain Trail

At the top of the ridge, there is a junction with the Zigzag Mountain Trail. To quickly reach the best viewpoint in the area, turn left for 0.1 mile, and then scramble a few yards to the top of an obvious high point to a first-rate lunch spot with an excellent view of bulky Mt. Hood, which is not far to the northeast. For details on a fine loop-trip possibility, see the description for the Cast Creek Trail (Trip 21).

TRIP 23 West Zigzag Mountain from Zigzag

Distance	11.0 miles, Out-and-back
Elevation Gain	3200 feet
Hiking Time	6 to 7 hours
Optional Map	Green Trails *Government Camp*
Usually Open	Late May to October
Best Times	June and July
Trail Use	Dogs OK
Agency	Zigzag Ranger District, Mt. Hood National Forest
Difficulty	Difficult

HIGHLIGHTS The trail up to the old lookout site atop West Zigzag Mountain has a lot in common with other ridge walks southwest of Mt. Hood. Like the others, it's quite a long way to the top of West Zigzag Mountain, so this is a good choice for a conditioning hike. Also like the other ridge walks, this one features fine views from the top, with lots of wildflowers and plenty of tasty huckleberries to enjoy along the way. Unlike most of the other ridge walks, however, this trail is rarely steep. It makes its way gradually up a long series of switchbacks, rather than charging directly up the wooded slopes. Another advantage of this trail is that its southern exposure allows it to open for hiking two or three weeks before most of the others. Bring plenty of water—none is available on the trail.

DIRECTIONS Drive U.S. Highway 26 to Zigzag, and turn north on E. Lolo Pass Road. You cross a bridge over Zigzag River, and 0.3 mile from Highway 26 turn right on pothole-covered E. Mountain Drive. After 0.7 mile the road ends at a gate.

◉ West Zigzag Mountain & Castle Canyon

The trail starts right beside the gate and immediately begins the steady uphill pace that will prevail for the first 4 miles. The grade is deceptively gentle, so you may be tempted to start out at too fast a pace. Don't use up all your energy here because the gentle grade is unrelenting and will eventually slow you down to a crawl if you don't conserve some energy.

The climb features no real highlights, as there aren't any good viewpoints, splashing creeks, or other reasons to make a stop. The entire route is heavily forested, a blessing for the welcome shade it provides on this long climb. To sustain your interest, you can just count switchbacks. More interesting is to study the subtle changes in vegetation that occur as you climb.

At the start are the usual forests of Douglas fir, western hemlock, and western red cedar, with vine maple, sword fern, Oregon grape, and salal being the dominant species on the forest floor. Farther up the ridge, Pacific silver fir and western white pine are added to the mix, and Pacific rhododendron is now the most abundant shrub. In June, this latter species puts on a marvelous show of pink blossoms. Higher still on the ridge, you encounter Alaska yellow cedar, Engelmann spruce, and mountain hemlock, together with beargrass and tough-limbed manzanita bushes. Also in this zone are huckleberry bushes, which become increasingly common as you near the top. These vegetative milestones track your uphill progress, encouraging you to keep on trudging.

The first 16 switchbacks take you close to a ridge crest, which you then follow on an uphill traverse to the east. After this, six more switchbacks draw you close to another ridgeline, which you ascend. By now, your thigh and calf muscles will recognize the pattern. Their complaints finally stop as you top out on the ridge, at a rather disappointing viewpoint near the high point of West Zigzag Mountain. Trees block most of the views, but you can peer through them to the east and

Mount Hood Area

northeast to East Zigzag Mountain and Mt. Hood.

If you aren't exhausted from the climb, continue southeast, along the mountain's ridge, to a series of much more satisfying viewpoints. The trail here goes up and down, working its way past rocky outcroppings and cliff edges, where you trade the views of Mt. Hood on one side for views of the Zigzag River Valley on the other. A switchback and a narrow ridge-crest traverse take you to a final dramatic viewpoint at the former site of the West Zigzag Lookout. Tiny alpine wildflowers like phlox, stonecrop, and larkspur cannot compete for your attention with the magnificence of the views.

Once you've soaked in all the scenery you and your camera can handle, brace your knees and return down all those switchbacks to your car.

TRIP 24 Castle Canyon

see map on p.351

Distance	1.8 miles, Out-and-back
Elevation Gain	800 feet
Hiking Time	1 hour
Optional Map	Green Trails *Government Camp*
Usually Open	March to December
Best Time	April to June
Trail Use	Dogs allowed, but not recommended.
Agency	Zigzag Ranger District, Mt. Hood National Forest
Difficulty	Moderate
Note	Good in cloudy weather

HIGHLIGHTS This short but rewarding leg-stretcher is close to busy U.S. Highway 26 but a world away from the hustle and bustle of that traffic-plagued thoroughfare. Here you will enjoy a quiet forest, fascinating geology and some reasonably good viewpoints. Another benefit is the good workout this short but rather strenuous path provides. It also will not take up too much of your time if you are on your way to more distant destinations.

DIRECTIONS For the shortest approach, drive U.S. Highway 26 for 1.8 miles east from Zigzag to Rhododendron. At the west end of town, turn sharply left (north) on E. Littlebrook Lane (which almost immediately becomes E. Arlie Mitchell Road), a narrow paved route that you should follow for 0.3 mile to a junction. Bear left here and follow signs for the BARLOW ROAD ROUTE. Drive 0.4 mile on a pothole-covered dirt road past driveways of summer homes to the Castle Canyon Trailhead on the right. Since there is virtually no legal parking here (all of the driveways are conspicuously signed to keep hikers from parking in or near them), you may be better off starting this hike 0.9 mile to the west at the West Zigzag Mountain Trailhead (see Trip 23).

From that parking area you simply walk the washed out and permanently closed road between the two trailheads. The additional 1.8 miles of round-trip walking is pleasant and doesn't make the overall hike too long, considering the shortness of the path up Castle Canyon.

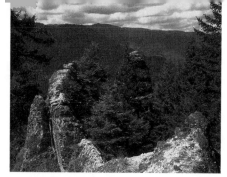
View from end of Castle Canyon Trail near Zigzag

From the Castle Canyon Trailhead, the trail climbs gradually in trees for a short distance to a wilderness permit station and then continues its gentle, woodsy ascent. A series of short switchbacks signals an increase in the grade, as you gain elevation rapidly up the spine of a little ridge. The slope is covered with trees but gradually provides a more open feeling with occasional glimpses of the steep sides of West Zigzag Mountain. The steep climb continues as you round the side of the rock pinnacles that give this trail its name. The ancient spires, part of an exposed volcanic dike, are covered with moss, ferns, and small shrubs that cling to the poor soil amid the rocks.

The trail ends with a final steep push to a rather disappointing overlook amid the rocks. Only very daring, sure-footed hikers should contemplate further exploration down the knife-edge spine of the rocky ridge. The route is dangerous but leads to some nice viewpoints of the Zigzag area. Although it is difficult to get a decent view of the rock pinnacles themselves, the looks at the valley below and the distant ridges in the Salmon-Huckleberry Wilderness are ample compensation.

TRIP 25 Burnt Lake & East Zigzag Mountain

Distance	9.6 miles, Out-and-back
Elevation Gain	2400 feet
Hiking Time	4½ to 6 hours
Optional Map	Green Trails *Government Camp*
Usually Open	Late June to October
Best Time	July
Trail Use	Dogs OK, backpacking option, fishing
Agency	Zigzag Ranger District, Mt. Hood National Forest
Difficulty	Difficult

HIGHLIGHTS Second only to Ramona Falls, Burnt Lake is the most popular hiking destination on the west side of Mt. Hood. This popularity is well deserved and not just because this it is one of the few lakes in the Mount Hood Wilderness. The view across the swimmable waters of this 8-acre pool is picture-perfect. The lake also has picnicking and camping spots that are ideal for an easy backpacking trip or for eating lunch while contemplating the glories of the outdoors.

Just don't expect to be lonesome. People have flocked here for years in numbers that recently led the U.S. Forest Service to consider restrictions on the number of hikers allowed to visit the lake. For the time being, land managers are relying on volunteers to enforce wilderness regulations designed to protect the land. Please be a good outdoor citizen, and do your part to keep these voluntary rules from becoming mandatory limits on our hiking options. You can enjoy a bit more solitude, as well as views that extend for hundreds of miles, by continuing your hike to East Zigzag Mountain.

Burnt Lake & East Zigzag Mountain

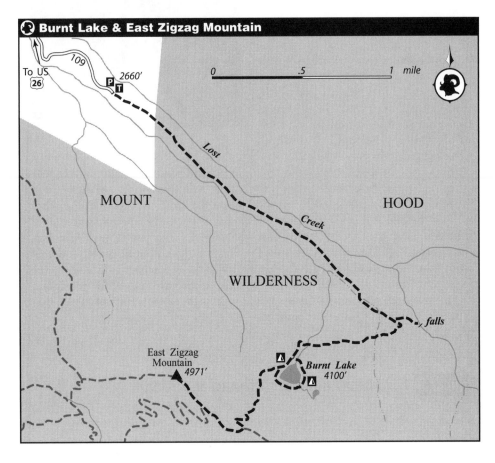

DIRECTIONS Follow U.S. Highway 26 to Zigzag, and turn north on E. Lolo Pass Road. After 4.3 miles, turn right onto paved Forest Road 1825, which you follow for 1.2 miles, over a bridge. Go left at a fork, still staying on Road 1825, and about 1.5 miles later, bear right at a junction where the road going left leads to Ramona Falls. Stay on the right-hand road (Forest Road 109) as it changes from pavement to rough gravel and climbs 1.6 miles to a trailhead and parking area at the end of the road. This road is very narrow and winding, so drive slowly and be on the lookout for oncoming traffic.

The first 1.8 miles of this hike are very gentle, as the trail gradually works its way up between two parallel creeks on either side of a narrow valley. The heavy forest cover provides lots of welcome shade, while tiny forest wildflowers add some color. It's a very pleasant forest walk, despite the absence of views.

Just after crossing a small creek, you start on a newly rerouted section of trail, which is much better graded than the old switchbacking route. The gentle uphill takes you to a junction with a 100-yard spur trail, which goes left to a cascading waterfall on Lost Creek and then makes a switchback. From here, you make a long, steadily ascending traverse on a shady hillside covered with fir and hemlock, whose shade helps to keep tired hikers from becoming overheated.

For views, you get only occasional glimpses, but that changes as you cross the clear outlet creek of Burnt Lake and come to the northwest shore of the lake a few hundred yards later. A trail circles the lake, and several designated campsites are set back from the shore. As always, avoid damaging the fragile shoreline vegetation by camping too close to the water. The most photogenic views of Mt. Hood are from the west and southwest shores.

To continue your hike to the viewpoint at East Zigzag Mountain, keep hiking on the main trail as it pulls away from the lake. The trail up to the ridgeline south of Burnt Lake has also been rerouted in recent years, changing what used to be a rather steep ascent into a longer but much more comfortable climb. The first part of the hike crosses relatively gentle terrain with lots of forest openings. The final part of the climb switchbacks up a steep, north-facing hillside, whose dense forests provide shade for lingering snow patches early in the season.

Turn right at a junction on the ridgeline and then climb a little farther to a second junction. Go straight, and climb quite steeply for the next 0.3 mile over increasingly rocky and open terrain to the top of East Zigzag Mountain. Views extend in all directions, but the best is to the east, over the basin that holds Burnt Lake and up to shining Mt. Hood.

TRIP 26 West Zigzag Mountain from Enola Hill

Distance	5.0 miles, Out-and-back or Loop
Elevation Gain	1300 feet
Hiking Time	3 hours
Optional Map	Green Trails *Government Camp*
Usually Open	June to October
Best Time	Mid-June to July
Trail Use	Dogs OK
Agency	Zigzag Ranger District, Mt. Hood National Forest
Difficulty	Moderate

HIGHLIGHTS The Enola Hill Road provides a sneaky sort of backdoor approach to the Zigzag Mountain area, avoiding the long uphill hikes that other trips require. Here, your car does most of the work, so you might think that most hikers would opt for this alternative. Relatively few do so because most hikers don't want to put their cars through the ordeal. The dirt road is passable for passenger cars, but it's a slow go and not much fun to drive. Take this approach only if you think your car is in better shape than you are!

DIRECTIONS Drive 1.5 miles east of Rhododendron on U.S. Highway 26, and turn left (north) onto paved Forest Road 27. After 0.6 mile, this narrow road turns to rough gravel, switchbacks sharply to the left, and climbs a heavily wooded hillside. The road affords you little room to pass oncoming traffic, so take it slow and be prepared to back up to the nearest pullout if you meet a car coming down the hill. Actually, you won't be going very fast anyway, as the road is miserably rutted with rocks, potholes, and deep mud holes.

At a major switchback to the left, take the time to get out of your car and enjoy the view of a tall waterfall in Devils Canyon. The road ends 5.2 miles from the highway at a small trailhead parking area.

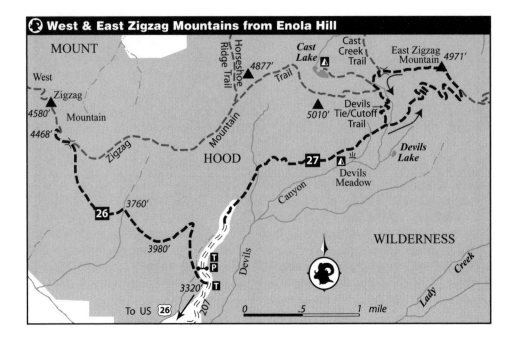

Two trails leave from this trailhead. By far the more popular follows a long-abandoned section of the Enola Hill Road heading northeast up Devils Canyon (see Trip 27). For the trail to West Zigzag Mountain, walk back down the road about 150 feet to a small sign for West Zigzag Trail #789. This trail is not maintained as regularly as most others in the Zigzag area, so you can expect to crawl over the occasional log. You can still easily follow the path, but it's a little overgrown with grasses, ferns, shrubs, and herbs. After a rain, this wet, overhanging vegetation will get you soaked, so bring along rain pants and, possibly, gaiters in order to stay comfortable.

The path drops briefly to cross a seasonal creek and then begins climbing a long switchback to the top of a woodsy ridge. From here you descend about 200 feet to a small creek whose banks are crowded with lots of ferns, monkeyflower, bleeding heart, and other water-loving plants. One of those plants is stinging nettle, so be careful about what you brush

up against. After hopping across the creek, you climb at an irregular pace on a trail that is often rocky, so watch your step. Beargrass and huckleberry become increasingly common as you approach a trail junction in a saddle on the top of the ridge forming Zigzag Mountain. To reach the dramatic viewpoint from the old lookout site on West Zigzag Mountain, you turn left and in just 0.2 mile reach the open viewpoint.

Hikers who want to tackle a long loop trip can turn right at the trail junction below West Zigzag Mountain and follow the increasingly open and spectacular ridgeline to the east. The up-and-down route passes massive wildflower meadows and lots of huckleberries, as well as stunning views of Mt. Hood as you pass junctions with the Horseshoe Ridge Trail (Trip 22) and the Cast Creek Trail (Trip 21) before coming to the final high viewpoint at East Zigzag Mountain. From there you return on the route down Devils Canyon (Trip 27) back to your car.

TRIP 27 East Zigzag Mountain from Enola Hill

Distance	8.0 miles, Semiloop
Elevation Gain	1700 feet
Hiking Time	4 to 5 hours
Optional Map	Green Trails *Government Camp*
Usually Open	Mid-June to October
Best Time	July
Trail Use	Dogs OK, backpacking option
Agency	Zigzag Ranger District, Mt. Hood National Forest
Difficulty	Moderate

HIGHLIGHTS Just as the Enola Hill Road provides a shortcut to West Zigzag Mountain (Trip 26), it provides a much easier approach to East Zigzag Mountain. And while this trip misses Burnt Lake, it does have better meadows and more flowers than the approach from the north. That's a reasonable tradeoff, and ambitious hikers can still visit Burnt Lake if they want to by taking a side trip off the main trail.

DIRECTIONS Drive 1.5 miles east of Rhododendron on U.S. Highway 26, and turn left (north) onto paved Forest Road 27. After 0.6 mile, this narrow road turns to rough gravel, switchbacks sharply to the left, and climbs a heavily wooded hillside. The road affords you little room to pass oncoming traffic, so take it slow and be prepared to back up to the nearest pullout if you meet a car coming down the hill. Actually, you won't be going very fast anyway, as the road is miserably rutted with rocks, potholes, and deep mud holes. The road ends 5.2 miles from the highway, at a small trailhead parking area.

The trail begins on a long-abandoned jeep route that was once the extension of the Enola Hill Road. While the width of this route identifies it as an old road, it has been so long since it was used by vehicles that it is now effectively an easy, gently graded trail. The vegetation along the route is lush and attractive, with lots of wildflowers, including some unusual varieties. Look for goatsbeard, beardtongue, devil's club, tiger lily, goldenrod, and aster.

After about 0.7 mile, you enter the wilderness. Soon thereafter you will leave the forest and begin to travel through increasingly lush and attractive meadows. The old road stays generally level all the way to its end in Devils Meadow, where a close inspection may reveal evidence of an old car campground. If you'd rather inspect something more attractive, spend your time identifying the profusion of wildflowers. There are lupine and paint-brush, of course, but also larkspur, beargrass, arnica, spiraea, bistort, valerian, and other colorful species.

Now a true footpath, the route crosses a trickling creek and arrives at a junction with the Devils Tie/Cutoff Trail. This marks the end of a recommended loop trip you can take on your return from East Zigzag Mountain. For now, go straight at this junction and climb the open meadowy slopes covered with huckleberry bushes and a few scattered trees. In mid- to late August, you will need to schedule extra time for feasting on huckleberries. Seven long switchbacks lead you up to a ridgetop junction, where you'll gain your first look at imposing Mt. Hood. If you want to visit Burnt Lake, turn right at this junction and then left at a second junction about 200 yards later. This switchbacking trail drops down a shady, north-facing slope to the shores of the popular lake.

Mount Hood Area

To reach East Zigzag Mountain, the high point of the trip, turn left at the ridgeline junction, and ascend a steep, rocky trail 0.3 mile to the summit. Views from here extend in all directions and include a look all the way south to distant Mt. Jefferson, but the main attraction is Mt. Hood. With binoculars you can even see the crevasses in Reid and Zigzag glaciers. Tiny alpine wildflowers such as lomatium, phlox, and cliff penstemon provide colorful foregrounds for pictures of the mountain.

To return by a different route, drop down the west side of the peak and come to a junction with the Cast Creek Trail, in a wooded saddle. You bear left at this junction and switchback down a little more to a second junction, this time with the Cast Lake Trail. This lake is worth a visit, even though it doesn't have a view of Mt. Hood. To close out the loop, go straight at the junction, and loop around a lovely little mountain meadow that is home to lots of spiraea, a small, pink-blooming shrub whose flowers have a wonderful aroma. Just past this meadow is a junction with the Devils Tie Trail. Turn left here and descend several short, steep switchbacks to the junction just above Devils Meadow.

TRIP 28 Paradise Park Trail

Distance	12.4 miles, Out-and-back
Elevation Gain	3100 feet
Hiking Time	7 to 8 hours
Optional Map	Green Trails *Government Camp, Mount Hood*
Usually Open	Mid-July to October
Best Times	Late July to early August
Trail Use	Dogs OK, backpacking option
Agency	Zigzag Ranger District, Mt. Hood National Forest
Difficulty	Difficult

HIGHLIGHTS The Paradise Park Trail is a quiet, but tiring approach to the extremely popular Paradise Park area. There are relatively few highlights on this trail, but you will enjoy lots of solitude, especially compared to the extremely busy approach from Timberline Lodge (Trip 36). By connecting this trail with the Hidden Lake Trail (Trip 29), you can make a long, strenuous dayhike or very enjoyable weekend backpacking trip.

DIRECTIONS Drive east on U.S. Highway 26 from Zigzag to Milepost 48.6, and then bear left onto paved Forest Road 39. Drive 1.3 miles, and then turn left on a dirt road with a sign for the Paradise Park Trail. This access road goes over a bridge and, about 100 yards later, comes to a parking and camping area beside the trailhead.

The trail starts in a dense western-hemlock and western-red-cedar forest amid mossy rocks on a gently sloping bench above the rushing Zigzag River. The serious climbing doesn't begin until you come to the permit and sign-in box, and the trail switchbacks to the left. Six long, moderately ascending switchbacks take you up a viewless, woodsy slope, where July-blooming rhododendrons add some color to the scene. The trail then climbs above the traffic sounds of Highway 26,

Paradise Park Trail & Hidden Lake

into the more soothing natural sounds of clicking juncos, rasping one-note red-breasted nuthatches, and the more varied songs of mountain chickadees. After the switchbacks end, the path comes to some open lodgepole-pine woods and goes along the edge of a precipitous cliff, with good views south to Tom Dick Mountain and Zigzag Canyon.

The grade of your climb picks up again as you enter thicker forests of noble and Pacific silver fir as well as Douglas fir. On the forest floor, look for beargrass blooms in July and the downward-facing flowers of pipsissewa later in the summer. There are a few short switchbacks along this section but no real landmarks as the path climbs steadily, but not overly steeply, through the trees. Eventually you reach a junction with the Zigzag Mountain

Trail coming in from the left. Go straight and almost immediately you will notice an improvement in the scenery. Most obvious are the abundant and colorful wildflowers, which peak in late July and include white valerian, blue lupine, green false hellebore, and yellow groundsel. Soon after you reach the junction a good view of the deeply eroded Zigzag Canyon and part of Mt. Hood appears.

Although the climbing isn't over yet, most of it is, and what little remains goes unnoticed because your attention will instead be turned to the scenery. Just 0.3 mile from the last junction, you go straight at a four-way junction with the equestrian bypass trail below Paradise Park. From here, you climb through increasingly open, flower-covered meadows to

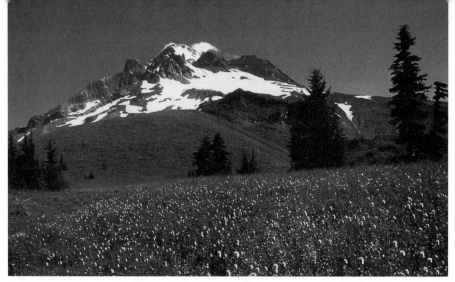

Mt. Hood from above Paradise Park

a junction with the Pacific Crest Trail (PCT).

The number and variety of flowers here are positively overwhelming. In addition to the previously mentioned species, you will enjoy bistort, Jacob's ladder, purple asters, pearly everlasting, and cat's ear. It's a riot of color in late July and early August—some of the best flower displays in the state of Oregon. If the summer has been cool and wet, then the flower show remains good all the way through Labor Day. The scattered trees at this altitude are mostly mountain hemlock and subalpine fir, which add to the magic of this alpine scene. It's probably impossible to resist the temptation to explore higher on the sloping meadows above the junction.

After satisfying your sense of adventure, return to the PCT and turn west for 0.3 mile to reach the many good camps and the dilapidated shelter at Paradise Park. Since this area is very popular, it is crucial that you camp only in official sites that have been used for years and can take the pounding—but don't build a fire.

To do the loop with the Hidden Lake Trail, turn east at the PCT junction and descend this route into Zigzag Canyon. Ford the stream a short distance below

an impressive waterfall. Then climb long switchbacks out of the canyon to the junction with the Hidden Lake Trail. Turn right on this relatively little-used trail and descend, often fairly steeply, on a forested hillside. There are few flowers or other things of interest along this route, but the setting is tranquil and the trail is quiet so the hiking is pleasant and the downhill miles go by quickly. The path goes through lots of huckleberries, but the shade here prohibits a bumper crop. About 0.2 mile after you hop over a splashing creek, the trail reaches tiny, marsh-rimmed Hidden Lake. This is a shallow pool with lots of bugs in July and little to recommend it other than solitude. The outlet creek does, however, have some impressive skunk cabbage with enormous leaves.

The path leaves Hidden Lake, climbs briefly, and then descends through western-hemlock forests with lots of rhododendrons blooming in mid-July. The last mile of this trail is always within earshot of busy U.S. Highway 26 as it descends four steep switchbacks and arrives at Forest Road 39 at a gravel trailhead pullout. The Paradise Park Trailhead is an easy 1.4-mile stroll down this road.

TRIP 29 Hidden Lake

Distance	4.2 miles, Out-and-back
Elevation Gain	700 feet
Hiking Time	2 to 3 hours
Optional Map	Green Trails *Government Camp*
Usually Open	May to early November
Best Time	June
Trail Use	Dogs OK, backpacking option
Agency	Zigzag Ranger District, Mt. Hood National Forest
Difficulty	Moderate
Note	Good in cloudy weather

see map on p.359

HIGHLIGHTS People are always drawn to lakes. It doesn't really matter if the lake isn't very scenic, doesn't have many fish, or is too brushy and muddy to provide good swimming. All those unexciting qualities describe Hidden Lake, the small mountain pool that is the goal of this hike. But the hike is worth your time, in part because it is relatively easy and in part because of the varied vegetation along the way, but mostly because at the destination you can lie back and enjoy the tranquility of a forest-rimmed mountain pool with few other hikers around to disturb your sense of solitude.

DIRECTIONS Drive east on U.S. Highway 26 from Zigzag to Milepost 48.6, and then bear left onto paved Forest Road 39. Follow this route 2.7 miles, and park in a gravel parking area on your left. If you reach the end of the road at the Little Zigzag Falls Trailhead, you have driven about 0.2 mile too far.

The most difficult part of the hike is right at the beginning, as you wind up a series of four short switchbacks. The route is generally well graded, although there is a short rocky section that is quite steep. After coming to the top of the switchbacks, the path follows a partly open ridgeline with some decent views of Tom Dick Mountain and the Zigzag Valley. Unfortunately, the tranquility of this scene is rudely broken by the sounds of traffic on busy Highway 26.

The trail gradually gains elevation as it winds through the trees and works away from the sounds of cars. The forests here support lots of rhododendrons, which fill the forest with pink blossoms from late June to mid-July. The trail eventually tops a low ridge and then goes briefly downhill to a crossing of a small creek, just downstream from Hidden Lake. A short spur trail goes through the brush to the shores of the lake, but it is also worth spending some time examining the outlet creek, which features an abundance of skunk cabbage. This plant loves wet environments and has enormous, shiny, green leaves. The large yellow flowers, which bloom in spring and early summer, are responsible for the unpleasant odor for which this plant is named.

The trail continues beyond Hidden Lake, crossing a splashing creek about 0.2 mile above the lake and climbing a rather monotonous, wooded ridge. The path has no real highlights, so it isn't really worth the hike on its own, but the often-steep path is sometimes used as the return route of a giant loop hike in combination with the Paradise Park Trail (see Trip 28).

Mount Hood Area

TRIP 30 Little Zigzag Falls & Enid Lake

Distance	4.0 miles, Out-and-back
Elevation Gain	600 feet
Hiking Time	2 hours
Optional Map	Green Trails *Government Camp*
Usually Open	Late May to early November
Best Times	June and October
Trail Use	Good for kids, partly wheelchair accessible, dogs OK
Agency	Zigzag Ranger District, Mt. Hood National Forest
Difficulty	Moderate
Note	Good in cloudy weather

HIGHLIGHTS The 0.7-mile round-trip hike to Little Zigzag Falls is short for a full dayhike, but it makes an excellent leg-stretcher for families with children. If you want a full day of hiking, you can add an enjoyable outing up the old Pioneer Bridle Trail to Enid Lake. Little Zigzag Falls is worth a visit because it is a pleasant cascade surrounded by deep woods. The setting makes the falls difficult to photograph, but that can't take away from the soothing tranquility of the scene. Enid Lake is little more than a marshy pond, but it has a pretty setting. Plus, from it you can see the top one-third of Mt. Hood, so it is worth a look.

DIRECTIONS Drive east on U.S. Highway 26 from Zigzag to Milepost 48.6, and then bear left off the highway onto paved Forest Road 39. Follow this route for 3.0 miles to the roadend turnaround and parking area.

The trail to Little Zigzag Falls leaves from the east end of the parking area and follows the north bank of the clear, splashing Little Zigzag River. The easy path travels through a lush forest composed mostly of western red cedar and western hemlock, while beside the creek such water-loving plants as devil's club, maidenhair and other ferns, skunk cabbage, and false Solomon's seal crowd the bank.

After a little more than 0.3 mile, the gentle uphill path comes to a small, open, bouldery slope and, immediately thereafter, a sturdy log bench at the base of Little Zigzag Falls, a twisting cataract that puts out a cool spray of water. This is a pleasant spot to eat lunch and enjoy the beauty of both falls and forest. From the bench, the path continues in two switchbacks to a disappointing overlook at the top of the falls, but this extra mileage is worthwhile only for the exercise.

The trail to Enid Lake leaves from the same trailhead and begins as a gated road taking off from the south side of the parking area. You cross the Little Zigzag River on a bridge and climb the road on a partially forested hillside. After 0.1 mile, look for a trail tunnel going under the road, and drop down to it. You are now on the Pioneer Bridle Trail, which, as you might guess from the name, is an historic section of the old Barlow Wagon Road. Turn east on this wide trail, follow the shoulder of Highway 26 for a few dozen yards, and then bear left back into the trees.

The trail soon leaves the traffic sounds behind and enters a quiet and lovely forest. The wide path is littered with the tiny needles and cones of hemlock trees and lined with huckleberry bushes laden with

🔍 Little Zigzag Falls, Enid Lake, & Laurel Hill Chute

To US 26

39

Little

Trail

Bridle

Pioneer

26

3150'

30

Little Zigzag
Falls

Zigzag

River

chute

3400'

31

3180'

Camp

Yocum Falls

Creek

26

30

ski   trail

3620'
Enid
Lake

Crosstown   Trail

P

0   .1   .2   .3   .4   .5   mile

delicious fruit in late August. Much of the route is marked by blue diamonds on trees, which identify this as a cross-country ski route in winter. You go straight at an unsigned junction with a spur trail, which goes to the right to the end of a closed section of the old highway.

The quiet trail now very gradually gains elevation and eventually follows a lovely little mountain creek. The joyous sounds of bubbling water join with the sight of mossy rocks and lush riparian vegetation to make a magical scene. The streambed is choked with skunk cabbage, a plant with huge, shiny, green leaves and showy yellow flowers. The trail crosses the creek on a wooden footbridge and then veers away from it to a junction with the Enid Lake Ski Trail. Despite the name, this path does not visit Enid Lake, so bear right and stay on the Pioneer Bridle Trail to a junction right beside an upper trailhead on a barricaded section of the old highway. You turn left here on the Crosstown Trail and, after 0.1 mile, look for a 20-yard side trail to the left that leads to the shore of shallow Enid Lake. The best pictures are from the south shore.

Little Zigzag Falls

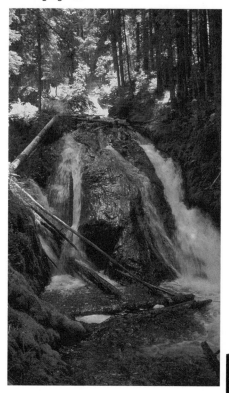

TRIP 31 Laurel Hill Chute Loop

Distance	1.3 miles, Loop
Elevation Gain	300 feet
Hiking Time	1 hour
Optional Map	Green Trails *Government Camp* (trail not shown)
Usually Open	Late April to November
Best Time	June
Trail Use	Good for kids, dogs OK
Agency	Zigzag Ranger District, Mt. Hood National Forest
Difficulty	Easy

HIGHLIGHTS This is a convenient option for hikers who want to mix a little exercise with a dose of history. The view from trail's end is good, but the real attraction is standing above a rocky precipice and visualizing the exploits of pioneers who somehow managed to negotiate this ruggedly steep terrain in covered wagons.

DIRECTIONS Drive U.S. Highway 26 about 9 miles east of Zigzag, and park in the small pullout on the right side of the road beside a historical marker.

The path begins by climbing a short flight of stone stairs to a junction with a section of old Highway 26. Turn right on this closed road. Then gradually climb past an interpretive sign and some openings that provide good views of Tom Dick Mountain and Zigzag Canyon. After about 150 yards, you bear left onto a signed footpath and slowly ascend five switchbacks through an open forest of Douglas fir, western hemlock, and western red cedar. The forest floor is dominated by bracken fern, some salal, and two plants with showy June flowers—beargrass and Pacific rhododendron.

The climb tops a rounded hill, where there is an unsigned junction. You go straight and descend a little to the viewpoint above Laurel Hill Chute. As you look down this very steep, rocky defile, it is hard to envision how the early pioneers made it through here. They tied ropes around trees at the top of the gorge and used muscle power to lower their wagons down the slope—an incredibly dangerous and difficult task and your admiration of their achievement will increase when you realize that, even today, it is too

dangerous for you to go down the chute of loose rocks on foot.

For some variety on the return trip, make a loop by turning left at the unsigned junction mentioned earlier. This path follows what is believed to be the actual route of the old wagon road for 0.1 mile and then comes to a junction with an upper section of the old paved highway. You turn right on it and then walk down this route, which is gradually being taken over by encroaching willows and lodgepole pines. You make one long, curving switchback before returning to the junction with the Laurel Hill Chute Trail and taking the stairs back to your car.

Tom Dick Mountain from Laurel Hill Chute Trail

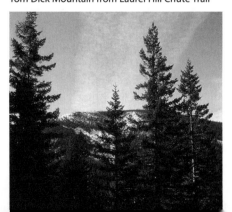

TRIP 32 Mirror Lake & Tom Dick Mountain

Distance	3.2 to 6.4 miles, Out-and-back
Elevation Gain	700 to 1500 feet
Hiking Time	2 to 4 hours
Optional Map	Green Trails *Government Camp*
Usually Open	June to October
Best Times	Late June and July
Trail Use	Good for kids, dogs OK, backpacking option, fishing
Agency	Zigzag Ranger District, Mt. Hood National Forest
Difficulty	Moderate

HIGHLIGHTS Mirror Lake has been a popular hiking destination for decades. With easy trail access and a classic view of Mt. Hood, it will likely remain popular for a long time. So don't come to Mirror Lake hoping for a quiet wilderness experience. On summer weekends hundreds of fellow admirers trek up this trail. It's best to visit on a weekday although even then you should be prepared to meet plenty of people. By extending the hike up the western spur of Tom Dick Mountain, you can get more exercise and reach a nice viewpoint above most of the crowds.

DIRECTIONS Drive U.S. Highway 26 east toward Government Camp. A little before Milepost 52, park in the large roadside pullout on the right side of the road. There is no trailhead sign here, but you can't miss the small trail bridge leaving from the parking area or the dozens of other cars already parked in the lot.

The trail starts by crossing a narrow bridge over Camp Creek a little upstream from unseen Yocum Falls. The wide, gently graded trail has been built to withstand the punishment of so many visitors. In places the U.S. Forest Service has installed wooden handrails to keep people on the official trail. To protect the land, it is important that you never cut switchbacks and, even better, chastise anyone who does.

The trail traverses a short distance, crosses a bridge over a tributary creek, and returns to the forested hillside. The forests are relatively open, with lots of vine maple and Pacific rhododendron beneath a mix of evergreens, including Douglas fir, western white pine, western hemlock, and western red cedar. You will make a long, gradual ascent to the base of a rockslide, before switchbacking to cross the slide higher on the slope. Look

for pikas here busily gathering grasses to store for the long winter ahead.

Above the rockslide, the trail enters slightly wetter forest and makes a fairly long traverse. After this, you ascend three quick switchbacks and come to a junction just below the lake. The trail to the left immediately crosses the outlet creek and then loops around the lake's east and south shores. Much of the lakeshore is crowded with thick brush, mostly salmonberry, rose, willow, and slide alder. From the south shore, your eyes are irresistibly drawn to the stunning view of Mt. Hood, which is best seen by getting off the main trail and visiting any of several lakeshore picnic sites. The best photographs are usually taken during the afternoon. Windless days are preferable because the water does indeed act like a mirror, although jumping fish often create circular ripples in the glassy stillness

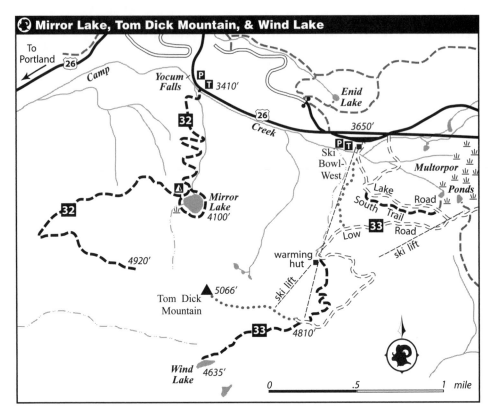

and temporarily disturb the reflecting properties that gave this lake its name. There is a fine meadow on the southwest shore of the lake, which in early summer has lots of blooming marsh marigolds and shooting stars. To protect these fragile meadows, please stay on the log planks marking the route of the trail. If you wish to camp at the lake, use the designated sites above the drier west shore.

To reach a quiet viewpoint, leave the lakeshore loop and climb a trail going southwest. The path travels through an open forest of lodgepole pine and mountain hemlock and then gradually climbs across an open hillside with lots of huckleberries and views to the town of Zig-

zag. When you reach a ridgeline, turn east, and slowly gain altitude. The trail becomes increasingly faint on this partly forested slope, but it is still easy to follow until it ends at an excellent viewpoint near a large cairn. From here you can look northeast to Mt. Hood and down on circular Mirror Lake, or spend your time picking out lesser landmarks tucked away in the Salmon-Huckleberry Wilderness to the south and west. In recent years, peregrine falcons have nested on the upper slopes of Tom Dick Mountain. To protect this endangered species, the U.S. Forest Service has restricted access beyond the viewpoint, so turn back here, well satisfied with what you have achieved.

TRIP 33 Wind Lake

Distance	6.4 miles, Out-and-back
Elevation Gain	1400 feet
Hiking Time	3 to 4 hours
Optional Map	Green Trails *Government Camp* (trail not shown)
Usually Open	Mid-June to October
Best Times	Late June and July and mid-August to September
Trail Use	Dogs OK, mountain biking, backpacking option, fishing
Agency	Zigzag Ranger District, Mt. Hood National Forest
Difficulty	Moderate

HIGHLIGHTS Forest-rimmed Wind Lake hides in a quiet basin on the back side of Tom Dick Mountain. The lake seems to be a world away from the unsightly hustle and bustle of the ski area on the other side of the mountain. Surprisingly, few hikers take the time to visit this little gem, perhaps because there is no mountain view across its waters. But while Wind Lake will never be featured on calendars, it is a good place to enjoy the kind of solitude that is no longer possible at nearby Mirror Lake.

DIRECTIONS Take U.S. Highway 26 up to a little past Milepost 52 near Government Camp, and then turn right into the huge parking lot for Mount Hood Ski Bowl-West.

Begin by walking south past the main ski lodge buildings. When you come to the base of the ski lift and the alpine slide, bear left on a gravel and dirt road. This road climbs steeply for about 0.1 mile and then comes to a junction, where you turn left on Lake Road. About 75 yards later, turn right at a sign for South Trail, and walk this pleasant footpath as it winds up and down through cedar and hemlock forests. The path parallels an unobtrusive dirt road for 0.5 mile and then meets and crosses that road. Instead of crossing, you turn right and walk on the road, under a ski lift, to a junction with a second jeep road signed LOW ROAD.

You turn sharply right on Low Road, which gradually climbs a hillside where the tree cover is occasionally broken by cleared ski runs. In late June and July, Pacific rhododendrons bloom here in profusion, helping to give the scene a wilder feeling. As you gain altitude, the open forests gradually change from mid-elevation species to higher-elevation varieties like lodgepole pine, Alaska yellow cedar, and mountain hemlock. After a little over 1 mile, the road hits the top of the main ski run above Ski Bowl-West and switchbacks to the left. Immediately after this switchback, you come to the warming hut for the ski area, where you will get terrific views of Mt. Hood.

At this point, you have a choice of routes. The longer and gentler alternative is to stay on the gravel road as it climbs in one long switchback to the top of a ridge. The steeper and more direct route veers to the right at the hut and steeply climbs an open hillside. This mountain biking trail uses a series of switchbacks to gain elevation and with every step provides increasingly far-ranging views. At the top of the ridge, you rejoin the road and turn right.

After just 100 yards, bear left onto a wide, but unsigned, footpath, which gently descends through an open forest of scraggly lodgepole pines for 0.5

Mount Hood Area

mile to the shores of shallow Wind Lake. Although it lacks mountain views, this lake is quiet and very attractive. One of the nicest times to visit is in mid- to late summer, when the shallow waters have warmed enough for a pleasant swim. During cold winters the lake may freeze almost all the way to the bottom, killing most of the brook trout that are planted here. As a result, fishing is only medio-

cre. Since very few anglers come here, however, it may be worthwhile to give it a try.

You can return the way you came, or, for variety, you could walk directly from the warming hut down ski slopes back to the lodge. Although quite steep, the route is obvious, and the goal is always in sight.

TRIP 34 Multorpor Mountain View & Loop

Distance	5.1 miles (combined), Loop
Elevation Gain	1700 feet
Hiking Time	3 hours
Optional Map	Green Trails *Government Camp, Mount Hood* (trail not shown)
Usually Open	June to October
Best Time	Mid-June to mid-July
Trail Use	Dogs OK, mountain biking
Agency	Zigzag Ranger District, Mt. Hood National Forest
Difficulty	Moderate

HIGHLIGHTS The little-known summit of Multorpor Mountain provides a classic view of Mt. Hood and the busy ski town of Government Camp. The steep, unsigned trail to the top is rarely hiked, but it is well worth the effort for adventurous hikers who like good views. By combining this climb with the trail around the base of the mountain, you can enjoy a full day of scenic hiking.

DIRECTIONS Drive U.S. Highway 26 east to Government Camp, and park in the lot for the Summit Rest Area on the north side of the highway. To reach the trailhead, you must walk across the highway, something that is easier said than done on summer weekends when the traffic is very heavy.

For a bit of history, start by walking down a dirt road next to a gray post with an OREGON TRAIL marker. The road is about 80 yards east of the Milepost 54 sign. This route immediately passes a cluster of wooden buildings near the highway and then comes to a trail-maintenance donation box and a trail sign. This sign, like most of the others along this route, is over 12 feet high in order to ensure that cross-country skiers can see it when traveling over deep snow. In sum-

mer, however, the average hiker needs to crane his neck, and possibly squint, to make out the small lettering on the lofty signs.

You bear left at the sign and follow the Barlow Trail, which immediately becomes either a very narrow abandoned jeep road or a very wide foot trail, depending on your point of view. You are now literally walking in the footsteps of pioneers, as this is a portion of the historic Barlow Wagon Road traveled by many of the

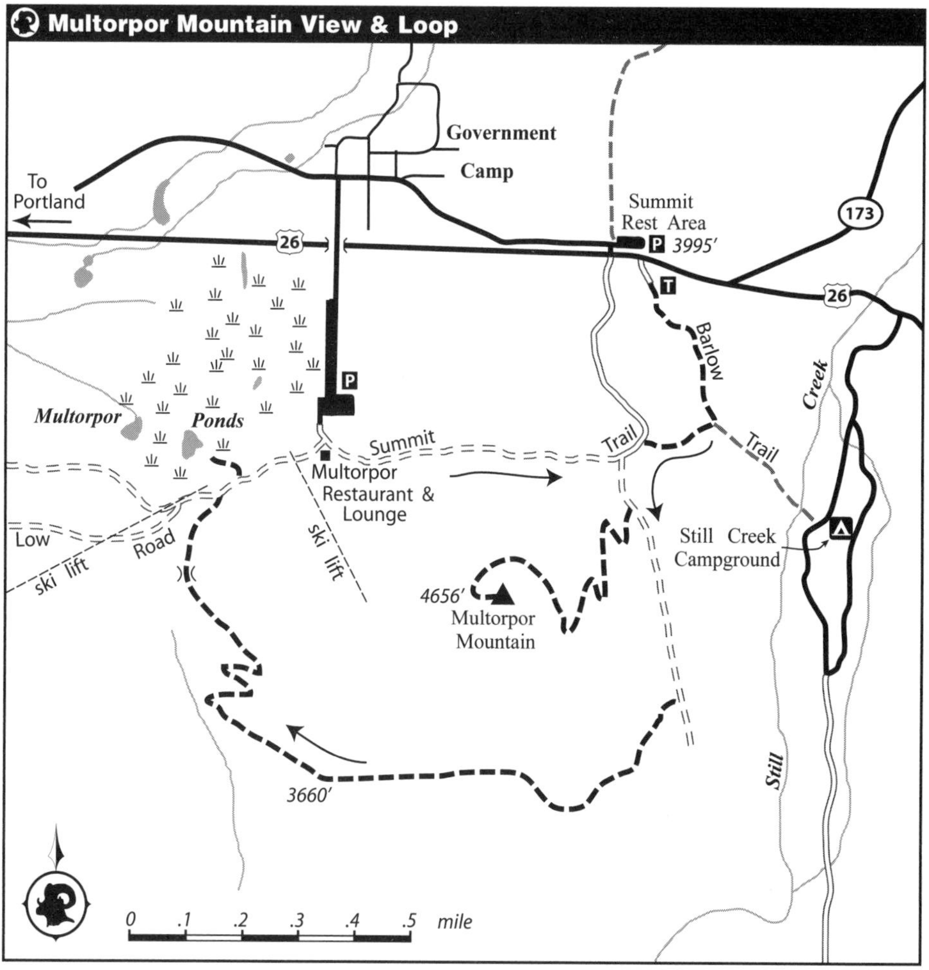

Multorpor Mountain View & Loop

Government
Camp

To
Portland

Summit
Rest Area
P 3995'

173

26

26

Barlow

Creek

Summit   Trail   Trail

Multorpor   Ponds

P

Multorpor
Restaurant &
Lounge

Still Creek
Campground

Low

ski lift   Road

ski lift

4656'
Multorpor
Mountain

3660'

Still

0   .1   .2   .3   .4   .5   mile

early pioneers on the Oregon Trail. The surrounding forests are mostly mountain hemlocks with a few firs and Alaska yellow cedars for variety. The forest floor is sprinkled with beargrass, young evergreens, and huckleberry bushes.

A maze of cross-country ski trails and mountain biking routes lace these forests, and they can get very confusing, so follow these directions carefully. About 0.1 mile from the highway, go straight at a signed junction with the Barlow Trail, and a few hundred yards later turn right at a sign saying TO SUMMIT TRAIL. Follow this short footpath to a dirt road, which doubles

as the Summit Trail, and turn left on the road. About 50 yards later, at an unsigned junction next to a small power line, you turn left again, and climb a jeep track in the trees beneath the power line.

Only 100 yards from the last junction, where the jeep route crests a small hill and begins to descend, look for an unsigned but obvious foot trail going up the steep hillside on your right. To visit the summit of Multorpor Mountain, turn right and follow this often-steep trail up a wooded hillside. In late June and July, lots of blooming Pacific rhododendron make for a nice visual treat. Even though it is obvious on the ground, this trail is not part of the U.S. Forest Service's trail inventory. Do your part to help maintain it by removing any rocks, limbs, or debris that block the path. The 0.7-mile trail tops out at the rocky summit of Multorpor Mountain.

The view here is one of the best in the area. In addition to the main attraction of Mt. Hood to your immediate north, you will also be able to pick out partially obstructed Mt. Jefferson in the distance to the south and Mt. St. Helens peeking over a western spur ridge of Mt. Hood. Lesser summits include the talus slopes of Tom Dick Mountain to the west, forested Eureka Peak to the south, and rounded Barlow Butte to the east. The woodsy valley of Still Creek curves away to the southwest.

To do the loop around Multorpor Mountain, go back down the steep trail to the jeep route and turn right. This rocky jeep track goes steeply downhill and then veers away from the power line and meanders through the woods at a much gentler grade. About 0.1 mile later, you turn right onto a trail that is marked with a sign stating that the path is open to hikers, mountain bikers, and skiers. This trail was constructed for the benefit of mountain bikers, so watch for two-wheeled travelers and let them pass unimpeded. This pleasant path alternates between dense woods and miniature forest openings as it takes a circuitous route across the south side of Multorpor Mountain. Many different birds, including thrushes, warblers, kinglets, and flycatchers, provide treats for your ears, while a variety of wildflowers are a feast for the eyes.

The trail eventually descends about 200 feet, curves right, and regains that lost altitude (and more) by ascending a series of nicely graded switchbacks. At the top of this ascent, the trail makes an extended contour of a hillside covered with a very attractive forest. The path goes through a saddle, where you go straight at an unsigned junction, and then almost immediately comes to a confusion of roads and ski runs in Mount Hood Ski Bowl. Your best bet is to go generally to the right staying on the lowest of several roads. From this road you should take the opportunity to bushwhack a few dozen feet through the trees and brush on your left, to visit the marshy Multorpor Ponds. These pools feature lovely reflections of Mt. Hood, but they also host abundant mosquitoes in late June and July.

To finish the loop, you need to find the dirt jeep road that serves as the Summit Trail. This is most easily done by simply making your way east, past a confusion of ski runs and maintenance sheds, to the Multorpor Restaurant & Lounge at Ski Bowl-East. The signed Summit Trail takes off about 70 yards southeast of this building. Follow this quiet jeep track for about 0.5 mile back to the Multorpor Mountain turnoff you passed earlier in the day. For variety on the way back, skip the connecting path to the Barlow Trail and simply stay on the main Summit Trail. This road takes you through open woods back to Highway 26 about 90 yards west of where you started. Carefully cross the highway to get back to your car.

Mt. Hood over Multopor Ponds

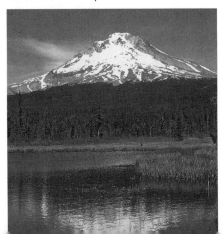

TRIP 35 West Fork Falls

Distance	2.8 miles, Out-and-back
Elevation Gain	500 feet
Hiking Time	1 to 2 hours
Optional Map	Green Trails *Mount Hood*
Usually Open	Late June to October
Best Times	July and August
Trail Use	Good for kids, dogs OK
Agency	Zigzag Ranger District, Mt. Hood National Forest
Difficulty	Moderate
Note	Good in cloudy weather

HIGHLIGHTS This quiet forest hike is the perfect complement to the more spectacular mountain trails in the Mt. Hood area. Views aren't an issue on this hike, so if you are in Government Camp and the skies have turned cloudy, consider this little-known outing. The destination is a pretty little falls in a mossy canyon, but since the trail is unmarked, few people ever come to visit. Thus, in addition to a lovely setting, you will enjoy plenty of solitude.

DIRECTIONS Turn north off U.S. Highway 26, just east of Government Camp, onto the Timberline Lodge Road (State Highway 173). After just 0.2 mile, turn left on a narrow, one-way road that goes west past some summer homes and lodges. Just 30 yards before this road rejoins Highway 26, turn right on unsigned West Leg Road. Follow this single-lane, paved road 1.6 miles to a sharp left-hand switchback, and look for a tall sign marking the East Leg Cross-Country Ski Trail. There is room to park about three cars here.

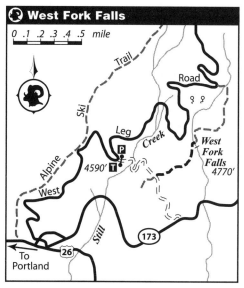

Walk east on an old road through a cool forest mostly composed of mountain hemlock and lodgepole pine with some Engelmann spruce and subalpine fir. Just 200 yards from the start, a road culvert takes you over splashing Still Creek, and then you go very gradually downhill. Where the road makes a slow turn to the right about 0.8 mile from the trailhead, look carefully for an unsigned foot trail crossing the route. Turn left (uphill) and climb steadily, but not too steeply, on this trail, which is lined with beargrass and huckleberries that provide blossoms to enjoy in mid-July and fruit to eat in late August.

The trail goes about 0.6 mile and then it bears slightly to the right and drops gradually to a viewpoint on the slope beside West Fork Falls. The falls isn't a

Mount Hood Area

towering drop on the order of Mult-nomah Falls, but it has subtle charms as it cascades about 40 feet over cliffs and rocks covered with bright green mosses and then tumbles into a shady canyon. The trail crosses the creek above the falls on slippery and unstable logs, and then it follows the cascading creek upstream and eventually takes you back to West Leg Road. The falls is the main attraction, however, so most hikers simply turn around there.

TRIP 36 Timberline Lodge to Paradise Park

Distance	10.1 miles, Out-and-back
Elevation Gain	2100 feet
Hiking Time	5 hours
Optional Map	Green Trails *Mount Hood*
Usually Open	Mid-July to October
Best Time	Late July to early August
Trail Use	Dogs OK, backpacking option, horseback riding
Agency	Zigzag Ranger District, Mt. Hood National Forest
Difficulty	Difficult

HIGHLIGHTS Several trails converge on Paradise Park. Deciding which one is best for you depends on your preferences, your fitness level, and the time of year. The shortest, easiest, and most scenic approach follows the Pacific Crest Trail (PCT) from Timberline Lodge. Not surprisingly, this is also the most crowded route. If you can get away on a weekday or don't mind sharing your outdoor experience with packs of out-of-state tourists, then this is the trail for you.

DIRECTIONS Turn north off U.S. Highway 26 just east of Government Camp onto the Timberline Lodge Road (State Highway 173). Climb this winding paved road 5.5 miles to the historic lodge with its acres of parking.

From the back side of the lodge pick up a paved footpath marked with a small sign saying TIMBERLINE TRAIL. This route climbs briefly amid midsummer wildflowers to a junction with the PCT. Turn left, go under a ski lift, and then gradually wander at a slight downhill grade through open timberline meadows with good views south to Mt. Jefferson and the Three Sisters in the distant haze. You go straight at a four-way junction with the Mountaineer Trail and then soon reach the lip of the small canyon holding Little Zigzag River. The trail then drops to the "river" (nothing more than a small creek), crosses it on rocks, and climbs out of the little canyon. From here you travel in open subalpine forests to a junction with the little-used Hidden Lake Trail. Go straight on the PCT and then gradually lose elevation, first in the trees and then across open meadowy slopes where the soil is loose and sandy. After a couple of small zigs and zags, you reach the lip of, appropriately enough, Zigzag Canyon, where there is a stunning viewpoint. Mt. Hood towers above the scene on your right, while directly below are the rocky and sandy canyon slopes and the rushing waters of the river.

The path briefly follows the edge of the canyon, ducks into the trees, and

Timberline Lodge to Paradise Park & Mountaineer Trail Loop

makes three long switchbacks down a cool, forested slope. There are several small creeks and springs on this segment that provide habitat for water-loving plants, including both yellow monkeyflower and pink Lewis' monkeyflower. At the bottom of the 1000-foot descent is a bridgeless crossing of Zigzag River. In early summer this ford can be wet and a little tricky, but by mid-August it's a fairly simple rock hop. About 0.1 mile upstream from the crossing is an impressive waterfall, which is visible from the

trail and can be reached by those willing to scramble over the loose rocks beside the stream. Once on the opposite bank, follow the PCT as it climbs in and out of a small tributary gully to a switchback and a junction with the equestrian bypass trail below Paradise Park.

The much more scenic hiker's trail turns back to the right and continues uphill as you regain all of the elevation you lost in reaching the Zigzag River. At first this route ascends through trees, and then it crosses open slopes and switchbacks up a wide ravine with pleasant scenery but very little shade. Shortly after you finally reach the top of the canyon, there is a junction with the Paradise Park Trail (Trip 28). Explorations up the flower-covered meadow slopes to your right are highly recommended and very rewarding.

After doing some exploring, go west on the PCT to a crossing of Lost Creek in a gully that positively bursts with wildflowers, and reach the camp area at Paradise Park just 0.3 mile from the last junction. Since this area is extremely popular, it is crucial that you camp only in official sites that have been used for years and can take the pounding—but don't build a fire.

It is hard to pass up the many additional exploration options available in this area. The most rewarding one goes cross-country up and around a bluff northeast of Paradise Park and wanders

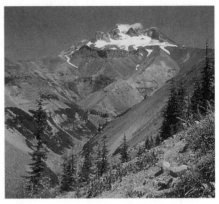

Mt. Hood over Zigzag Canyon on the Pacific Crest Trail

up sloping meadows toward the rocks and glaciers on Mt. Hood's higher slopes. A somewhat easier option continues north on the PCT for 0.5 mile to some great above-timberline meadows with lots of delicate heather and views of the wide bulk of Mt. Hood's southwest flank.

TRIP 37 Mountaineer Trail Loop

Distance	2.2 miles, Loop
Elevation Gain	1100 feet
Hiking Time	1 to 2 hours
Optional Map	Green Trails *Mount Hood*
Usually Open	Late July to late September
Best Time	August
Trail Use	Dogs allowed but not recommended.
Agency	Zigzag Ranger District, Mt. Hood National Forest
Difficulty	Moderate

see map on p.373

HIGHLIGHTS The great diversity of landscapes that you can reach with just a single-hour's drive from Portland is truly amazing. From the sea-level flats on Sauvie Island to the glaciers on Mt. Hood, this area has scenery to meet the preferences of any outdoor lover. This path, for example, climbs into the alpine zone, well above timberline, through a harsh land of permanent snowfields and rocks. Views extend for hundreds of miles, and tiny wildflowers brighten the rocky crevices.

Travel in this harsh environment involves some difficulties not encountered on most hikes. For one thing, the weather at these altitudes can be harsh and unpredictable. Blizzards can occur in any season, and there is nothing to slow the fierce winds. Save this trip for a clear, calm day. You might also notice that the air is slightly thinner up here—not enough to give you altitude sickness, perhaps, but enough to slow your progress while hiking. Finally, there is no shade above treeline, and at these altitudes it is very easy to get a sunburn. Put on sunscreen and wear a hat.

DIRECTIONS Turn north off U.S. Highway 26 just east of Government Camp onto the Timberline Lodge Road (State Highway 173). Climb this winding, paved road 5.5 miles to the historic lodge with its acres of parking.

Walk west on the paved road past the south side of the lodge, and then go under the start of the Magic Mile Ski Lift to a dirt road. Turn left when the road splits, and walk about 50 yards to a sign for Mountaineer Trail 798. Walk west on this sandy path through an open forest of mountain hemlock and subalpine fir that struggle to survive at these high altitudes. Clark's nutcrackers, striking gray, black, and white birds who caw at you like small crows, are one of the few avian species that live at these altitudes. Flowers such as lupine, western pasqueflower, phlox, lomatium, arnica, and partridge foot abound in the open forests and meadows, but they don't bloom until late summer.

The trail goes gradually up and down through this harsh environment, often crossing small gullies, which are usually filled with snow until mid-August. These openings also afford some terrific views to the south of Trillium Lake, Mt. Jefferson, and the Three Sisters. After about 0.4 mile, you go under a second ski lift, which, unlike the Magic Mile lift, is quiet because it is not used during the summer. The trail passes the marked site of the old Timberline cabin and then comes to a junction with the Pacific Crest Trail. You cross this route, staying on the Mountaineer Trail, and head steeply uphill. You soon enter a region where the subalpine firs cannot survive. They are replaced by hardier whitebark pines, which manage to survive in this windy environment because their branches are so flexible they can literally be tied in knots. As you

climb, you might hear the distant rattle from the working Magic Mile lift, but otherwise things are amazingly quiet.

You reach the last of the ground-hugging trees and bleached snags about halfway up to your goal, the metal building at the top of the Magic Mile lift, and enter an area with unrestricted views. Towering above you is craggy Mt. Hood, with its glaciers shimmering in the summer sun. To the southeast are the semidesert country of central Oregon and the dark, rounded forms of the distant Ochoco Mountains. To the west are the hazy lowlands of Portland and the Willamette Valley. Finally, to the south is the Ski Bowl development, Government Camp, Tom Dick Mountain, and a multitude of small, forest-covered peaks. Things get more crowded and busy as you approach the top of the Magic Mile lift, where you are treated to the peculiar sight in August of downhill skiers headed for the permanent snowfields on Palmer Glacier. Mt. Hood is the only place in North America, in fact, where it is possible to ski in a developed ski area year-round.

Once you reach the top of the lift, make your way east over groomed snowfields for a short distance to the Silcox Hut, an old stone building constructed as a warming hut for skiers in the winter. To return to Timberline Lodge, pick up the old access road to this hut, which is now closed and serves as a wide, sandy trail, and follow it downhill. About halfway down this rather steep route, bear to the right onto an unsigned trail traveling above a snow-filled gully, which is often used as a summer ski run. Timberline Lodge and your car are always in sight as you reenter the zone of twisted trees and return to the parking lot. Watch your step as you approach the lodge because the ground seems to come alive with chubby little golden-mantled ground squirrels. Sadly, these cute native residents now rely more on tourist handouts than their natural foods. Don't add to the problem by offering them anything.

Before heading home, take some time to tour the old lodge. It's worth taking the time to admire its magnificent architecture, massive stone fireplace, and wonderful wood carvings. Interpretive signs discuss the building's interesting history.

TRIP 38 Mount Hood Climb

Distance	8.0 miles, Out-and-back
Elevation Gain	5320 feet
Hiking Time	4 to 9 hours
Optional Map	USGS *Mount Hood South*
Usually Open	Late May and June
Best Time	May
Trail Use	No dogs
Agency	Zigzag Ranger District, Mt. Hood National Forest
Difficulty	Very strenuous

HIGHLIGHTS Okay, campers, let's be clear here—this trip is not a "hike." It's a mountain climb, requiring all the things a major mountain climb entails, including experience, special equipment, lots of stamina, and good judgment. If you do not have all of those things, then do not take this trip! I have included it in a hiking guide because the climb is extremely popular and many Portland area residents have a strong desire to reach the top of the area's dominant landmark. In fact, Mount Hood is the second most climbed major mountain in the world (after Japan's Mt. Fuji). The appeal is certainly understanding. Making it to the top of a major mountain—the highest point in the entire state of Oregon—is great for the ego, a perfect conversation starter, and absolutely terrific for the soul. And that doesn't even mention the unbelievable view!

DIRECTIONS Turn north off U.S. Highway 26 just east of Government Camp onto the Timberline Lodge Road (State Highway 173). Climb this winding, paved road 5.5 miles to the historic lodge with its acres of parking. Stop in at the Wy'East Day Lodge, just south of the main lodge building, to obtain the required wilderness permit and to sign the climber's register.

Even though a lot of people climb Mt. Hood, every year some people try and never come back. We've all seen the news stories on television of dramatic rescues and sad scenes of body bags being transported off the mountain. Generally these tragedies result from people who are unprepared, don't pay attention to the weather, and fail to bring the right gear. But the mountain is a tough and fickle place. Sometimes even the best prepared and most experienced climbers get caught in an unexpected blizzard or fall into a crevasse. Overconfidence can be a

Mount Hood Climb

MOUNT HOOD

MOUNT

Hogback

11,237'

Newton

Reid

Glacier

Hot Rocks

Crater Rock

Clark

Illumination
Rock 9543'

10,560'

Glacier

Glacier

Steel Cliff

HOOD

Zigzag

WILDERNESS

White River Glacier

Palmer Glacier

ski lift

Silcox
Hut
6940'

lift

ski

5920'

Timberline
Lodge

P

173 To US 26

0   .5   1 mile

how to, for example, put on crampons or self arrest with an ice axe, then you'd better be prepared to do a lot of learning. But, if you are up for the challenge and great rewards of a major adventure, here is a quick overview of the climb to whet your appetite.

To obtain the necessary experience, gear, and climbing partners (never attempt a climb like this alone), a little research and legwork is in order. The best place to start is to contact a well-established and experienced climbing group, such as the Mazamas (see Appendix 3) to learn about resources, where to rent the right gear, what classes are available, and when climbs are scheduled. The value of this expertise cannot be overstated.

For all but the most experienced climbers, the best time to attempt the mountain is in May and early June. At that time there is usually still plenty of snow filling the crevasses and the climb is much safer and easier. (Those are relative terms. Compared to any other trip in this book, it is still extremely difficult). Of course, at that time you can also expect plenty of snow to be piled up at the parking lot, which means that all those convenient trailhead signs and landmarks you enjoy on other trips won't help you here.

The second unusual timing issue for this trip has to do with the time of day, or, should I say, the time of night. For safety reasons, most people begin their climb in the wee hours of the morning (typically between midnight and 3 AM). This precaution generally ensures that the ice will be more solid so that your crampons will get better traction and that conditions won't become dangerously slushy on the return trip. A bonus of this timing is that it allows you to reach the summit at around dawn, when you can enjoy a fabulous view of the sunrise. With enough moonlight and plenty of snow reflecting

killer on Mt. Hood, which has earned its reputation as one of the country's most dangerous mountains.

As a hiking rather than a climbing guide, this book makes no attempt to go into detail about all the special equipment and skills necessary for mountain climbing. Put simply, if you don't already know

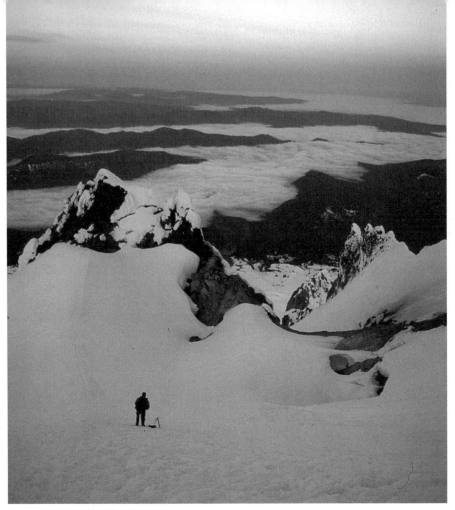

Near the summit of Mt. Hood

the available light, it is often surprisingly bright during the climb. Nonetheless, a headlamp is required gear, and most people use them for at least part of the climb.

Finally, in addition to all the usual climbing paraphernalia, a more recent high-tech piece of equipment that climbers are strongly encouraged to bring is a mountain locator unit. Mountain locator units can be rented in Portland from the Mountain Shop, which can be contacted at (503) 228-6768, as well as at the REI stores in Portland and Tualatin (see Appendix 3). You can also rent them from the Mount Hood Inn in Government Camp, which you can reach at (503) 272-3205. As of 2007 the rental cost was about $5 per unit. If a member of your party becomes injured, stranded, or lost, one of these units—along with a cell phone to call for assistance—might mean the difference between life and death.

Once all the preliminary arrangements, conditioning, and planning have been accomplished, the climb, though strenuous, is fairly straightforward. In good weather (and only attempt this climb in good weather) the goal is generally obvious and the route apparent. Even so, first-time climbers should always go with an experienced individual who is familiar with the route and the idiosyncrasies of Mt. Hood's weather.

Leave from the north end of the parking lot at Timberline Lodge, and head almost directly north climbing over snow at a steady but not overly steep grade for 1 mile to the small Silcox Hut. Most climbers stop here to put on crampons and take a quick breather. Although it is possible to take the ski lift to this point, doing so requires that you wait for daylight when the lift begins operation. Since this means a much later start and potentially dangerous ice conditions above, it is not recommended.

From the hut you ascend at a much steeper grade, maintaining a fairly steady five-degree compass bearing for almost 2 miles as you head for the low area between prominent Crater Rock and Steel Cliff. This hike places you at about 10,200 feet in elevation (easily the highest in this book), so the air is noticeably thinner, something that is especially obvious to Portlanders who live close to sea level. Take it easy and watch for signs of altitude sickness in your group. If anyone starts to have problems, turn around and get to lower elevations as quickly as possible. Also here are the Hot Rocks, a geothermal feature that includes intermittent hot sulfur emissions, providing proof that while Mt. Hood is classified as a "dormant" volcano, it is far from extinct—something to keep in mind given the activity at nearby Mt. St. Helens in the last few decades.

Above Crater Rock is the Hogback, a narrow ridge of snow that leads up about 0.2 mile to the summit wall of Mt. Hood. Here is where most climbing groups elect to rope up. It is likely that other climbers will be here, waiting in line to make the traverse across the top of the Hogback, which is only wide enough for groups to go across single file. Near the top of the Hogback, as the slope gets noticeably steeper, is a deep crevasse, or bergschrund, directly across your route. If snow completely fills this crevasse you might be able to safely cross, but snow bridges sometimes collapse, so most climbers choose to go around the bergschrund.

Above the bergschrund is a wall of snow and ice leading to the summit. It can be very steep and requires solid ice conditions to ascend safely. The obvious narrow opening at the top of the wall (usually where you can see several other climbers, or at least their footprints) is called the Pearly Gates. On the other side of the Pearly Gates is the much sought after "Heaven" of the summit. The actual high point is easy to reach about 150 yards to the east. Do not expect to be alone here. On a weekend with ideal weather conditions there will typically be dozens (even hundreds) of other climbers sharing the view. And what a view to share! From the seemingly endless dry plains of eastern Oregon to the buildings of downtown Portland, from Washington's Alpine Lakes country and Mt. Rainier to Oregon's distant Three Sisters and Diamond Peak, the view seems to extend forever. Snap plenty of pictures, not only of the view, but of yourself, to commemorate your accomplishment.

Don't overstay your welcome, however, because you need to get back down while ice conditions remain favorable. Also remember that going down the steep headwall and the Hogback is often more dangerous than going up because the ice is less stable and climbers are often tired, overconfident, and go too quickly. Finally, be very careful to navigate correctly on the return route. Poor visibility as a result of clouds moving in has caused hundreds of climbers over the years to mistakenly follow a route that looks to be "straight down" but actually leads southwest into Zigzag Canyon, well to the west of Timberline Lodge and a potential danger zone.

TRIP 39 Veda Lake

Distance	2.8 miles, Out-and-back
Elevation Gain	750 feet
Hiking Time	1½ to 2 hours
Optional Map	Green Trails *Government Camp, High Rock*
Usually Open	Mid-June to October
Best Times	July and late August
Trail Use	Good for kids, dogs OK, backpacking option, fishing
Agency	Zigzag Ranger District, Mt. Hood National Forest
Difficulty	Moderate

HIGHLIGHTS In 1917, two locals named Vern Rogers and Dave Donaldson took it upon themselves to pack in a load of trout to a small, unnamed lake south of Government Camp, probably hoping to create a private fishing hole. Much to their surprise, their efforts garnered them a sort of immortality. To honor their achievement, the local forest ranger named the lake by combining the first two letters of each man's first name.

The offspring of the original fish can still be caught today. On their way to the lake's shores, visitors can also enjoy fine views of nearby Mt. Hood. This short but very satisfying little hike is well worth the lousy road access to the trailhead.

DIRECTIONS Take U.S. Highway 26 about 0.7 mile east of Government Camp, and then turn south on the road to Still Creek Campground. Drive through the campground for another 0.7 mile, and then keep straight at a junction where the campground loop road goes left. Following signs for Trillium Lake, you drive south on a pothole-covered gravel road for 0.4 mile to a junction where you turn right onto E. Chimney Rock Road.

This road goes past several private cabins for 0.4 mile to a four-way junction. You go straight on Forest Road 2613 and slow down because this soon becomes a miserably rutted and bumpy dirt road. After 3.7 carefully negotiated miles, pull into a poorly marked parking area on the left, just opposite the trailhead.

The trail starts on the north side of the road next to a small brown sign and then climbs in a forest of Pacific silver fir and mountain hemlock. Tall red huckleberry bushes crowd the forest and provide a treat for the taste buds in late August. After gaining about 250 feet, you top a viewless ridge and then begin to gradually descend. About 200 yards later, you reach an excellent viewpoint of Mt. Hood, almost perfectly framed by the forested valley of Still Creek, with round Veda Lake sparkling in the basin directly below.

You switchback down past three more good viewpoints, at openings that pro-

Veda Lake

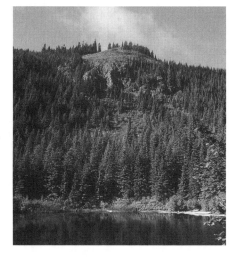

Veda Lake

vide sunshine for early to mid-July wildflowers like lupine, paintbrush, beargrass, arnica, and showy Washington lily. The final descent is made on one long switchback down a partly forested hillside to the north shore of three-acre Veda Lake. Ever since Vern and Dave stocked this lake, it has produced catchable brook trout. If fishing isn't your goal, the lake is also a good place to swim, camp, or just relax and enjoy a peaceful mountain setting.

TRIP 40 Trillium Lake Loop

Distance	2.0 miles, Loop
Elevation Gain	Negligible
Hiking Time	1 to 2 hours
Optional Map	Green Trails *Mount Hood* (trail not shown)
Usually Open	Very late May to October
Best Times	Late May and September
Trail Use	Good for kids, dogs OK, wheelchair accessible, fishing
Agency	Zigzag Ranger District, Mt. Hood National Forest
Difficulty	Easy

HIGHLIGHTS Trillium Lake is an extremely popular destination for campers, picnickers, photographers, skiers, anglers, and just about any other outdoor-oriented "-ers" in the Portland area. That popularity is understandable, and since the lake boasts such a gorgeous view of Mount Hood, the place is frequently featured in national calendars and photo books. Until recently, however, hikers have not been among the lake's many admirers, kept away by the crowds and the lack of a shoreline trail. Well, it may be time to change that opinion, because a wonderful trail now circles this mountain gem, and as for the crowds, you can avoid those too, with good timing and a little luck.

In an average snow year the road to the lake opens just before Memorial Day, when the U.S. Forest Service tries to have the campground open for the holiday weekend. The ideal time to visit is immediately after the road opens on a weekday just before Memorial Day. It is wise to call ahead to check on the status of the road (no sense in wasting a trip), but with luck there may be only a dozen or so other admirers to share the view. If this plan doesn't work, the lake is still a must visit; just try to come early on a weekday.

DIRECTIONS Drive U.S. Highway 26 east from Government Camp to the signed junction with Trillium Lake Road (Forest Road 2656) near Milepost 56.7. Turn right (south), drive 1.8 miles, and then turn right into the day-use area. Proceed 0.2 mile and park in any of the available lots near the boat ramp.

Stroll down to the boat ramp and spend time admiring the postcard-perfect views over the lake of snowy Mt. Hood. After snapping plenty of photos, put on your pack and head north on the gravel Trillium Lake Trail. Since this loop trail is designed to be wheelchair accessible, the entire route is virtually level and has either a packed gravel surface or consists of boardwalks over wet areas. These circumstances make for very easy hiking and allow you to concentrate on the scenery. When you can take your eyes off the mountain views, it is interesting to look at the forest. Since the lake lies in the transition zone between low- and high-elevation environments, the mix of trees is quite varied. You will see both western red and Alaska yellow cedars, mountain hemlocks growing beside western hemlocks, and lodgepole pines mixed with western white pines. On the forest floor are upper-elevation plants, such as huckleberry and beargrass, as well as lower-elevation species like wood violet and Oregon grape. In late May, the forests are awash with the blossoms of, appropriate enough, trillium. Botanists will have a field day.

The trail makes its way north along the east side of the tranquil lake (motor-boats are not allowed) and soon follows the shore in a loop around the lake's busy campground. Keep left at junctions with a series of side paths that lead to car campsites and eventually walk past the campground amphitheatre. Soon thereafter, you leave the bustling campground and follow a much quieter path around the marshy northeast arm of the lake. Look here for vegetation adapted to wetlands, such as skunk cabbage, marsh

Mt. Hood over Trillium Lake

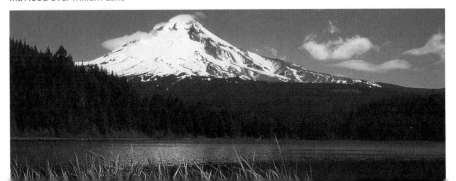

marigolds, and pond lilies. As it curves around the north shore, the trail comes to an unsigned junction with a boardwalk-covered trail going left (south). This path dead-ends after just 60 yards but leads to a nice viewpoint of a large marsh.

The main trail continues around the lake, never straying very far from the shore, all the way to the lake's southwest end. Here you reach a junction with the paved road over the lake's dam. Cross the dam by following the road shoulder, watching for traffic while simultaneously gawking at the amazing views of Mt. Hood. At the dam's east end turn left where the trail resumes, and hug the lakeshore for 0.2 mile, past a series of idyllic picnic sites and back to the boat ramp and the close of the loop.

TRIP 41 Upper Salmon River Trail

Distance	11.0 miles, Out-and-back
Elevation Gain	1400 feet
Hiking Time	5 to 6 hours
Optional Map	Green Trails *High Rock*
Usually Open	Late May to October
Best Time	Late May to October
Trail Use	Dogs OK, backpacking option, horseback riding, fishing
Agency	Zigzag Ranger District, Mt. Hood National Forest
Difficulty	Difficult
Note	Good in cloudy weather

HIGHLIGHTS Unlike the famous lower portion of the Salmon River Trail (Trip 7), the upper part of this canyon has no waterfalls and no spectacular views, but it's also a lot less crowded. Solitude seekers come here, not only for the quiet, but also to explore pretty side creeks and interesting, diverse forests that hikers on the lower trail miss.

DIRECTIONS Drive 1.8 miles east of Government Camp on U.S. Highway 26, and then turn right (south) at the Trillium Lake junction. Follow paved Forest Road 2656 for 1.7 miles, passing the lake's campground and day-use area, to a junction near the southeast corner of the lake. You bear left, staying on Road 2656, and after 1.1 miles, you will come to a fork where you bear right. The pavement ends as you continue on a good gravel road for 0.7 mile to another fork. Bear right once again on Forest Road 309, and drive a final 2.0 miles to a trailhead sign. Park on the shoulder of the road about 20 yards past the sign.

Two trails depart from this trailhead. For this loop, take the Salmon River Trail, which starts about 15 yards west of the parking area, off of a turnaround loop road.

This hiker-only trail descends through a relatively open forest to a log footbridge over misnamed Mud Creek, which is actually a lovely trout stream. After this, climb up and over a little ridge, hop across trickling Fir Tree Creek, and come to a junction with Dry Lake Trail at 0.5 mile. Although officially abandoned by the U.S. Forest Service, the Dry Lake Trail is still signed and the path is in reasonably good condition.

Go left, still on the Salmon River Trail, recross Fir Tree Creek soon, and begin a

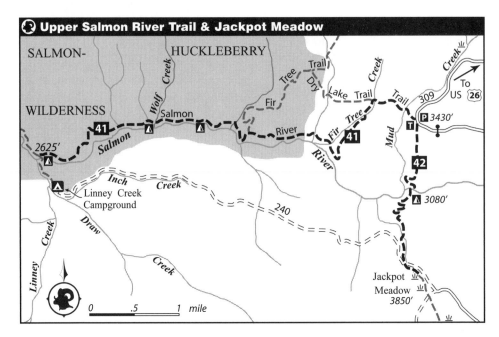

long gentle descent into the Salmon River Canyon. The relatively dry slopes here support unusually high concentrations of western white pine, a lovely tree with soft, 3-inch-long needles and oversized cones. Also common here are chubby western toads, which resemble wart-covered rocks. They are very slow of foot, so be careful not to step on one.

The trail makes a long downhill switchback and then crosses Fir Tree Creek a final time. Shortly thereafter you hop across an unnamed creek, pass the base of a large talus slope, and then come to a possibly unsigned junction with Fir Tree Trail at 2.5 miles. Like the Dry Lake Trail, this path has been abandoned by the U.S. Forest Service, but it is still hikable. On the return trip you can follow this steep path uphill for 1.6 miles, and then turn right and follow the Dry Lake Trail for 1 mile back to its junction with the Salmon River Trail.

For now, go straight on the Salmon River Trail, and continue your gentle downhill walk. At 3 miles you pass above a nice campsite along the river, and then at 3.6 miles you splash across Wolf Creek and come to another good campsite. Although this section of the trail offers very few opportunities to visit the river, the hiking is easy and the forest scenery attractive. At 4.5 miles the trail climbs away from the river onto the slopes above and then drops back down to a junction at 5.5 miles.

The main trail goes straight, but you turn sharply left on the Linney Creek Trail and walk 50 yards down to the river. There used to be a log bridge across the river here, but it is now gone. The ford that remains is always cold and often dangerous. Most hikers should not attempt it. Fortunately there is an excellent campsite nearby, just upstream and on your side of the river. This comfortable camp, situated under the shade of some large cedar and fir trees, makes a fine lunch spot for dayhikers or a good place for backpackers to spend the night savoring the sounds of a rushing mountain stream.

TRIP 42 Jackpot Meadow

Distance	5.8 miles, Out-and-back
Elevation Gain	1200 feet
Hiking Time	3 hours
Optional Map	Green Trails *High Rock*
Usually Open	May to October
Best Times	June and July
Trail Use	Good for kids, dogs OK, backpacking option
Agency	Zigzag Ranger District, Mt. Hood National Forest
Difficulty	Moderate
Note	Good in cloudy weather

HIGHLIGHTS This quiet trail is a good choice when you want to get away from the crowds. Even on the busiest summer weekends, this path remains lonesome, making it ideal for seekers of solitude. In addition to solitude, this trail provides hikers with a pleasant forest walk, visiting a beautiful spot along the upper reaches of the Salmon River, and giving you the chance to explore a lush mountain meadow. There may be no grand views, lakes, or any of the other attributes that tend to draw crowds, but the more subtle charms of the Oregon Cascades are nowhere on better display.

DIRECTIONS Drive 1.8 miles east of Government Camp on U.S. Highway 26, and then turn right (south) at the Trillium Lake junction. Follow paved Forest Road 2656 for 1.7 miles, passing the lake's campground and day-use area, to a junction near the southeast corner of the lake. Bear left, staying on Road 2656, and after 1.1 miles, come to a fork where you bear right. The pavement ends as you continue on a good gravel road for 0.7 mile to another fork. Bear right once again on Forest Road 309, and drive a final 2.0 miles to a trailhead sign. Park on the shoulder of the road about 20 yards past the sign.

Two trails depart from this trailhead. You take the path to Jackpot Meadow, going downhill to the south, from just below the parking area. For the first mile, the easy trail gradually descends through an exceptionally interesting and diverse forest of western white pine, lodgepole pine, western hemlock, Alaska yellow cedar, Douglas fir, and both Pacific silver and noble fir.

Once you reach the edge of the Salmon River Canyon, you descend two gentle switchbacks to a log footbridge over the clear, rushing stream. You'll probably have this spot all to yourself, so take some time to enjoy the waters and contemplate the subtle beauties of a mountain stream.

Once across the bridge, the trail goes upstream, past a small campsite, switch-backs to the right, and begins climbing moderately steeply away from the water. In three long and then three short switchbacks to the south rim of the canyon, the trail ascends a forested hillside with unusually high concentrations of low-growing Pacific yew and slow-moving western toads. Now on a forested plateau, you gradually ascend to a small tributary creek, hop across the flow, and then wander uphill to a trailhead on a dirt road.

To visit lovely Jackpot Meadow, with its little creek, grassy openings, scenic tree islands, and abundant wildflowers, you cross the road at a diagonal and then follow an unmaintained but obvious trail. This path crosses a sluggish creek and then travels around the east side of the meadow, just a few yards through the trees on the right. Take the time to go over to the meadow and explore. You will be rewarded with lots of wildflowers, especially camas, dandelion, shooting star, and aster. You may even be lucky enough to spot one of the sandhill cranes that occasionally nest here.

Jackpot Meadow is the recommended turnaround point for this hike. If you want more exercise, however, the main trail continues around the east side of Jackpot Meadow, crosses a gravel road, and then reaches Dry Meadow. After looping around the west side of that meadow, the trail crosses a paved road and comes to a junction with the Pacific Crest Trail north of Little Crater Lake (see Trip 49).

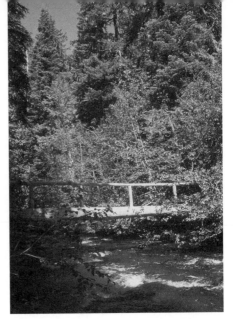

Log bridge over the Salmon River, the Jackpot Meadow Trail

TRIP 43 Barlow Butte

Distance	3.7 miles, Out-and-back
Elevation Gain	1100 feet
Hiking Time	2 hours
Optional Map	Green Trails *Mount Hood*
Usually Open	Mid-June to October
Best Time	July
Trail Use	Dogs OK
Agency	Zigzag Ranger District, Mt. Hood National Forest
Difficulty	Moderate

HIGHLIGHTS This generally overlooked hike offers the outdoor lover two outstanding features. First, you start the trip literally in the ruts of the wagon route of the old Oregon Trail. History buffs will get a kick out of following the tracks of the old-time immigrants. Second, the hike ends with a superb view of Mt. Hood. Despite these attributes, you are likely to have this trail all to yourself even on busy summer weekends. Add the short distance and good workout, and this route should be considered a "must do" hike for every Portland-area outdoor lover.

DIRECTIONS Drive U.S. Highway 26 a short distance east from Government Camp, and then exit onto State Highway 35, following signs to Hood River. Just 2.7 miles later, you'll come to Barlow Pass. Turn right here, and drive 0.2 mile on single-lane, paved Barlow Road (Forest Road 3531) to the signed trailhead for the Pacific Crest Trail.

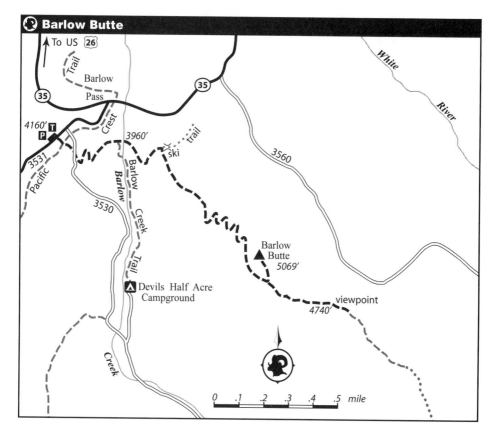

Barlow Butte

To US 26

Barlow Pass

Trail

Crest

35

35

4160'

P T

3531

3530

Pacific

Barlow

3960'

ski trail

Creek

Trail

Devils Half Acre Campground

Barlow Butte 5069'

3560

White

River

viewpoint

4740'

Creek

0 .1 .2 .3 .4 .5 mile

From the north end of the parking lot, hike due east on the signed tracks of the Oregon Trail, and then, after a few yards, cross the Pacific Crest Trail and go straight, staying on the historic wagon route. About 200 yards later, go diagonally across a dirt road and gradually lose elevation for 0.2 mile to a junction with the Barlow Creek Trail. You turn left, leaving the wagon road, and cross tiny Barlow Creek on a plank bridge. This trail climbs through a typical high-Cascades forest, mostly composed of Pacific silver fir and mountain hemlock. The sparse undergrowth, kept small by being smothered in snowdrifts for most of the year, is principally beargrass and huckleberry, with the white blooms of vanilla leaf, anemone, queen's cup, and bunchberry adding their bright faces in July. Just before reaching a

forested saddle, turn right at the marked junction with the Mineral Jane Ski Trail.

Now on a narrow footpath, you gradually ascend to the corner of a human-made clearing, where you can briefly glimpse the top half of Mt. Hood, before you return to the trees and climb. Your pace slows considerably as the trail angles sharply uphill and several short switchbacks guide you up a shady, north-facing slope. Eventually, you reach a ridgetop and an unsigned junction at a tiny opening in the trees. To the left, a sketchy track climbs for about 200 yards to the rocky summit of Barlow Butte. Unfortunately, the view of Mt. Hood from this high point is entirely blocked by trees.

To reach a more satisfying reward, turn right at the ridgetop junction and lose about 150 feet of elevation as you go

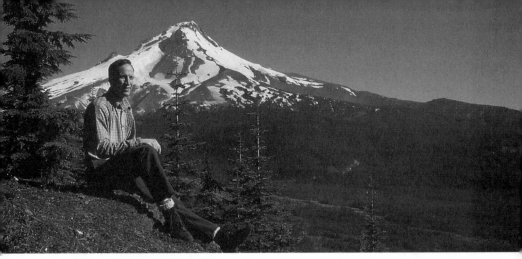

Mt. Hood from a ridge south of Barlow Butte

through a scenic rock garden with lots of July blossoms. Look for stonecrop, lomatium, yarrow, groundsel, cats ear, penstemon, and many other species. You probably still won't be satisfied with the partially obstructed view of Mt. Hood though, so continue hiking through trees. Then climb for another 200 yards to a second open area with great views of towering Mt. Hood and the glacial out-wash of the White River Valley to the north and the snowy landmark of Mt. Jefferson to the south. The best photos are from a rocky outcrop above the trail on the right. The trail continues along the wooded ridge to the south, but the views along that path are disappointing—it gets little or no maintenance, so turn back and return to your car.

TRIP 44 Pacific Crest Trail: North of Barlow Pass

Distance	7.4 miles, Out-and-back
Elevation Gain	1100 feet
Hiking Time	4 hours
Optional Map	Green Trails *Mount Hood*
Usually Open	July to October
Best Time	July
Trail Use	Dogs OK, horseback riding
Agency	Zigzag Ranger District, Mt. Hood National Forest
Difficulty	Moderate

HIGHLIGHTS This convenient segment of the Pacific Crest Trail (PCT) is not noticed by most hikers, who typically head for the more popular destinations on Mt. Hood. The thinking seems to be that if it is possible to drive to both ends of a trail then there isn't much point in hiking it. Nonsense! Granted, you might not want to drive four or five hours out of your way to take this hike, but for a simple one-hour stint in the car, the scenery and exercise are ample compensation.

DIRECTIONS Drive U.S. Highway 26 a short distance east from Government Camp, and then exit onto State Highway 35, following signs to Hood River. Just 2.7 miles later, you'll come to Barlow Pass. The PCT crosses the highway about 0.2 mile beyond the pass, but it is quieter and safer to park at the Barlow Pass Sno-Park. To reach it, turn south on single-lane, paved road Barlow Road (Forest Road 3531), and drive 0.2 mile to the signed trailhead for the PCT.

From the north end of the parking lot hike due east on the signed tracks of the Oregon Trail, and then, after a few yards, come to a junction with the PCT. Turn left on this gentle path, which wanders through a dense forest of mountain hemlock, Douglas fir, and noble fir on an old roadbed for 0.1 mile before arriving at Highway 35. You cross the highway and pick up the well-marked trail on the other side.

The road is a noisy intrusion, but you soon leave its sight and, a little later, its sounds behind as you climb west across a woodsy hillside. The trail rounds a ridge marking the crest of the Cascade Divide and then curves north as it continues its ascent. There are no views along the way, but the forests are pleasant, with a few shade-loving wildflowers in July and some huckleberries in late August. The trees become generally smaller in size as the trail curves west to reach a small campsite beside a tiny creek in a gully. As you continue to gain elevation, the flowers become increasingly abundant, and the views improve, making for very enjoyable hiking throughout the summer. Shortly after reaching the edge of a meadow, you come to a junction with the Timberline Trail.

You now have a choice. Those looking for a good workout should continue straight on the PCT to historic Timberline Lodge. This often exposed path stays in timberline meadows for most of the next 1.4 miles on a tiring, sandy ascent overlooking the glacial and volcanic mudflow material in White River Canyon. The scenery along this path is very good, but it is no better than what you can obtain without this extra effort. If you've had enough exercise (or you simply have no desire to fight the tourist crowds at Timberline Lodge), turn right at the Timberline Trail junction, and walk for a couple hundred yards to a lovely, flower-filled meadow with a view of Mt. Hood.

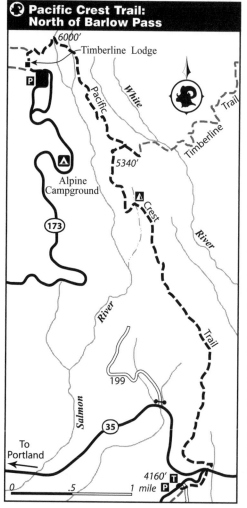

Pacific Crest Trail: North of Barlow Pass

6000'

Timberline Lodge

P

Pacific

White

Trail

Timberline

5340'

Alpine Campground

173

Crest

River

River

River

Trail

199

Salmon

35

Trail

To Portland

4160'

0   .5   1 mile   P

Mount Hood Area

TRIP 45 Twin Lakes & Palmateer Point Loop

Distance	7.8 miles, Semiloop
Elevation Gain	1100 feet
Hiking Time	3½ to 4 hours
Optional Map	Green Trails *Mt. Hood & Mt. Wilson*
Usually Open	June to October
Best Time	Mid- to late August
Trail Use	Dogs OK, backpacking option, horseback riding, fishing
Agency	Zigzag Ranger District, Mt. Hood National Forest
Difficulty	Moderate

HIGHLIGHTS This popular outing has just about everything you can ask from a hike in the Oregon Cascades. There are two sparkling lakes, lots of attractive forests, acres of berries to pick, and a smashing view of Mt. Hood. About the only thing missing is a wildflower-filled meadow, but to complain about that would really be getting picky. The easy trail makes this an ideal family backpacking trip, with enough to keep both children and adults happy, while not excessively tiring young legs.

DIRECTIONS Drive U.S. Highway 26 a short distance east from Government Camp, and then exit onto State Highway 35, following signs for Hood River. Just 2.7 miles later, you'll come to Barlow Pass. Turn right here, and drive 0.2 mile on single-lane, paved Barlow Road (Forest Road 3531) to the signed trailhead for the Pacific Crest Trail (PCT).

Pick up the PCT just a few feet east of the parking lot and turn right (south). The wide, gently graded trail gradually gains elevation as it passes through a viewless mountain-hemlock forest. The miles go by quickly as you climb into more open terrain and reach a junction with the return route of the loop. Go straight, sticking with the PCT, and gradually go down through open forests with lots of huckleberries lining the trail. The delicious fruit of these plants ripens in the second half of August, a particularly good time for this hike. Just 0.6 mile later is a second junction, where you once again go straight on the PCT. After

Mt. Hood from a viewpoint northeast of Upper Twin Lake

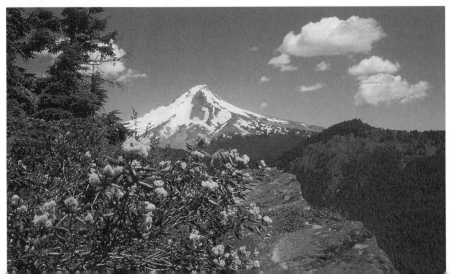

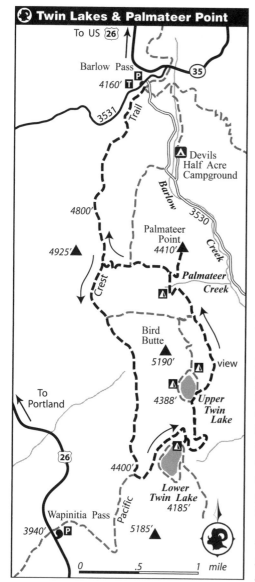

Twin Lakes & Palmateer Point

To US 26
Barlow Pass
4160' T
35
3531 Trail
Devils
Half Acre
Campground
Barlow
3530
Creek
4800'
Palmateer
Point
4410'
4925'
Palmateer
Creek
Crest
Bird
Butte
5190'
view
To
Portland
4388' Upper
Twin
Lake
26
4400'
Lower
Twin Lake
4185'
Wapinitia Pass
Pacific
3940' P
5185'
0   .5   1 mile

To continue the loop, bear left at a junction just above the lake and loop back to the north, climbing two switchbacks, to shallow Upper Twin Lake. This tranquil pool has adequate camps, lots of huckleberries, and a view of the top of Mt. Hood. You go right at a junction at the south end of the lake, follow the east shore for 100 yards, and then bear right at a junction with the Palmateer View Trail. After about 0.4 mile, don't miss visiting a superb viewpoint at a small rock outcropping atop the cliffs on your right. The view from here of Barlow Butte, the Barlow Creek Valley, and towering Mt. Hood is classic. If you stop for lunch, you may also be rewarded with a visit from friendly rufous hummingbirds feasting on the pink cliff penstemon that clings to these rocks.

After reluctantly leaving this idyllic location, you soon hit a junction where you go right and drop to a lush little meadow with adequate camps and a nice creek. Shortly after the easy creek crossing, you have the option of turning right on a 0.3-mile side trail leading to the fine view from Palmateer Point. This is worth a visit, even though the view is not as photogenic as that at the trailside location described above.

The main loop goes left at the Palmateer Point junction and climbs a gentle slope in an interesting forest of mixed conifers. Unlike the rather monotonous mountain-hemlock forests in most of the Cascades, here there are open woods of Alaska yellow cedar, western white pine, lodgepole pine, Douglas fir, Pacific silver fir, and Engelmann spruce, along with the hemlocks. Partway up the slope, you go straight at the junction with a trail to the right, which leads to Devils Half Acre, and continue uphill to close the loop at the junction with the PCT.

another 1.4 viewless miles you arrive at a third junction. Turn left to climb this path over a low rise, and then drop gradually to some excellent camps at the north end of lovely Lower Twin Lake. Even though it is crowded on weekends, this is a good place to spend the night, partly because the greenish waters of this deep lake are great for swimming.

TRIP 46 Twin Lakes from Wapinitia Pass

Distance	5.6 miles (to Upper Twin Lake), Out-and-back
Elevation Gain	900 feet
Hiking Time	2½ hours
Optional Map	Green Trails *Mt. Hood, Mt. Wilson*
Usually Open	June to October
Best Time	Mid- to late August
Trail Use	Good for kids, dogs OK, backpacking option, horseback riding, fishing
Agency	Zigzag Ranger District, Mt. Hood National Forest
Difficulty	Easy
Note	Good in cloudy weather

HIGHLIGHTS This is a good option for hikers with children or pedestrians who just want to visit the Twin Lakes without the added miles of the approach from Barlow Pass (Trip 45). By starting from Wapinitia Pass, your drive is a little longer, but since you save almost two hours of hiking, that is a reasonable tradeoff. This approach is less scenic than the one from the north, but this is the superior choice if your goal is to spend more time fishing or swimming at the lakes.

DIRECTIONS From the junction of U.S. Highway 26 and State Highway 35 east of Government Camp, go 6 miles southeast on Highway 26 (toward Bend), and then turn left into the large Frog Lake Sno-Park and trailhead.

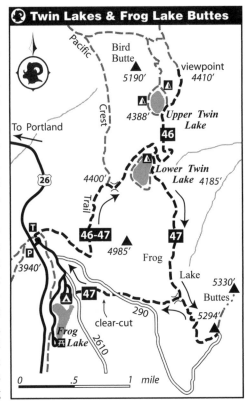

You will find the Pacific Crest Trail (PCT) a few feet north of the lot, near a brown marker for skiers. You turn right on the PCT and, in 120 yards, go straight at the junction with a trail that heads south to the busy car campground at Frog Lake (Trip 47). The gently graded PCT climbs gradually, in one very long switchback, up a slope covered with mountain hemlocks and firs. Nearer at hand are dense thickets of huckleberries, which ripen nicely in late August.

After 1.3 miles, you reach a trail junction where you leave the PCT and turn right. Follow this path as it crosses a saddle and begins a gradual descent toward Lower Twin Lake, which is visible through the trees on the right. Just after crossing the often-dry inlet creek, a signed trail drops to the right and leads to some large camps at the north end of the lake. A fisherman's path goes around the lake, while the trail to Frog

Lake Buttes climbs away from the lake's eastern shore. To reach Upper Twin Lake, which has poorer camps but fewer people and a partial view of Mt. Hood, hike past the signed turnoff to Lower Twin Lake, round a ridge, and climb two well-graded switchbacks to the shallow upper lake.

Views from both lakes are limited, so hikers who want to see Mt. Hood, or who simply want more exercise, must take one of two options. Most hikers head south from Lower Twin Lake to Frog Lake Buttes on a rather dull, woodsy route that tops out at a decent viewpoint but one whose immediate surroundings are rather ugly. A much better and quieter option follows the Palmateer View Trail from the eastern shores of Upper Twin Lake. After 0.4 mile, you reach an unmarked viewpoint just a few feet off the trail with outstanding views of the Barlow Creek Valley and Mt. Hood.

TRIP **47** Frog Lake Buttes Loop

Distance	6.3 miles, Loop
Elevation Gain	1600 feet
Hiking Time	3 hours
Optional Map	Green Trails *Mount Wilson*
Usually Open	Mid-June to October
Best Time	Any time it's open
Trail Use	Dogs OK
Agency	Zigzag Ranger District, Mt. Hood National Forest
Difficulty	Difficult

see map on p.392

HIGHLIGHTS The Frog Lake Buttes are a cluster of forested peaks not far east of their namesake lake that provide a nice getaway for hikers looking for a relatively uncrowded destination near Mt. Hood. The view from the top is a little disappointing, with small trees blocking most of the scene, but when you combine the buttes in a loop that visits Lower Twin Lake, you can enjoy a scenic and diverse mix of mountain landscapes in an unusually compact package.

DIRECTIONS From the junction of U.S. Highway 26 and State Highway 35 east of Government Camp, go 6 miles southeast on Highway 26 (toward Bend), and then turn left into the large Frog Lake Sno-Park and trailhead.

From the north end of the parking lot take a short spur trail to a junction with the Pacific Crest Trail (PCT), and turn right (northbound) on this famous route. Just 120 yards later you go straight at a junction and ascend the wide, gently graded PCT in one long switchback to a junction at 1.3 miles. Turn right, leaving the PCT, soon go through a wide saddle, and then make a gentle woodsy descent to a junction above the north-east end of sparkling Lower Twin Lake. Turn right (downhill) and soon reach the large camping area above the north shore of this deep, green-tinged, 15-acre pool.

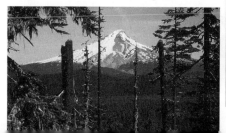

Mt. Hood from the trail below Frog Lake Buttes

There is a nice view south over the lake of one of the forested Frog Lake Buttes.

To continue the loop, follow the shoreline trail around the east side of Lower Twin Lake for 0.1 mile, and then turn left at a sign for Frog Lake Buttes. This narrow trail, which is lined with an abundance of huckleberries (bring your appetite in late August), makes an irregular climb through fairly dense hemlock and fir forests to a junction in a saddle at 3.7 miles. The return route of the recommended loop goes right, but to reach the summit of Frog Lake Buttes, you turn left and rapidly ascend a forested ridge with tantalizing glimpses of Mt. Hood through the trees. After five steep, rounded switchbacks you reach the partial openings and beargrass meadows just below the summit of the middle Frog Lake Butte. The top of this peak sports the all-too-common eyesores of a road and a com-

munications tower, but the setting is still attractive, with lots of perky little evergreens scattered about and a profusion of wildflowers in the open areas. Unfortunately, most of the views are blocked by trees. Somewhat more open views are available by following a wide trail to the northeast that soon grows faint as it heads toward the highest of the Frog Lake Buttes about 0.4 mile away.

To finish the recommended loop, return to the junction in the saddle 0.6 mile below the summit and turn left. This moderately steep trail descends 0.7 mile to a crossing of gravel Road 290 and then passes through the top of a recovering clear-cut. After reentering forest, the path descends to cross gravel Road 2610 and then continues another 80 yards to the trail's end at the paved loop road in Frog Lake Campground. Turn right and walk the road 0.4 mile back to your car.

TRIP 48 Clear Lake

Distance	7.8 miles, Out-and-back
Elevation Gain	1750 feet
Hiking Time	4 hours
Optional Map	Green Trails *Mount Wilson*
Usually Open	June to November
Best Time	Any
Trail Use	Dogs OK, horseback riding, fishing
Agency	Zigzag Ranger District, Mt. Hood National Forest
Difficulty	Difficult

HIGHLIGHTS Clear Lake is a large human-made lake surrounded by forested hills and ridges in the heart of the Mount Hood National Forest. The lake's water level is often drawn down for irrigation, which significantly reduces its scenic appeal, but it is still worth a visit, especially for anglers looking to catch big rainbow and brook trout. There is a nice car campground on the lake's eastern shore, but for hikers it is more fun to follow this pleasant trail that wanders over a forested hill before dropping steeply to the remote north shore of Clear Lake.

DIRECTIONS From the junction of U.S. Highway 26 and State Highway 35 east of Government Camp, go 6 miles southeast on Highway 26 (toward Bend), and then turn left into the large Frog Lake Sno-Park and trailhead.

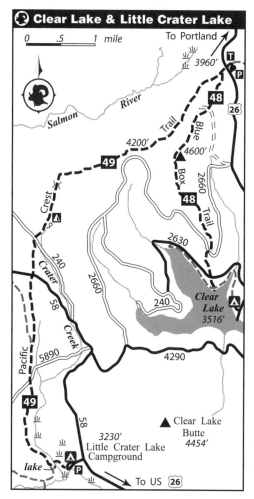

Clear Lake & Little Crater Lake

0   .5   1 mile   To Portland

3960'

T
P

48

26

Salmon River

Trail

4200'

Crest

4600'

Blue

Box

48

49

2660

Trail

2630

240

2660

Crater

Creek

58

240

Clear
Lake
3516'

Pacific

5890

4290

49

58

3230'
Little Crater Lake
Campground

▲ Clear Lake
Butte
4454'

lake

P

To US 26

and begin an irregular, often steep, climb in a dense viewless forest of Douglas firs, western hemlocks, grand firs, and noble firs. Except for a smattering of huckleberry bushes and beargrass plants, the forest here has almost no undergrowth.

At 0.9 mile the trail's grade evens out somewhat shortly before the path crosses a narrow dirt road. At 1.7 miles the trail tops an unnamed butte and passes through two recovering clear-cuts. The first of these openings provides decent views to the north of Mt. Hood, while the second gives you a look at rounded Frog Lake Buttes to the east. After returning to unlogged forest, the trail begins going downhill. At times the route is a little sketchy, especially in a few rocky and brushy spots, but it remains reasonably easy to follow.

The downhill becomes considerably steeper as you drop to a crossing of gravel Road 2660 at 3.2 miles and then continues steeply down to a crossing of paved Road 2630. After that it's a gradual 0.2-mile descent to an unsigned junction with a shoreline all-terrain vehicle trail just above the waters of Clear Lake. This north-shore location is well away from the crowded campground, so wildlife is often present. Look for Canada geese and ospreys, as well as deer and several small mammals. There is a nice view of Clear Lake Butte over the water to the south. Sharp-eyed hikers might even be able to make out the short lookout tower at the top.

From the north end of the parking lot take a short spur trail to a junction with the Pacific Crest Trail, and turn left (southbound) on that famous path. You soon cross Highway 26 (watching carefully for traffic), and walk 75 yards to a junction. Turn left on the Blue Box Trail,

Mt. Hood from a clear-cut along the Blue Box Trail to Clear Lake

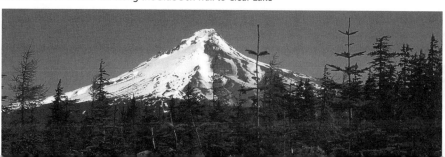

TRIP *49* Pacific Crest Trail: South to Little Crater Lake

see map on p.395

Distance	8.2 miles, Point-to-point; 16.3 miles, Out-and-back
Elevation Gain	350 feet, Point-to-point; 1350 feet, Out-and-back
Hiking Time	4 to 8 hours
Optional Map	Green Trails *High Rock, Mount Wilson*
Usually Open	Late May to November
Best Time	June
Trail Use	Dogs OK, horseback riding
Agency	Zigzag Ranger District, Mt. Hood National Forest
Difficulty	Moderate to Difficult

HIGHLIGHTS A deep, blue artesian spring situated in an absolutely gorgeous mountain meadow, Little Crater Lake is one of Oregon's great hidden treasures. A paved road takes you to a campground within 0.1 mile of the lake, but it is well worth the time to hike there instead, with the lake as the icing on the cake of a fun day on the trail. The Pacific Crest Trail leads to within 150 yards of the lake, so following that famous path is the ideal hiking option. With a car shuttle, you can make this into a fun, mostly downhill, one-way adventure.

DIRECTIONS From the junction of U.S. Highway 26 and State Highway 35 east of Government Camp, go 6 miles southeast on Highway 26 (toward Bend), and then turn left into the large Frog Lake Sno-Park and trailhead.

If you are leaving a second car at Little Crater Lake, continue 4.5 miles southeast on Highway 26, and then turn right (southwest) at a sign for Skyline Road/Forest Road 42. Drive 4.2 miles, and then turn right onto Road 58. Follow this one-lane paved road for 2.4 miles, and then turn left into Little Crater Lake Campground. Parking for the trailhead is at the far end of the campground loop, about 0.2 mile from Road 58.

From the north end of the Frog Lake parking lot take a short spur trail to a junction with the Pacific Crest Trail (PCT), and turn left (southbound) on that famous path. You soon cross Highway 26 (watch carefully for traffic) and walk 75 yards to a junction.

Continue straight on the PCT, and follow this well-graded route as it gradually goes up and down in a long southwesterly traverse through a lovely forest of western and mountain hemlock and Douglas firs. Pacific rhododendrons are common along this section, blooming profusely in late June and early July. Most of the way is viewless, but from time to time you gain tantalizing glimpses to the north of large Salmon River Meadows with snowy Mt. Hood towering behind. After about 3.5

miles the trail turns south, goes through a low, forested saddle and soon comes to a small campsite next to a tiny spring.

About 0.3 mile past the campsite is a crossing of gravel Road 240 and then a nearly level section mostly in a lodgepole-pine forest to a crossing of paved Road 58. Still going south, you begin gradually losing elevation to a junction with a faint trail going sharply right toward Jackpot Meadow. Keep straight on the PCT, cross gravel Road 5890, and soon level out. You should now begin to notice marshy Little Crater Meadow through the trees to the left (east). If the mosquitoes aren't too bad (they often are in June and July), it is worth going over to this lush meadow to take a look. There aren't any views, but the water-loving flowers, especially

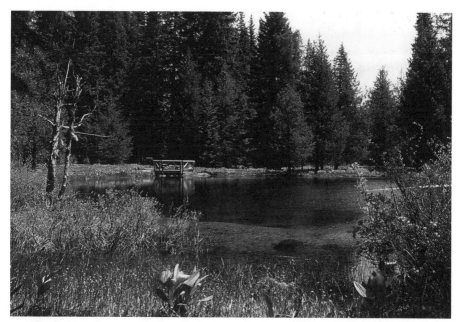

Little Crater Lake

shooting stars, false hellebores, and buttercups put on a fine show.

At 8 miles is a junction. Turn left, leaving the PCT, and follow a short trail that goes over a small creek and through the wet meadow to Little Crater Lake. This clear 45-foot-deep artesian spring boasts a striking blue color and an absolutely gorgeous meadowy setting. The water is a chilly 40 degrees year-round, so swimming is not only officially discouraged but also dangerously cold. Beyond the lake, the now-paved trail goes 0.1 mile through more of the spectacular meadow and then to the road at Little Crater Lake Campground.

Chapter 7
Clackamas River Area

Rising in the forested highlands and wilderness areas of the Cascade Mountains, the strikingly beautiful Clackamas River is perhaps the loveliest stream in the Portland/Vancouver region—and that's a category with lots of competition. Everything seems designed to add to this river's scenic attributes. With no glaciers in its watershed, the river's water is free of any glacial silt and incredibly clear. Over the millennia the river has cut a twisting canyon that screens the stream from the clear-cuts on surrounding ridges and provides close-up looks at many scenic basalt cliffs and densely forested slopes. The forests right beside the river have escaped the chain saw, and represent some of the most impressive, and acces-

sible, old-growth forests in the region. Rollicking rapids between glassy eddies give the stream a wide variety of moods, all of which put visitors in a perpetually good mood.

To give visitors the chance to enjoy these attributes, the U.S. Forest Service has developed several comfortable campgrounds and picnic areas along the river. There are also developed launch sites for rafters and kayakers, and even a fishing pier specifically designed for the disabled. And, of course, most relevant to this book, there are trails. You will find easy paths beside the river's waters and, in the surrounding hills, more challenging trails that lead to viewpoints on ridgetops and to sparkling mountain lakes. While

A fisherman on the Clackamas River, Milo McIver State Park (Trip 2)

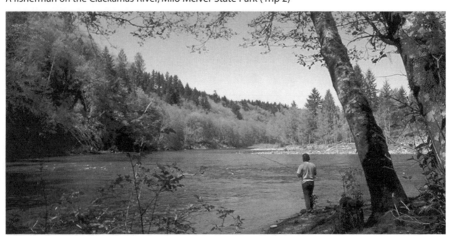

it is true that compared to Mt. Hood or the Columbia River Gorge these trails are relatively few in number, every trail here is worth hiking and, for that matter, rehiking. What more could you ask for?

Like so many other place names in our region, the name *Clackamas* has Native American origins. The Clackamas Indians were once a large tribe who lived along the banks of this stream. Meriwether Lewis and William Clark became familiar with them (spelling the name *Clacka-mus*) during their 1803–1806 expedition, and most other early explorers and settlers had friendly contact with this tribe. Unfortunately, repeating the sad history of Native Americans throughout this continent, most of the tribe was wiped out by disease or pushed off their homeland by white settlers. The remnants of the tribe were relocated to the Grande Ronde Reservation in the Oregon Coast Range.

Most people also assume that the town of Estacada, which serves as the gateway to the Clackamas River region, also has a

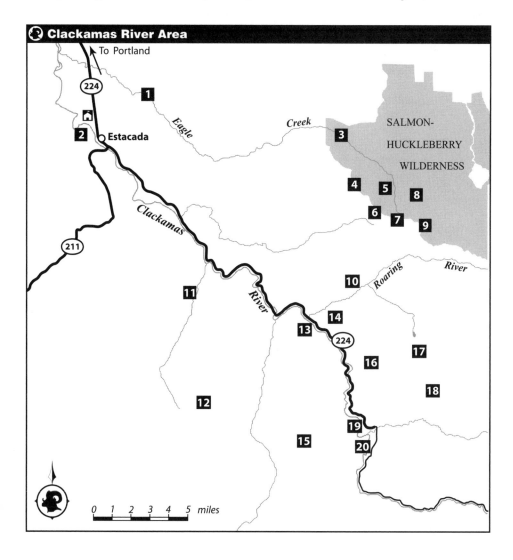

Native American name. Actually *estacada* is a Spanish word meaning something like "marked with stakes." This name was chosen for this town for no better reason than that the early residents thought it had a pleasing sound.

State Highway 224 provides the principal access to the Clackamas River Area, paralleling the river from Estacada nearly to the stream's source. Trailheads are usually located along one of the dozens of Forest Service roads that branch off the state highway. Portland area residents typically reach Highway 224 by leaving Interstate 205 at Exit 12, driving 3.2 miles east on State Highway 212, and then branching right (southeast) on State Highway 224, following signs to Estacada.

TRIP 1 Eagle-Fern County Park Loop

Distance	1.3 miles, Loop
Elevation Gain	350 feet
Hiking Time	1 hour
Optional Map	USGS *Estacada* (trail not shown)
Usually Open	All year (except during winter storms)
Best Time	Any
Trail Use	Good for kids, dogs OK, partly wheelchair accessible, fishing
Agency	Clackamas County Parks
Difficulty	Easy
Note	Good in cloudy weather

HIGHLIGHTS Eagle-Fern County Park is a 171-acre preserve in the hills northeast of Estacada. Although the popular park offers only a few trails, they are well worth exploring. The main scenic attractions are a magnificent old-growth forest and the beautiful clear waters of Eagle Creek. In addition to being lovely to look at, this clear-flowing stream is a popular fishery for trout, salmon, and steelhead.

DIRECTIONS Take Exit 12A off Interstate 205, and then drive east and south on State Highways 212 and 224 following signs to Estacada. At Milepost 19, turn left (east) on Wildcat Mountain Road and drive 0.2 mile to a four-way junction. Go straight and proceed 1.8 miles to a junction with Eagle-Fern Road. Veer right, drive 2.3 miles, and then turn right into Eagle-Fern Park. Immediately after entering the park, turn right and park in the small trailhead parking lot. A fee of $3 per vehicle is collected on weekends and holidays.

The trail departs from the north end of the parking lot and immediately crosses a large bridge over the clear, rushing waters of Eagle Creek. In winter you can expect to see several anglers along this lovely stream hoping to catch some of the winter steelhead and coho salmon that spawn here. The trail forks on the other side of the bridge.

You turn right on a nearly level hard-packed gravel nature trail. This wheelchair-accessible loop trail passes many numbered posts and interpretive signs explaining the natural history of the stream and the spectacular low-elevation old-growth forest protected in the park. Magnificent western red cedars tower overhead, while smaller specimens of

⊙ Eagle-Fern County Park Loop

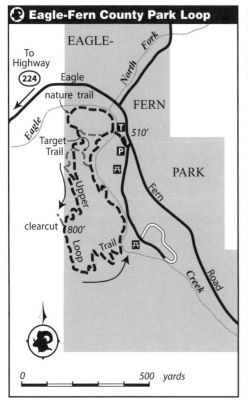

EAGLE-

To Highway

(224)

Eagle

North Fork

nature trail

FERN

Eagle

Target Trail

T 510'

P

PARK

Upper

Fern

clearcut 800'

Loop

Trail

Creek

Road

Creek

0   500   yards

clear-cut. The trees on the edge of this logged area are exposed to the wind and particularly susceptible to winter blow-down, so off-season hikers should expect to crawl over downed logs.

At a junction with a short spur trail that goes sharply right, you go straight and descend 13 mostly short and often steep switchbacks to the banks of Eagle Creek. The path then turns downstream winding along the forest-covered stream bank a little above the cascading waters. Several short spur paths lead to fishing or picnicking spots beside the creek. Shortly after the trail passes a large overhanging rock formation, you climb two switchbacks and come to a junction. The Target Trail goes left, but you turn right and descend past an excellent lunch spot atop a rock formation above the creek to a junction with the nature trail loop you left earlier in the hike. Turn right, and walk 80 yards to the trail bridge over the creek and to your car.

Rain forest in Eagle-Fern County Park

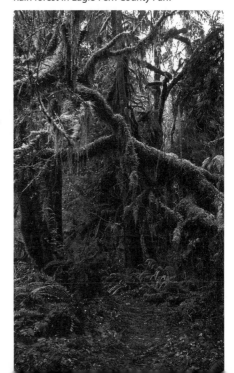

Douglas fir, western hemlock, and red alder fill out the canopy. The forest floor is dominated by salmonberry bushes and sword fern although a variety of small forest wildflowers, such as oxalis, also grace the area in the spring. Moss is draped over almost everything in sight, and epiphytic licorice ferns grow out of the trees and rocks.

At 0.15 mile you leave the nature trail, veering right on a narrower trail that in one switchback ascends to a flat area with a four-way junction. The Target Trail goes left, but you should go straight on the Upper Loop Trail, which briefly ambles through a red-alder woodland before ascending a heavily wooded hillside in one switchback to another junction. Go left and climb four gentle switchbacks to the park boundary and the edge of a

TRIP 2 Milo McIver State Park Loop

Distance	4.3 miles, Loop
Elevation Gain	250 feet
Hiking Time	2 hours
Optional Map	Use park brochure.
Usually Open	All year
Best Time	Late October to mid-November
Trail Use	Good for kids, dogs OK, horseback riding, fishing
Agency	Milo McIver State Park
Difficulty	Easy
Note	Good in cloudy weather

HIGHLIGHTS Milo McIver State Park is a quiet tract of land along the Clackamas River near Estacada. The park is surrounded by farms and woodlands that give the area a tranquil, rural setting rather than the feeling of true wilderness. The state parks department has developed an extensive network of trails in the park, although hikers generally have to take a backseat to equestrians, picnickers, and disc golfers. The best way to appreciate the wilder parts of this park is to follow the outer equestrian loop, which explores the forests, riverbanks, and open fields in the southern part of the park. The heavy emphasis on hooves makes the recommended path wide and easy to follow, but it also turns the trail into a chewed-up quagmire during the rainy season. Summer and fall are better; in the latter the many deciduous trees add color and a bed of fallen leaves on the trail.

DIRECTIONS To reach the park from the Portland area, take Exit 12 off Interstate 205, and drive east on State Highway 224/212. Turn right (south) where these roads split, following Highway 224 and signs to Estacada. About 1.5 miles later, bear right at the town of Carver and cross a bridge. At a junction on the other side of the bridge, turn left, and then simply follow the signs for the next 10 miles directing you to McIver Park. Once you turn into the park, pass the entrance station, where a $3 day-use fee is charged, and follow the signs to the Fish Hatchery at the south end of the park. Leave your car in the large equestrian overflow lot near the hatchery.

The horse trail departs from the Fish Hatchery directly across from the parking area. A slightly longer hiker approach, however, is worth the extra 0.1 mile of walking. To find it, follow a well-beaten path from the southwest end of the parking lot, and walk past mixed conifer and deciduous woods to a short spur trail, which leads to a river-bend fishing hole on the Clackamas River. The main loop goes left from the short spur to the river and immediately crosses a culvert over the outlet creek from the hatchery. In spring, expect thickets of tall, pink corydalis blooms to brighten the woodsy scene of moss-draped red alder, black cottonwood, western red cedar, and bigleaf maple.

You cross a bridged tributary creek as you loop around the hatchery and then pick up the horse route at a junction. Turn right and go uphill on a wide trail that is pleasant despite being chopped up by hooves and made aromatic by horse apples. The loop route goes right at the next junction, following the small posted markers for the horse loop. Hummingbirds, warblers, sparrows, chickadees, and other birds twitter away, taking the edge off the quiet of the open woods.

The horse trail travels near the park's access road for a short stretch, veers away, and follows the edge of some bluffs overlooking a large bend in the Clackamas River. You'll enjoy occasional glimpses through the trees down to the stream and out to the surrounding rural landscape, as the wide trail makes one long switchback up an embankment covered by red alder, bigleaf maple, and sword fern. Partway up this short climb, you keep straight at a junction with the Vortex Trail, which is often closed due to landslides. At the top of the 100-foot ascent, you reach a wooden bench and scenic overlook of the river. This is a nice lunch or rest stop, with the snowy foothills of the Cascade Mountains providing a scenic backdrop

for the raging river. You may hear trains in the distance and see a few farms and homes, but none of this really detracts from the scene.

Shortly after the bench, the path emerges from trees and follows the edge of a mowed grassy area, where you can see a nearby highway and farmhouses outside of the park. Your trail goes in and out of forested areas and through more lawns and then crosses the entrance road to the park maintenance buildings. After this, you pass through a wet area, which is home to false hellebore, and cross the park access road.

About 100 yards after crossing the road you come to yet another junction, where you bear right and soon arrive at a spot where the trail is regularly closed for the wet season. An alternate, drier route

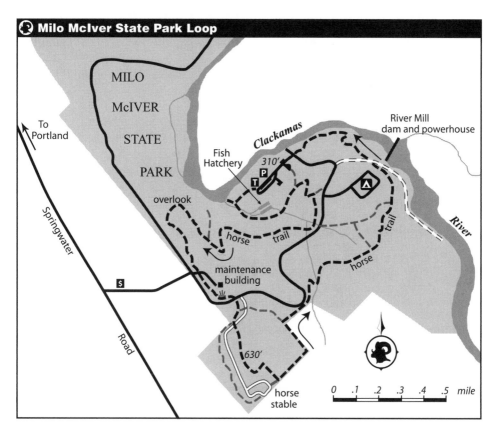

Milo McIver State Park Loop

goes left, crosses a gravel access road, and passes through a huge grassy area as it works toward a large barn. You turn left a little before reaching the barn—a private facility providing horse-riding opportunities—and enjoy nice looks at Mt. Hood over the wild grassy expanse directly ahead of you. After looping around the barn, the obvious, but not terribly wild, route turns left to follow a fence line at the edge of the park. The trail turns 90 degrees to the left, following a hedgerow along a property boundary, and then comes to a T-junction, where you turn right and walk through stunted woods and brushy areas popular with nesting birds.

The pleasant path winds downhill in deciduous woods to a bridge over a small creek and then levels off in lovely deciduous forests taking you to a junction. Go right again and pass through a semi-open area with very tall Oregon grape plants, which bloom from mid-April into May. You pass several junctions with hiker

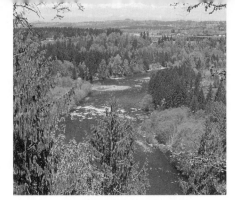

Clackamas River from a scenic overlook

trails and then once more follow a fence with the commercial activity of a dam and powerhouse on your right and car campsites on your left.

After leaving the campground area, cross a confusing old road at a left diagonal and then saunter through more mixed woods. The trail now drops to the banks of the Clackamas River, where you can enjoy the soothing sounds of rushing water or take any of several short, tempting side paths to the riverbank. The final short portion of this loop leads through deep woods near the river before arriving back at the road and parking lot.

TRIP 3 Eagle Creek

Distance	6.4 miles (with longer options), Out-and-back
Elevation Gain	900 feet
Hiking Time	3 to 5 hours
Optional Map	Green Trails *Cherryville*
Usually Open	March to December
Best Time	May to November
Trail Use	Dogs OK, backpacking option, horseback riding, fishing
Agency	Clackamas River Ranger District, Mt. Hood National Forest
Difficulty	Moderate
Note	Good in cloudy weather

HIGHLIGHTS Some trails you hike because the trailhead is nearby and easy to reach. Others you hike because they provide spectacular views or great mountain scenery. The Eagle Creek Trail gives you neither of these, and that's probably why so few people hike it. On this trip, just finding the trailhead is something of an adventure, and the only views feature rather ugly cut-over slopes near the trailhead. So what's the attraction? The answer is a beautiful rain forest and solitude.

DIRECTIONS Take Exit 12 off Interstate 205, and drive east on State Highway 224/212. Turn right (south) where these roads split, following Highway 224 and signs for Estacada. Near Milepost 19, at a junction 1.1 miles past the intersection with State Highway 211, turn left at a sign for Eagle Fern Park and the Eagle Creek Fish Hatchery. After 0.2 mile, go straight at a stop sign, now traveling on S.E. Wildcat Mountain Drive. Exactly 1.8 miles later, bear right on S.E. Eagle Fern Road. Follow this paved route for 9.1 miles, staying straight at several minor intersections, and then turn right on S.E. Harvey Road.

This narrow road soon turns to rough gravel with lots of lurking potholes, each with a sinister plan to ambush your car's suspension system, so take it slow. The road travels through ugly clear-cuts and past several side roads, most of which are blocked by berms. The only questionable junctions are at 1.3 miles, where you bear left, and at 2.0 miles, where you go straight. Exactly 2.5 miles from the start of S.E. Harvey Road, park beside an unsigned jeep track angling down to the right. Do not try to drive down this "road"—your car will never forgive you.

Walk downhill on the jeep route for about 1 mile, through rather unattractive, partially logged woods, into the canyon of Eagle Creek. Eventually, the road narrows to a footpath, and you come to a signboard for the Eagle Creek Trail. Up to this point, you probably were wondering why anyone would consider this hike to be worthwhile, but now things dramatically improve.

From here on, you walk through an impressive old-growth rain forest, composed mostly of western hemlock and western red cedar, with hanging mosses draping from nearly every limb. Old snags and downed nurse logs provide space for young trees to grow and homes for wildlife. On the forest floor, brambles of salmonberry show off their dark pink blossoms in the spring and edible salmon-colored berries in late summer. In open areas, the ground is carpeted in May with oxalis, with its shamrock-shaped leaves and five-petaled white blossoms. On the often muddy trail, you will probably see few boot prints but lots

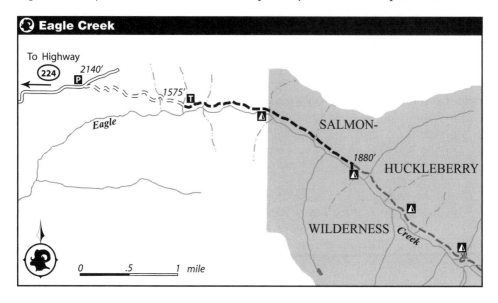

Eagle Creek

of dainty, crescent-shaped hoofprints of deer and the more substantial oval tracks of elk. From the forest, you will hear the raspy calls of chestnut-backed chickadees and the loud rollicking songs of winter wrens, who possess a decibel-to-body-weight ratio that would make an air horn jealous. A more soothing and constant sound comes from unseen Eagle Creek on your right. Overall, this is one of the nicest cathedral forests in the Portland/Vancouver area.

The easy path makes several gentle ups and downs but never works too hard as it wanders slowly up the canyon. Just before you reach a wooden sign announcing your entry into the Salmon-Huckleberry Wilderness, you encounter the first of many nice campsites along this trail. You splash across a dozen or so little side creeks but never come close to Eagle Creek itself until about 3.2 miles from your car when the trail forks. The smaller path to the right goes 80 yards to a spacious creekside camp. The strikingly beautiful waters of Eagle Creek flow right past the camp as they rush over boulders and under logs spanning the flow.

This point makes a very attractive and satisfactory goal, but to enjoy additional awe-inspiring forest scenery, go upstream as far as time and energy allow. You will discover more splashing tributary creeks, lots of big trees, a small marshy meadow, and plenty of places for quiet contemplation. Eventually, the muddy, overgrown trail crosses the creek and switchbacks up the ridge to the south. See Trip 5 for a description of that part of the trail.

TRIP 4 Old Baldy

Distance	7.6 miles, Out-and-back
Elevation Gain	1200 feet
Hiking Time	3 to 4 hours
Optional Map	Green Trails *Fish Creek Mtn, Cherryville*
Usually Open	Mid-May to October
Best Times	June and July
Trail Use	Dogs OK, horseback riding
Agency	Clackamas River Ranger District, Mt. Hood National Forest
Difficulty	Moderate

HIGHLIGHTS Although the view from Old Baldy is not as dramatic as that from nearby Squaw Mountain, this old lookout site is still well worth visiting because it provides a different perspective of Mt. Hood and a fine view of the green depths of Eagle Creek Canyon, which you can't see at all from Squaw Mountain. Another big advantage of Old Baldy is that, unlike on Squaw Mountain, you won't have to deal with noisy motorcycles disturbing the peace and quiet of your hike.

DIRECTIONS From the junction of State Highways 224 and 211 at the south end of Estacada, go southeast on Highway 224 for 1.6 miles, and then turn left on Surface Road. Proceed 1.2 miles to a T-junction, and then turn right on Squaw Mountain Road. Stay on this paved road for 13.2 miles to where it narrows to one lane; continue another 1.7 miles and park in a small unsigned pull-out on the right 0.1 mile after the road begins to go downhill.

Pick up the trail a few yards north of the road pull-out, and turn left (northwest) on the Old Baldy Trail. For a little less than 1 mile the trail steadily ascends a ridgeline heavily wooded with hemlocks and firs and then contours around the upper slopes of small Githens Mountain. Bear right at the unsigned junction with an abandoned trail in a small opening on the western shoulder of this peak, and then contour over to a saddle on the rim overlooking Eagle Creek

Canyon. Trees generally hide the view, but you can catch some nice looks into the canyon and north to the area around Wildcat Mountain. Closer to your feet are the moss-covered rock formations on the edge of the drop-off.

The trail travels up and down close to the rim all the way to a high point, just before the trail turns left. For the best viewpoint on the trip, leave the trail and head cross-country for about 15 yards to a clifftop opening visible through the

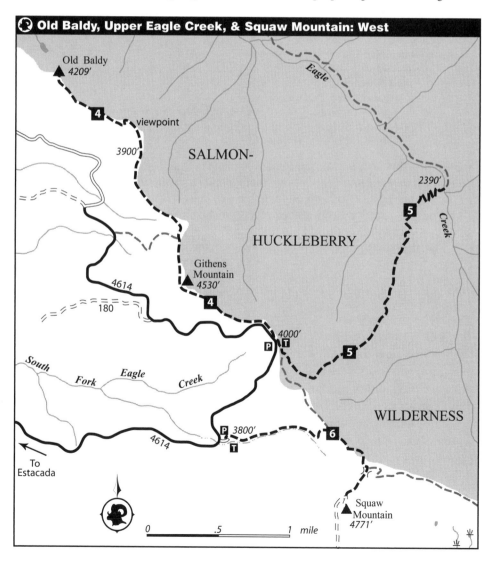

Old Baldy, Upper Eagle Creek, & Squaw Mountain: West

trees on your right. From this dramatic location you can see over the deep, forested depths of Eagle Creek Canyon and up to Mt. Hood rising in the northeast, with part of Mt. Adams visible over a shoulder of the closer volcano. From this viewpoint, the trail makes two downhill switchbacks and then goes up and down on a wooded traverse, before climbing a final time to the summit of Old Baldy. The foundations of the old lookout site are still visible to the careful observer, but trees have grown to block most of the former views.

TRIP 5 Upper Eagle Creek

Distance	5.8 miles, Out-and-back
Elevation Gain	1750 feet
Hiking Time	3 to 4 hours
Optional Map	Green Trails *Cherryville, Fish Creek Mountain*
Usually Open	June to November
Best Time	Any
Trail Use	Dogs OK, fishing
Agency	Clackamas River Ranger District, Mt. Hood National Forest
Difficulty	Difficult
Note	Good in cloudy weather

see map on p.407

HIGHLIGHTS This rarely traveled trail is the reverse of the typical hike in our area. Instead of climbing from a creek bottom to a high viewpoint, this trail descends from a high ridgeline into the depths of a remote wilderness canyon. The hike is terrific for solitude seekers, but be sure to reserve plenty of energy for the tough hike back up to your car.

DIRECTIONS From the junction of State Highways 224 and 211 at the south end of Estacada, go 1.6 miles southeast on Highway 224, and then turn left on Surface Road. Proceed 1.2 miles to a T-junction, and then turn right on Squaw Mountain Road. Stay on this paved road for 13.2 miles to where it narrows to one lane, continue another 1.7 miles, and park in a small unsigned pull-out on the right 0.1 mile after the road begins to go downhill.

Walk a few yards north into the woods from the parking area, and then turn right (east) on an obvious trail. After just 100 yards, veer left at a fork at a small sign for Eagle Creek. This trail goes up and down through forest and small openings for 0.3 mile and then turns left (northeast) following the top of a minor ridge. The path stays near the top of this ridge for 0.6 mile to a partially obstructed view of the heavily forested canyon of upper Eagle Creek. You can also see part of Squaw Mountain to the south.

After the viewpoint, the trail winds slowly downhill, remaining faithful to the rapidly diminishing ridge. With the loss in elevation the vegetation changes from the usual higher-elevation mix of true firs, beargrass, and Pacific rhododendrons to the typical lower-elevation zone featuring western hemlocks, western red cedars, and sword ferns. The trail's final 0.7 mile gives up any pretense of a gentle descent and plunges steeply downhill in 18 short switchbacks to Eagle Creek.

The trail immediately crosses the creek, requiring either a tricky rock hop on dangerously slippery rocks or a chilly but safer ford. The recommended course of action, however, is to sit back and enjoy the stream and then return the way you came. There is no campsite at the creek crossing, but backpackers can find

sites by crossing the stream and following the trail that goes downstream. It is also possible to turn this into a one-way hike, by exiting at the remote lower Eagle Creek Trailhead. See Trip 3: Eagle Creek for details.

TRIP 6 Squaw Mountain: West

Distance	3.2 miles, Out-and-back
Elevation Gain	1000 feet
Hiking Time	2 hours
Optional Map	Green Trails *Fish Creek Mountain*
Usually Open	Mid-May to October
Best Times	June and July
Trail Use	Good for kids, dogs OK, horseback riding
Agency	Clackamas River Ranger District, Mt. Hood National Forest
Difficulty	Moderate

see map on p.407

HIGHLIGHTS Squaw Mountain is the most dramatic destination in the southwest Salmon-Huckleberry Wilderness, with expansive views extending over the heavily clear-cut slopes to the south and west, and the more natural hillsides in the adjoining wilderness area to the north. At the summit of this generally overlooked little peak, you can also see distant high points, from Olallie Butte and Mt. Jefferson to the towering landmark for all of northwest Oregon, Mt. Hood. The short trail to the summit is easy enough for almost any hiker, making this one of the best viewpoint trips in our area for hikers not ready for the long, difficult climbs to other viewpoint destinations.

DIRECTIONS From the junction of State Highways 224 and 211 at the south end of Estacada, go 1.6 miles southeast on Highway 224, and then turn left on Surface Road. Proceed 1.2 miles to a T-junction, and then turn right on Squaw Mountain Road. Stay on this paved road for 13.2 miles to where it narrows to one lane, and then continue another 0.7 mile to where the road makes a sweeping curve to the left. Turn right on a bumpy, unsigned road that goes about 250 yards to a gravel turnaround in a clear-cut. The trail, marked only with a tiny wooden sign that reads "505," goes up the road bank about 100 feet before you get to the turnaround.

The trail slowly makes its way uphill in a mountain-hemlock and noble-fir forest beside a trickling creek. The lush riparian vegetation near the water is dominated by salmonberry, with its bland-tasting, orange-colored berries, and thimbleberry, which has a more powerful red fruit. There is also an unusually high concentration of baneberry, which

in midsummer features delicate clusters of white flowers. As the trail veers away from the creek, it climbs more steeply, and in July the forest opens up with lots of beargrass and beardtongue blooming.

Just before the top of a forested ridge is a junction with the Old Baldy Trail, coming in from the left. You go straight and ascend at a steady, moderate grade for 0.5 mile in dense forest to a junction in the saddle of a spur ridge that goes to the south. To reach Squaw Mountain, bear right and hike along the scenic, partially forested ridge for 0.3 mile to where the trail ends at a closed jeep road. Turn left and walk 100 yards up this road to the summit.

The excellent view from the rocky summit of Squaw Mountain includes the marshy Squaw Lakes to the east, hundreds of square miles of forested ridges to the south and west, and, most prominently, snow-capped Mt. Hood, which rises beautifully over the ridge to the northeast. Motorcyclists often visit Squaw Mountain by riding the closed jeep road that connects with a logging road to the south, so you may have to share this view with some noisy machines.

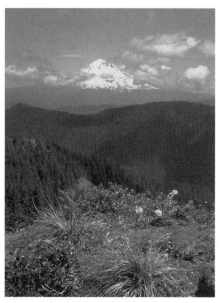

Mt. Hood from Squaw Mountain

TRIP 7 Squaw Mountain: East

Distance	4.0 miles, Out-and-back
Elevation Gain	1200 feet
Hiking Time	2 hours
Optional Map	Green Trails *Fish Creek Mountain*
Usually Open	Mid-June to October
Best Time	Any
Trail Use	Dogs OK, horseback riding
Agency	Clackamas River Ranger District, Mt. Hood National Forest
Difficulty	Moderate

HIGHLIGHTS No matter how you get there, the view from Squaw Mountain is well worth the effort. The approach from the west (Trip 6) has the advantage of paved road access and a slightly shorter trail. But the hike from the east has the edge in scenery with excellent views along the way of the swampy Squaw Lakes and the rocky summit of Squaw Mountain. The best plan is to take both trails, enjoying those fine summit views more than once.

DIRECTIONS From Estacada go 6.5 miles southeast on State Highway 224 to a junction directly opposite the entrance to Promontory Park. Turn left onto unsigned Forest Road 4610, a narrow winding road that is paved for the first 2.4 miles and then turns to gravel. Exactly 7.2 miles from Highway 224 is an obvious but poorly signed junction. Make a hard left, still on Road 4610, proceed 0.9 mile to another poorly signed junction, this time with Road 4613, and make a sharp right. From here you stay on Road 4610 at several minor intersections as the road becomes progressively rougher with encroaching brush, potholes, and numerous rocks. Exactly 10.6 miles from the junction with Road 4613, just as the road begins a wide curve to the right, is a small trailhead sign on the left for the Plaza Trail. There is no room to park here, but just 50 yards past the trailhead a road branches to the right into the former Twin Springs Campground, where there is plenty of parking.

Walk 12 yards north on the Plaza Trail to a T-junction, where you turn left, following signs to Old Baldy. The trail parallels Road 4610 for the first 150 yards, angles to the right, and climbs through forest to the top of a minor ridge at 0.3 mile. From here the path makes a sharp left turn, briefly descends, and then contours across a steep, heavily forested hillside for the next 0.2 mile.

When the trail curves to the right, it leaves the hillside and descends gradually along the north side of a small ridge. Here the scenery dramatically improves as the forest opens up and you are treated to excellent views over the marshy expanse of the Squaw Lakes in the basin to your left. Towering above this basin to the west is the rocky, multi-summit ridge of Squaw Mountain. In the distance to the south is hulking Fish Creek Mountain. Although the Squaw Lakes are 400 feet below the trail, you can still hear a surprisingly loud chorus from the thousands of frogs that call this swamp home.

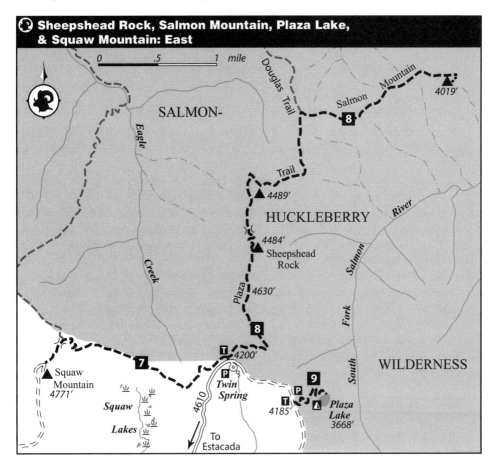

Sheepshead Rock, Salmon Mountain, Plaza Lake, & Squaw Mountain: East

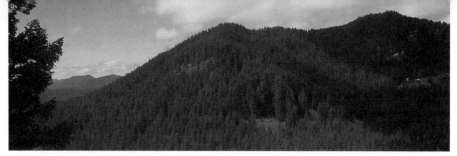

Squaw Mountain from the east

After dropping to the low point of the scenic ridge, the trail climbs a set of short, moderately steep switchbacks to a junction in a saddle. Turn left and hike along a scenic, partially forested ridge for 0.3 mile to trail's end at a closed jeep road. Turn left and walk 100 yards up the road to Squaw Mountain's rocky summit with its expansive views over the Salmon-Huckleberry Wilderness to the snow-capped splendor of Mt. Hood.

TRIP 8 Sheepshead Rock & Salmon Mountain

Distance	2.8 miles to Sheepshead Rock, Out-and-back;
	10.2 miles to Salmon Mountain, Out-and-back
Elevation Gain	550 feet to Sheepshead Rock,
	1800 feet to Salmon Mountain
Hiking Time	1½ to 6 hours
Optional Map	Green Trails *Cherryville, Fish Creek Mountain, Government Camp*
Usually Open	Mid-June to October
Best Time	Late June to mid-July
Trail Use	Dogs OK, horseback riding
Agency	Clackamas River Ranger District, Mt. Hood National Forest
Difficulty	Moderate to Difficult

see map on p.411

HIGHLIGHTS Tucked away in the central part of the Salmon-Huckleberry Wilderness is a little traveled ridge with terrific views of Mt. Hood towering over a remote roadless landscape. The full hike out to the former lookout site at Salmon Mountain is rather challenging, in part because the trail is overgrown and rather faint in places, but a much shorter option to the equally good viewpoint at Sheepshead Rock is more than adequate compensation for the rough drive to the trailhead.

DIRECTIONS From Estacada go 6.5 miles southeast on State Highway 224 to a junction directly opposite the entrance to Promontory Park. Turn left onto unsigned Forest Road 4610, a narrow winding road that is paved for the first 2.4 miles, and then turns to gravel. Exactly 7.2 miles from Highway 224 is an obvious but poorly signed junction. Make a hard left, still on Road 4610, proceed 0.9 mile to another poorly signed junction, this time with Road 4613, and make a sharp right. From here you stay on Road 4610 at several minor intersections as the road becomes progressively rougher with encroaching brush, pot-holes, and numerous rocks. Exactly 10.6 miles from the junction with Road 4613, just as the road begins a wide curve to the right, is a small trailhead sign on the left for the Plaza Trail. There is no room to park here, but just 50 yards past the trailhead a road branches to the right into the former Twin Springs Campground, where there is plenty of parking.

Walk 12 yards north from the trailhead to a T-junction, turn right on the Plaza Trail, and go up and down through a dense forest of mountain hemlocks and true firs. At 0.3 mile you reach the site of the long dismantled Plaza Guard Station, and then turn north and gradually climb, still in dense forest. At 1.1 miles the trail goes sharply downhill near the top of a narrow ridge. At 1.4 miles, shortly before the trail starts a series of downhill switchbacks, look for an unmarked path to the right. This route climbs a short distance to the top of the prominent rocky buttress called Sheepshead Rock. The views from this spot are superb, up to Mt. Hood, almost straight down into the canyon of South Fork Salmon River, and northeast to Salmon Mountain's long forested ridge. The viewpoint also supports an abundance of the usual flowers found at rocky mountain locations, including cliff penstemon, wallflower, and stonecrop.

If you are continuing to Salmon Mountain, return to the main trail, switchback down to a saddle, and then loop around the west and north sides of a high point in the ridgeline. From here the trail remains on the west side of the ridge, with occasional views down the long canyon of Eagle Creek, and comes to a junction at 3.1 miles. Turn right and then go up and down along a mostly forested ridge on an increasingly sketchy and brushy route for 1.8 miles to its end at a minor saddle on the side of Salmon Mountain. From here it is a straightforward scramble up a mostly open ridge to the top of the peak, with its wide views over this little-known wilderness.

Mt. Hood from Salmon Mountain

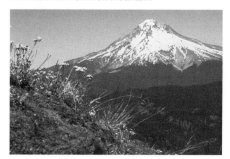

TRIP 9 Plaza Lake

Distance	1.7 miles, Out-and-back
Elevation Gain	500 feet
Hiking Time	1½ hours
Optional Map	Green Trails *High Rock*
Usually Open	Mid-June to October
Best Time	Any
Trail Use	Good for kids, dogs OK, backpacking option, fishing
Agency	Clackamas River Ranger District, Mt. Hood National Forest
Difficulty	Moderate

see map on p.411

HIGHLIGHTS On summer weekends people flock to mountain lakes, sometimes in numbers that rival the mosquitoes. So it's rare to find a mountain lake where you have a better than even chance of being alone. Plaza Lake is one such place. Protected from crowds by a rough road and an unsigned trailhead, this lovely pool has plenty of solitude, but it also boasts many of the qualities that cause people to come to mountain lakes in the first place—hungry trout, nice scenery, and a place to camp.

DIRECTIONS From Estacada go 6.5 miles southeast on State Highway 224 to a junction directly opposite the entrance to Promontory Park. Turn left onto unsigned Forest Road 4610, a narrow winding road that is paved for the first 2.4 miles, and then turns to gravel. Exactly 7.2 miles from Highway 224 is an obvious but poorly signed junction. Make a hard left, still on Road 4610, proceed 0.9 mile to another poorly signed junction, this time with Road 4613, and make a sharp right. From here you stay on Road 4610 at several minor intersections as the road becomes progressively rougher with encroaching brush, potholes, and numerous rocks. Exactly 10.6 miles from the junction with Road 4613 is a small trailhead sign on the left for the Plaza Trail. Continue driving another 0.7 mile, and look for a short, unsigned jeep road to the left. Park here.

Walk 15 yards up the jeep road to where it curves to the right and ends. The unsigned trail begins here, initially going northeast into the forest on the north side of a prominent rim. The path is well built and easy to follow as it goes gradually down a hillside covered with a dense old-growth forest of mountain hemlock, true firs, western white pines, and Douglas firs. The forest floor is crowded with Pacific rhododendrons, which has lovely pink blossoms in late June; huckleberries, which have delicious berries in late August; and beargrass, which has white blooms on tall stalks in mid- to late June. Most of the descent is in viewless forest although at two points you pass near talus slopes that provide partial views to the northeast.

After 17 gently graded switchbacks the trail ends at the shores of shallow, 5-acre Plaza Lake. There is a small but comfortable campsite on the west shore just before the end of the trail. The serene little lake lacks calendar-cover scenery, but the setting is attractive in a forested bowl that was carved out by ice age glaciers. Although the shore is a little brushy, the lake is up to 10 feet deep so swimming is an option in late summer. Anglers can try their luck going after small brook trout.

TRIP 10 Huxley Lake & Roaring River

Distance	2.7 miles to Huxley Lake, Out-and-back; 2.4 miles to Roaring River, Out-and-back; 5.1 miles total (The distances may be greater, depending on how far you can drive.)
Elevation Gain	650 feet to Huxley Lake, 900 feet to Roaring River, 1550 feet total
Hiking Time	3 hours total
Optional Map	Green Trails *Fish Creek Mountain* (some trails aren't shown and trail locations are inaccurate)
Usually Open	April to November
Best Times	May and June
Trail Use	Dogs OK, backpacking option, fishing
Agency	Clackamas River Ranger District, Mt. Hood National Forest
Difficulty	Difficult
Note	Good in cloudy weather

HIGHLIGHTS This trip takes you into a remote and difficult-to-access area that adventure-some types will really enjoy—others . . . maybe not so much. The attraction is the fine scenery, with nice forests, a small forest-rimmed lake, and an absolutely gorgeous river in a wild canyon. On the downside, the road access is confusing and rough, and once you get there the trails are either chewed up by all-terrain vehicles (ATVs) or are very steep and tiring. With the right attitude and a good sense of direction, you will probably love this trip. Without those qualities, you might return with strong doubts about the sanity of a certain guidebook author.

DIRECTIONS From Estacada go 6.5 miles southeast on State Highway 224 to a junction directly opposite the entrance to Promontory Park. Turn left onto unsigned Forest Road 4610, a narrow winding road that is paved for the first 2.4 miles, and then turns to gravel. Exactly 7.2 miles from Highway 224 is an obvious but poorly signed junction. Veer slightly right on Road 4611 and stay on the main road through numerous junctions with minor, unsigned roads. At several places there are major unsigned forks where you face a choice. The correct choices are to go left at a junction after 1.6 miles, right at a three-way split in the road just 0.6 mile later, right again at a fork in another 1.2 miles, and right a final time after 0.7 mile. Throughout this process you have stayed on Road 4611, but it has gotten progressively worse—now it becomes a test for most passenger cars. Continue driving as long as your car and your caution permit, and then park. You will come to the signed trail-head for Huxley Lake about 3 miles from the last major fork or 14.3 miles from Highway 224. There is only limited parking here, but that doesn't really matter since you probably weren't able to drive this far anyway.

Having survived the drive, you can now enjoy the rewards. The trail to Huxley Lake goes uphill from the left (north) side of the road and ascends through a lovely forest comprised mostly of drooping western hemlocks. Although

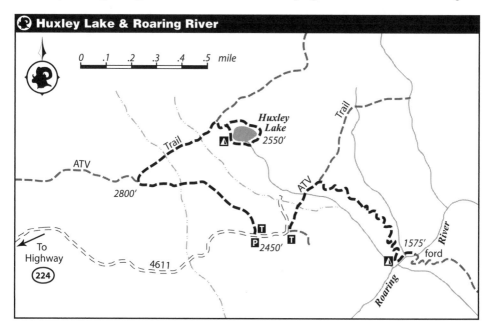

⊕ Huxley Lake & Roaring River

0 .1 .2 .3 .4 .5 *mile*

Huxley Lake 2550'

Trail

ATV

2800'

Trail

ATV

2450'

1575'

ford

Roaring River

To Highway **224**

4611

wide and heavily used by ATVs, the trail is fun to hike and, when the machines aren't around, both quiet and attractive.

After 0.6 mile of climbing, you come to a junction with an ATV trail not shown on either the U.S. Geological Survey or Green Trails maps. You turn sharply right and then go gently downhill, crossing a couple of small seasonal creeks before coming to a tiny clearing and another fork in the trail at 1.1 miles. The official trail goes left, climbing to abandoned Lookout Springs Campground in about 2 miles. A better option is to turn right on a more heavily used trail (not shown on most maps), which descends 0.15 mile to a possible campsite above the northwest shore of Huxley Lake. Skunk cabbage grows profusely along the shore of this shallow lake displaying large yellow blossoms in April. You can also expect to see both bufflehead and goldeneye ducks swimming and diving in the lake's waters. ATV riders have carved a trail around the lake that is worth exploring.

If you want to visit Roaring River, return to the trailhead, and walk 0.1 mile east on Road 4611 to a three-way split. What is left of the road goes left, while ATV trails go straight and right. Take the middle trail, which is badly chewed up by ATVs and therefore muddy early in the season. After a little less than 0.2 mile, look carefully for small sign marking a foot trail that goes downhill to the right. Turn onto this path and immediately leave the machines behind. The trail winds downhill, sometimes rather steeply, through an attractive and relatively open forest where you gain occasional glimpses of Grouse Point, a high point on the ridge to the south. At first you will hear a small creek tumbling down a gully on your right, but this is eventually drowned out by the cascading sounds of aptly named Roaring River in the canyon below.

The last 0.5 mile descends dozens of short but very steep switchbacks to a rarely used little campsite just above a brushy flat next to Roaring River. This isolated spot is great for solitude lovers, anglers, and anyone who loves wild streams. From the camp, the trail goes upstream about 100 yards to a ford of the river. The crossing is cold and potentially difficult before midsummer but provides access to an often faint trail that climbs steeply to Grouse Point. Easier access to that viewpoint is described in Trip 14.

TRIP 11 South Fork Clackamas River

Distance	3.2 miles, Out-and-back
Elevation Gain	900 feet
Hiking Time	2 hours
Optional Map	Green Trails *Fish Creek Mountain*
Usually Open	Mid-March to December
Best Time	Any
Trail Use	Good for kids, dogs OK, mountain biking, backpacking option, fishing
Agency	Clackamas River Ranger District, Mt. Hood National Forest
Difficulty	Moderate
Note	Good in cloudy weather

HIGHLIGHTS The beautiful South Fork Clackamas River is one of the most remote large streams in the state of Oregon. Situated in a deep, roadless canyon, this clear-flowing stream was once the water source for Oregon City and was, therefore, closed to all fishing. The river is now open for catch-and-release trout fishing, but its remoteness keeps most anglers away. The only decent access to the stream is on the Hillockburn Trail, which despite being unsigned and rarely hiked, is well maintained and features a paved road all the way to the trailhead.

DIRECTIONS From the junction of State Highways 211 and 224 at the south end of Estacada, turn southwest on Highway 211. Drive 4.8 miles, and then turn left on Hillockburn Road, following signs to Dodge. After 5.1 miles the road enters national forest land, goes through a yellow gate, and becomes Forest Road 45. Exactly 1.8 miles later, or 0.1 mile after the road goes through a minor saddle, pull into an unsigned gravel parking area on the left.

The trail starts as a long abandoned road, now often used by all-terrain vehicles (ATVs), that goes south-southeast across a heavily forested hillside. The forest here is typical of lower elevations in the western Cascades with a mix of Douglas firs and western hemlocks and an understory dominated by salal, sword fern, and Oregon grape. Smaller groundcover flowers such as false lily-of-the-valley and oxalis are also common. After 0.15 mile the tread narrows to become a foot trail, although the route is sometimes used by motorcycles.

After 0.7 mile of very gentle downhill, the trail turns sharply left in the first of 11 switchbacks that wind down the viewless hillside. Fortunately, the switchbacks are well graded so the downhill is easy on the knees. At 1.6 miles the trail ends at a mediocre campsite beside the South Fork Clackamas River. This is a great spot to do some fly fishing or to simply lay back and enjoy the soothing sounds of gently rushing water.

A long abandoned trail crosses the river and goes upstream on the opposite bank. This trail is not recommended, however, because it is hard to find, extremely rough, and can only be accessed by fording the river, a difficult task before mid-June.

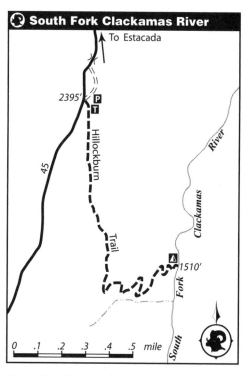

South Fork Clackamas River

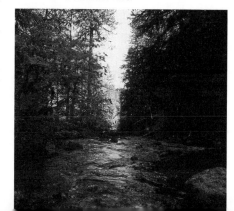

TRIP 12 Memaloose Lake & South Fork Mountain

Distance	4.6 miles, Out-and-back
Elevation Gain	1350 feet
Hiking Time	2 to 3 hours
Optional Map	Green Trails *Fish Creek Mountain*
Usually Open	Mid-June to late October
Best Time	June
Trail Use	Good for kids, dogs OK, mountain biking, backpacking option, fishing
Agency	Clackamas River Ranger District, Mt. Hood National Forest
Difficulty	Moderate

HIGHLIGHTS The popular hike past Memaloose Lake to the top of South Fork Mountain is a simple, unassuming walk that has no single outstanding feature but many worthwhile attributes. Lovers of big trees will delight in traveling through an isolated stand of old-growth Douglas fir. People who enjoy mountain lakes (and who doesn't?) can relax by the shores of a clear pool tucked in a little basin beneath a scenic rockslide. Finally, those who revel in expansive views can take in the scene from an old lookout site. Other hikes in this book include better old-growth forests, better mountain lakes, and better viewpoints, but this hike is one of the few to include good, if not outstanding, examples of all three.

DIRECTIONS Drive State Highway 224 southeast from Estacada 9.4 miles, and then turn right on Memaloose Road 45, which immediately crosses a narrow bridge. Stay on paved Road 45 for 11.3 miles to the end of pavement and a junction, where you turn right and drive a final 0.9 mile to the trailhead.

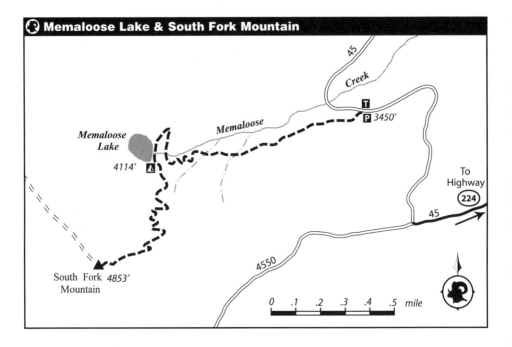

The gently graded trail makes a steady climb up a hillside above Memaloose Creek, where the trees are the most noteworthy feature and will impress even the most jaded hiker. Take the time to snap a photo of the kids next to one of these old-growth giants and use the occasion to teach them a lesson in both conservation and humility. The mostly open forest floor has very little brush but lots of low-growing wildflowers, including oxalis, vanilla leaf, and bunchberry. As it climbs, the path crosses several small creeklets and goes up a few short switchbacks before making a final series of longer switchbacks that takes you up to the shores of Memaloose Lake.

There are several good campsites near the lake for hikers who are looking to make this an easy overnight trip. In late summer, this shallow, 5-acre pool is also good for swimming. If you prefer more exercise, go straight through the camping area and pick up the 0.9-mile path that climbs 16 switchbacks to the top of South Fork Mountain. The views along this trail are limited by trees. The last section of the climb is along a high ridge leading to the summit. You may have to share the view with car-bound travelers, who can access this high point via a rough dirt road, but console yourself with the knowledge that these "cheaters" missed the lovely forest and lake below. From the summit, you can see Cascade snow peaks from Mt. Rainier to the Three Sisters, and look west to the Willamette Valley and the rolling green hills of the Coast Range. On perfectly clear days, those with binoculars can even pick out the familiar skyscrapers of downtown Portland.

TRIP 13 Clackamas River Trail

Distance	7.8 miles, Point-to-point
Elevation Gain	1300 feet
Hiking Time	4 hours
Optional Map	Green Trails *Fish Creek Mountain*
Usually Open	All year
Best Time	All year
Trail Use	Good for kids, dogs OK, backpacking option, fishing
Agency	Clackamas River Ranger District, Mt. Hood National Forest
Difficulty	Difficult
Note	Good in cloudy weather

HIGHLIGHTS The best way for hikers to enjoy the beauties of the Clackamas River is to take an extended walk along its shores. There is no better option for that than the segment of the Clackamas River Trail that goes upstream from Fish Creek. With easy road access to both ends, this hike is ideal for a car or bicycle shuttle. The hike is probably most enjoyable in late winter and early spring when the trees lack their summer leaves and allow you to see the many wispy seasonal waterfalls dropping from trailside cliffs. Unfortunately, the path gets very little sunshine in winter, which makes for chilly temperatures, so bring a coat.

DIRECTIONS Drive State Highway 224 southeast from Estacada 15 miles to the junction with Fish Creek Road (Forest Road 54). Turn right on this road, cross a bridge, and reach the large trailhead parking lot on the right. The newly rerouted start of the trail is across Fish Creek Road from the south end of the parking lot.

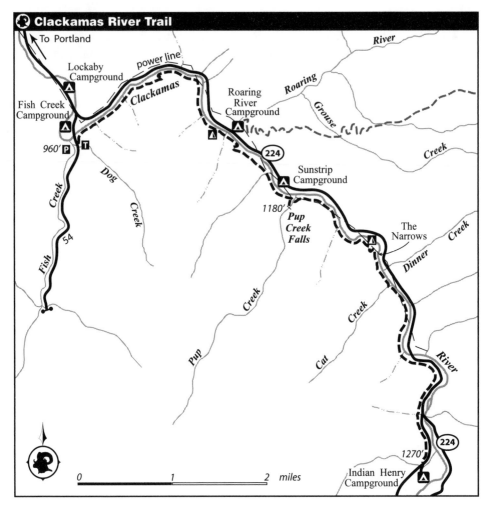

Clackamas River Trail

To Portland

Lockaby Campground

power line

Fish Creek Campground

Clackamas

Roaring River Campground

Roaring

River

Grouse

Creek

960' P T

224

Sunstrip Campground

Dog

Creek

Creek

Fish

54

1180'

Pup Creek Falls

The Narrows

Creek

Dinner

Pup

Creek

Cat

Creek

River

224

1270'

Indian Henry Campground

0   1   2 *miles*

If you are doing the trip one-way, you can leave a second car (or bicycle) at the Indian Henry Trailhead. To reach it, continue on Highway 224 another 7 miles, and then turn right off the main road just before it crosses a bridge. Drive this route 0.6 mile to the trailhead on the right.

From the Fish Creek Trailhead, the wide path begins by going through a forest of western hemlock and western red cedar. The forest floor is covered by sword fern, various mosses, salal, and lots of April-blooming oxalis. In a few hundred yards you bear right at a junction with the old trail coming in from the left and hike a wide, smooth path up the Clackamas River Canyon. Unless you are an angler, you can ignore the several side trails that drop to fishing spots on the river.

The trail crosses a small feeder creek and then begins a series of miniature ups and downs. Although the highway is never far away across the river, the intervening sounds of rushing water and the rollicking songs of small birds provide a more pleasant experience for the ears. If you are lucky, you may get a glimpse of the source of these songs, the diminutive, brown, winter wren. Be prepared to be surprised by the small size of this amazingly powerful songster.

To avoid mossy, river-level rocks and cliffs, the trail takes you up a slope almost 200 feet above the water. It then contours briefly before using two short switchbacks to descend to a camp on the riverbank. The road's sights and sounds are more intrusive for the next 0.6 mile, as the river is more placid and the road is especially close. More ups and downs

Pup Creek Falls along the Clackamas River Trail

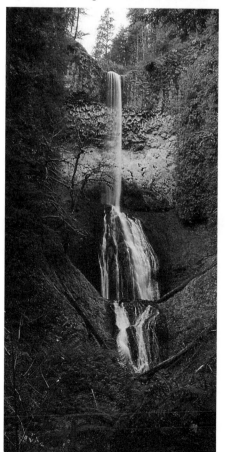

takes you past a tiny sloping falls, just above the trail, and then you descend to a comfortable riverside camp in a nice grove of cedars. Past this camp, you climb two steep switchbacks to a viewpoint of the Roaring River Canyon to the northeast. Here you stay high for a while. Then you will come close to a set of power lines, which follow the Clackamas River up the canyon. You will play hide and seek with this power line for much of the rest of the hike.

When you reach the power lines a second time, there is a well-signed junction with a 0.1-mile side trail to Pup Creek Falls. Don't miss the chance to visit this impressive 100-foot-tall falls, which is set in a dramatic grotto. Unfortunately, the falls is almost perpetually in the shade, so photographers will need either a tripod or very fast film.

Back on the main trail, you cross Pup Creek on a set of strategically placed stepping stones. Then you go through a partially cleared area near the power lines to a junction with a short side trail to a good riverside beach and campsite. From here, you climb over a small knoll and then descend in small switchbacks back to river level. At this point, a short side trail goes left to the river at the Narrows. The name isn't very original, but it is an accurate description of this place, where the river cuts through a 20-foot-wide chasm between large mossy rocks. The Narrows are ideal for sunbathing, and they make a great place to eat your lunch while watching rafters pass through the narrow opening. Beyond this point, the trail is less interesting as it either stays in heavy forest or goes beneath the power lines for about 1 mile. You then pass through a cavelike grotto that has been carved out of a cliffside and travel along a hillside above a paved road before the trail ends at Indian Henry Campground.

TRIP 14 Dry Ridge to Grouse Point

Distance	12.2 miles, Out-and-back
Elevation Gain	3600 feet
Hiking Time	7 hours
Optional Map	Green Trails *Fish Creek Mountain*
Usually Open	June to mid-October
Best Time	Mid-June to mid-July
Trail Use	Dogs OK
Agency	Clackamas River Ranger District, Mt. Hood National Forest
Difficulty	Difficult
Note	Good in cloudy weather

HIGHLIGHTS The most popular trails in the Clackamas River country stay at low elevations right along the river, but there are options for hikers looking for more exercise. The attractive trail up Dry Ridge is a good workout for any hiker. While most of the long climb is in viewless woods, those up for the challenge can end the hike at a good viewpoint, featuring part of Mt. Hood and the many wooded ridges of the Clackamas River country.

DIRECTIONS Drive State Highway 224 southeast from Estacada for 17.5 miles to Roaring River Campground. Turn left into this camp, and find the signed trailhead at the end of the campground loop near Campsite 8. This campground is closed until about June, so if you are visiting before then, you will have to park along Highway 224 and walk about 0.1 mile to the trailhead.

The trail begins by briefly following the bank of the sparkling Roaring River and then it cuts back to the right away from the water. Almost immediately thereafter, you cross beneath a set of power lines, the last human-made intrusion on the hike. The forest canopy here is almost uniformly Douglas fir, with some massive old-growth specimens to admire. Below the firs are the more shade-tolerant western hemlock, which, given a few more centuries of undisturbed growth,

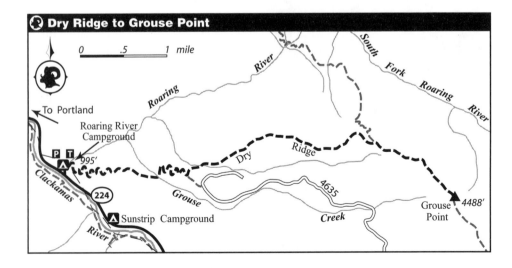

will take over as the dominant species. The forest floor is more varied than the trees, with lots of vanilla leaf, both sword and bracken fern, moss-covered rocks, and an abundance of white, five-petaled anemones.

After the power lines, the trail begins switchbacking on a relentlessly steady but not overly steep climb. The ascent is best done in the morning, when the weather is cooler and the trail is well shaded. Near the top of the first 12 switchbacks, the trail reaches a small grassy glade, where tiny white irises bloom in early summer. Above this glade the trail makes a final turn and takes you to the top of a rocky slope with a good view of the Clackamas River Canyon. This viewpoint is about 1.5 miles from the start, and it makes a good stopping point for off-season hikers because the trail is usually snow-free until this point for most of the winter.

Those continuing beyond this point must make an uneven, but generally uphill, traverse on the north side of Dry Ridge to a crossing of splashing Grouse Creek, which may get your boots wet in early summer. Beyond the crossing the trail continues its generally uphill traverse to the base of a small rockslide and the start of a second set of switchbacks. There are eight this time, which lead you up to a rockslide and to a trail junction. Going straight at this junction takes you 0.3 mile to Forest Road 4635, a possible starting point for hikers who care only about the view from Grouse Point.

The main trail turns left at this junction and soon demonstrates that most of the climbing is over. The grade of the ascent is much more gradual now, with many level sections mixed in with the uphills. You step over a small, seasonal creek and follow the edge where Dry Ridge's gentle slope suddenly drops off to your left. Views are limited by the forest cover, which is now made up of much smaller hemlock, cedar, and fir trees. The mostly open forest floor features scattered beargrass and rhododendrons, both of which bloom nicely from mid-June into July.

You bear slightly right at the signed junction with a sketchy, unmaintained trail that goes back to the left and then steadily ascend in forest for about another mile. Eventually you break out of the trees and reach the partially obstructed views from the beargrass meadows atop Grouse Point. For the best views, leave the trail and bushwhack a few dozen feet to the left. From here, you can sit and enjoy a marvelously wild landscape featuring the South Fork Roaring River Canyon and the top third of Mt. Hood peeking over Indian Ridge. Best of all, there isn't a road or a logging scar in sight.

Backpackers can extend this outing another 2 miles to scenic Serene Lake. This area is easier to reach, however, by shorter routes, such as that described in Trip 17.

TRIP 15 Fish Creek Mountain

Distance	7.2 miles with side trip to High Lake, Out-and-back
Elevation Gain	2500 feet
Hiking Time	2½ hours
Optional Map	Green Trails *Fish Creek Mountain* (part of trail not shown)
Usually Open	June to October
Best Time	Mid- to late June
Trail Use	Dogs OK (but the trail is rough for them in spots), backpacking option
Agency	Clackamas River Ranger District, Mt. Hood National Forest
Difficulty	Difficult

HIGHLIGHTS After the devastating floods of February 1996 wiped out many roads in the Mount Hood National Forest, the land managers decided for both cost and environmental reasons to permanently close some of the damaged roads rather than spend the money to repair them. Environmentalists applauded this decision, even though many lamented the resulting loss of access to some of their favorite hiking areas. One formerly popular location that hikers could no longer reach was Fish Creek Mountain. In the last few years, however, volunteers have worked to clear an old trail that accesses the mountain from an open road on the east side of the peak, so hikers can once again enjoy this beautiful area. The new trail is steep and is still rough in places, but it is a lot of fun. As for the destination, the view from atop Fish Creek Mountain is just as good as old timers remember, and nearby High Lake is an enchanting location for either a lunch stop or a quiet night in the wilderness.

DIRECTIONS From Estacada take State Highway 224 for 22 miles to the junction with Forest Road 4620 just before a highway bridge over the Clackamas River. Turn right, soon pass Indian Henry Campground, and drive 5.4 miles to the end of pavement. Continue on gravel another 2.7 miles and park where an unsigned road, which is blocked by rocks, goes to the left. (If you need a landmark, this road is exactly 0.4 mile after you pass a side road, also going left, that is a strange reddish/pink color.)

Start by walking up an unsigned trail that angles uphill to the right on the north side of the blocked side road. This path takes you through the usual west-side forest mix of western hemlock, Douglas fir, and various deciduous trees with a thick understory of Pacific rhododendrons and a variety of smaller shrubs. On the forest floor is a thick mat of vanilla leaf, queen's cup, white-blooming anemone, and other wildflowers. After 100 yards the trail angles uphill to the right and begins climbing, sometimes steeply, in dense forest. The trail is faint in spots (work continues to improve matters), but any reasonably experienced hiker should have no trouble.

After climbing through and around some deadfall, the trail makes several short switchbacks and then tops a wooded ridge at 0.8 mile before dropping briefly to a junction with an old road. A small rock cairn marks this junction so you can find it on the return trip. Turn right (north) on the abandoned road, which has a rough surface because the U.S. Forest Service covered it with jumbles of rocks and berms after the road was closed in 1996. Grasses, shrubs, and other vegetation are rapidly taking over the sur-

⊙ Fish Creek Mountain

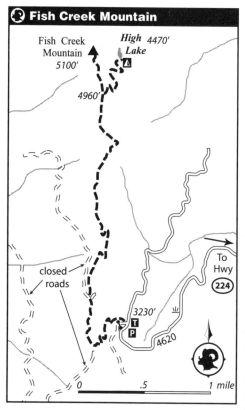

Fish Creek Mountain 5100'

High Lake 4470'

4960'

closed roads

3230'
T P

4620

To Hwy 224

0 .5 1 mile

Fish Creek Mountain over High Lake

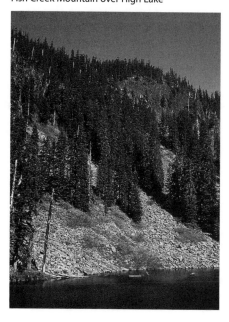

face. After 0.4 mile you come to a fork in the road. The trail goes up the middle of a rocky rib directly between the two forks.

The trail, which is now obvious and in good shape, generally remains near the top of the ridge as it gradually gains elevations. A few irregularly spaced switchbacks help to ensure a relatively gentle grade. Most of the way is in forest, but occasional breaks in the tree cover open up good views especially southwest to pointed Mt. Jefferson. A few tiny meadows provide enough sunshine for wildflowers to put on a nice show. Look for dark blue larkspur, red columbine, bright yellow arnica, and light pink phlox. The main highlight along the way comes from a pair of impressive rock formations that jut up from the ridgetop and host many colorful wildflowers, especially cliff penstemon, cats ear, and lomatium.

The path remains loyal to the ridgetop, sometimes ambling along with almost no elevation gain, to a junction at 2.6 miles. The trail to the right switchbacks down 500 feet in 0.7 mile to High Lake, a very scenic 2-acre pool backed by a talus slope and with excellent views of the hulking mass of Fish Creek Mountain. Backpackers will find a very comfortable campsite above the lake's south shore.

The Fish Creek Mountain Trail goes straight (south) from the junction with the High Lake Trail and in 0.3 mile climbs over a false summit and then loses a little elevation before making the final ascent to the top of the 5100-foot mountain. Rapidly growing hemlock and fir trees are starting to block the views from this former lookout site, but the vistas are still first-rate. Especially noteworthy is the look west into the Fish Creek drainage and southwest to snowy Mt. Jefferson. In late June and July beargrass often blooms profusely at the summit.

TRIP 16 Cripple Creek Trail

Distance	5.0 miles, Out-and-back
Elevation Gain	1400 feet
Hiking Time	2½ hours
Optional Map	Green Trails *Fish Creek Mountain*
Usually Open	March to December
Best Time	Mid-April to June
Trail Use	Dogs OK, horseback riding
Agency	Clackamas River Ranger District, Mt. Hood National Forest
Difficulty	Moderate

HIGHLIGHTS With easy road access and a tread that remains snow-free for most of the winter, this pleasant trail provides a nice alternative for late winter or early spring hikers looking for some scenic exercise. Since most of this trail is on relatively sunny south or southwest-facing slopes, it melts out much earlier than other trails in the area. By the same token, hikers who visit on a midsummer afternoon may struggle with the heat.

DIRECTIONS From Estacada, drive 20.5 miles southeast on State Highway 224 to a signed junction near Milepost 44.5 with the road to Three Lynx. Turn left on this one-lane paved road, and proceed 0.6 mile to a multiway junction in the small town of Three Lynx. Go straight on a narrow but good gravel road, drive 0.9 mile, and then park in a pull-out on the left immediately before a saddle where a large pipe goes under the road.

The trail, marked with a small sign on a tree, starts on the east side of the road and begins climbing immediately. In one moderately long switchback the trail gradually puts distance (or at least elevation) between you and the trailhead, taking you to a minor saddle and a junction with faint traces of an older alignment

for this trail. You bear left and continue steadily uphill through a Douglas-fir forest occasionally broken by talus slopes. These openings provide nice views to the southwest of hulking Fish Creek Mountain and the more distant peaks of the Bull of the Woods Wilderness. The open feeling is enhanced by the forests, which

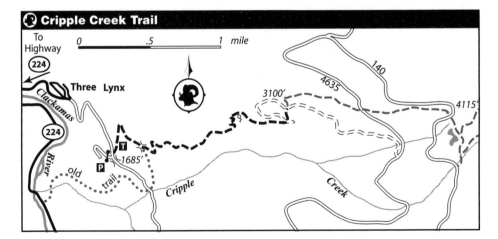

Cripple Creek Trail

have only limited undergrowth on this south-facing slope.

After a couple of switchbacks, the trail settles in for a lengthy traverse well above cascading Cripple Creek, which you can hear but not see in the canyon on your right. At the end of the traverse, four short switchbacks take you up to a small spring, which provides an opportunity for overheated hikers to dunk their heads in cool water. At 2.4 miles you cross a long abandoned logging road that is now completely overgrown with young trees. Listen in this area for the drumming of woodpeckers and the soft buzzing call of red-breasted nuthatches. Another 0.1 mile of uphill through a forest that is increasingly dominated by western hemlocks and western red cedars, takes you to a crossing of a second primi-

tive road. Although this road is still open to vehicles, it clearly receives very little use. Winter trail maintenance ends here, so this road makes a good turnaround point for off-season hikers. If you want a viewpoint to end your hike, backtrack about 30 yards, and then scramble south 50 yards to the top of a prominent basalt outcropping. From here there are decent but partially obstructed views of Fish Creek Mountain and the heavily forested Clackamas River Canyon.

For ambitious types, the Cripple Creek Trail continues climbing another 1.4 miles, crossing two logging roads along the way, before connecting with the start of Trip 17. This section is not as well maintained, however, and is easier to access from above.

TRIP 17 Cripple Creek & Serene Lake Loop

Distance	11.0 miles, Loop
Elevation Gain	1800 feet
Hiking Time	6 to 8 hours
Optional Map	Green Trails *Fish Creek Mountain, High Rock*
Usually Open	Mid-June to October
Best Times	Mid-June and late August to September
Trail Use	Dogs OK, backpacking option, horseback riding, fishing
Agency	Clackamas River Ranger District, Mt. Hood National Forest
Difficulty	Difficult

HIGHLIGHTS This outstandingly scenic loop includes a sampling of all the things that make hiking in the Cascade Mountains such a joy. There are scenic lakes tucked away in old glacial cirques, lush mountain meadows carpeted with wildflowers, lovely high-elevation forests, high viewpoints where you can look out to snow-capped volcanic peaks, and fields of huckleberries that provide tasty treats in late summer. The hike makes a perfect short backpacking trip, as all the lakes have good campsites. Wildlife enthusiasts might be interested to know that the author has been fortunate enough to observe both black bears and mountain lions in this area. Keep your eyes open and hope for similar luck.

In early summer, mosquitoes can be terrible around the high lakes. To avoid them, try to visit during a two-week window of opportunity in June just after the snowmelt and before the bugs hatch. Since it is difficult to time this exactly right, it may be easier to visit in late August or September, when most of the bugs are gone and the huckleberries are ripe.

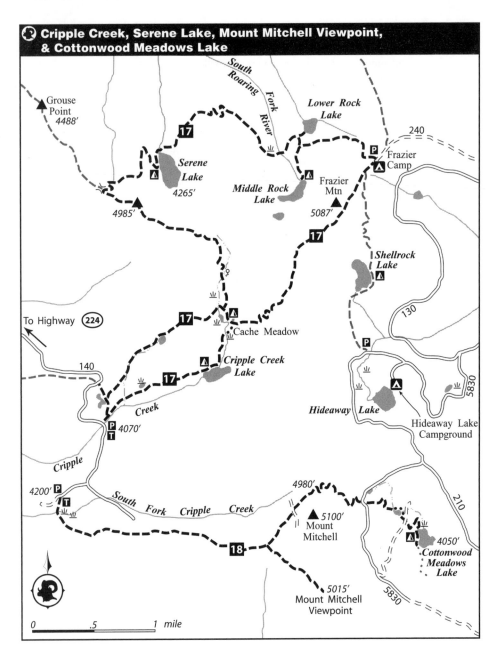

Cripple Creek, Serene Lake, Mount Mitchell Viewpoint, & Cottonwood Meadows Lake

DIRECTIONS From Estacada, drive 25.5 miles southeast on State Highway 224 to Ripplebrook Guard Station. Just past the station, turn left on paved Forest Road 4631, and drive 2.6 miles to a fork. Go right, soon come to the end of pavement, and continue 0.7 mile to a fork. Bear left onto Forest Road 4635, and climb 8.8 miles on this narrow, twisting, gravel road to a junction. Bear right on Road 140, and proceed 1.8 miles to a culvert over Cripple Creek. Park in a small pull-out on the left, immediately before the culvert.

The unsigned, but obvious, trail departs from the left side of the trailhead pull-out. Just 50 yards from your car, you come to an unsigned junction. Either route will get you to the destination, but it is slightly easier to navigate this loop if you go straight. This path gradually climbs through a lovely, high-elevation forest dominated by Pacific silver fir and mountain hemlock. On the generally open forest floor are beargrass and huckleberry bushes, with a few flowers like blue and white anemone and yellow wood violet for color. This general description of the flora holds true throughout this hike.

You pass a shallow, marshy lake and then continue slowly ascending in the open forest. The rarely used trail is reasonably easy to follow, but even if you temporarily lose it, you can quickly relocate the tread by using the yellow paint marks on trees along the route. After a little more than 1 mile, the trail arrives at shallow, 15-acre Cripple Creek Lake, where brook trout and roughskin newts rise to the surface, breaking the glassy stillness of this forest-rimmed lake. After working its way along the north shore of

the lake, and passing two good campsites, the trail curves left and goes gradually uphill beside the inlet creek. The path is a little sketchy, but experienced hikers can easily follow it, especially with the help of the many orange survey tapes tied to tree limbs along the route.

After about 0.3 mile, you arrive at the lower end of marshy Cache Meadow. Just as the snow melts in June, this meadow comes alive with white marsh marigolds, while a little later in the season pink shooting stars put on a nice show. Throughout the season you'll enjoy the serenade of frogs, which live in the shallow ponds of this meadow.

Although the trail seems to end at the meadow, to continue the hike, simply cross the seasonal creek that runs out of a pond and, 20 feet later, arrive at a campsite at the former site of Cache Meadow Shelter. The main loop trail passes through this campsite. To do a clockwise loop, turn left and walk 200 yards to a confusing junction. The loop trail, marked only with a tiny wooden sign that reads 517, turns right. You pass a couple of small meadows and a bubbling

Serene Lake and Roaring River country

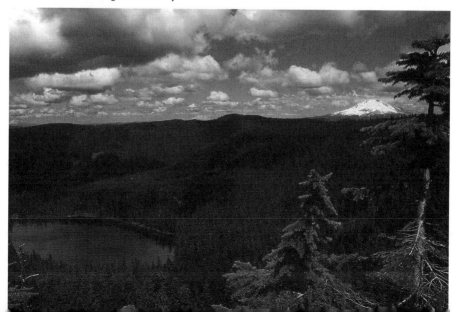

spring, before climbing fairly steeply for 0.8 mile to a wonderful clifftop viewpoint. The ancient glacial basin of Serene Lake spreads out below you like a geology classroom display. Easiest for the amateur to recognize are the old glacial features that are now filled by the Serene Lake or covered by forests. Towering in the distance are Mounts St. Helens, Adams, and Hood, where glaciers still do their work and the ice age continues.

To make the loop, continue hiking northwest across a high forested tableland, and then descend to a junction in a small saddle, where there are lots of rhododendron bushes. Going straight would take you to Grouse Point and Dry Ridge (Trip 14). For the loop, you turn right, descend four quick switchbacks, and then make a downhill traverse to lovely Serene Lake. This deep, 20-acre lake has several popular and comfortable camps, one of which includes a seemingly out-of-place wooden picnic table.

The trail curves around the northwest shore of the lake, crosses the outlet stream, and veers away from the water to go around a low, forested ridge. On the other side of this ridge, a series of switchbacks descends about 300 feet, elevation that you partially regain on a subsequent uphill traverse. You pass above a tiny pond, hop across the headwaters of South Fork Roaring River, and then come to a junction. To the left, a 0.1-mile spur trail goes to Lower Rock Lake, which is worth the trip, if you have the time. The main trail goes right and quickly meets a second spur trail, which goes straight and, in 0.2 mile, reaches Middle Rock Lake,

a large, swimmable mountain gem with nice camps.

To continue the loop, you turn left at this junction and gradually climb to a primitive and waterless car campground at Frazier Turnaround. This is where most people begin this hike, although the miserably rock-strewn dirt road you must drive to reach this trailhead would make you wonder why it is so popular. You turn right and follow a wide trail that leaves the camp area and gradually ascends a ridgeline. After 200 yards, a side trail drops to the left on its way to scenic Shellrock Lake. Backpackers with more time to do this loop, or very athletic day-hikers, will want to take the 1.1-mile side trip to this beautiful lake, which is backed by a scenic talus slope.

The main trail, actually an ancient jeep road, crosses an open rockslide with good views of pointed Mt. Jefferson, before topping out on a small forested plateau. A little after the almost straight old road begins going downhill, you turn left at a sign for Grouse Point Trail 517. This narrow foot trail winds fairly steeply downhill, all the way back to Cache Meadow.

For a slightly different route back to your car, go 200 yards past the shelter to the junction you passed earlier in the day, and veer left. This attractive trail lazily loses elevation for 1.7 miles, traveling through narrow meadows and along the rocky bottom of seasonal streambeds, where the trail is easy to lose. You pass a lovely lakelet, and then, just in front of a second shallow lakelet, turn left at an unsigned junction. About 0.1 mile later, you return to the junction just 50 yards from your car.

Clackamas River Area

TRIP 18 Mount Mitchell Viewpoint & Cottonwood Meadows Lake

Distance	5.0 miles to Mt. Mitchell Viewpoint, Out-and-back;
	8.2 miles to Cottonwood Meadows Lake, Out-and-back;
	9.4 miles combined
Elevation Gain	920 feet to Mt. Mitchell Viewpoint,
	1850 feet to Cottonwood Meadows Lake,
	2150 feet combined
Hiking Time	2½ to 5 hours
Optional Map	Green Trails *Fish Creek Mountain, High Rock* (trailhead shown incorrectly)
Usually Open	Mid-June to October
Best Times	Mid-June and mid-August to mid-September
Trail Use	Dogs OK, backpacking option, horseback riding, fishing
Agency	Clackamas River Ranger District, Mt. Hood National Forest
Difficulty	Difficult

see map on p.428

HIGHLIGHTS Sometimes it is a mystery why certain trails are crowded while others remain virtually deserted. Based solely on scenery, this hike to a pair of first-rate destinations in the upper Clackamas River country deserves rave reviews and legions of admiring hikers. But for some reason, most local hikers have not even heard of it. That was certainly true of me, when I discovered to my delight what a treasure had been overlooked by every other guidebook author and virtually every hiker in the Portland area. Check it out for yourself and add to your own delight.

DIRECTIONS From Estacada, drive 25.5 miles southeast on State Highway 224 to Ripplebrook Guard Station. Just past the station, turn left on paved Forest Road 4631, and drive 2.6 miles to a fork. Go right, soon come to the end of pavement, and continue 0.7 mile to a fork. Bear left onto Forest Road 4635, and climb 8.8 miles on this narrow, twisting, gravel road to a junction. Bear right on Road 140, and proceed 2.3 miles to a junction. Turn right at a small sign for Rimrock Trail #704, drive 0.2 mile, and park just as the road leaves an old clear-cut.

Follow the unsigned trail that goes left (south) into a lichen-draped forest of old hemlocks and firs, and descend 0.1 mile to the lower end of a brushy swamp. The trail is often flooded here in early summer. Once across the outlet creek, you climb gradually through dense forest to a faint junction with an unsigned spur trail at 0.4 mile. This 20-yard spur trail leads to the top of a rocky buttress, where you gain excellent views of the forested hills and valleys of the Clackamas River country south to Olallie Butte and the glacier-draped sentinel of Mt. Jefferson.

After the viewpoint, the main trail continues very gradually uphill, generally remaining in dense forest where there are no views. The forest, however, is quite attractive, with some unusually large mountain hemlocks and a groundcover of huckleberries and beargrass. At 1.9 miles is a signed junction and a choice of destinations.

The trail to the right goes to Mount Mitchell Viewpoint and really should not be missed. This 0.6-mile path climbs at a steady but moderate grade to an incredibly dramatic clifftop viewpoint at the end of a ridge. The setting is spectacular and the view is a real jaw-dropper, extending north to Mt. Rainier in Washington and south to central Oregon's Three Sisters. Adding color to the scene are several rock-garden wildflowers, such as paintbrush, cliff penstemon, beargrass, and ground-hugging manzanita. The fact that you will almost certainly have this tremendous scene all to yourself is hard to understand but also hard to complain about.

The main trail goes straight at the Mt. Mitchell junction and soon begins climbing more noticeably. After 0.3 mile you reach an abandoned road that has been deliberately covered with boulders and berms to keep vehicles out. Go left on the old road, walk about 10 yards, and then relocate the trail going uphill to the right. In another 0.3 mile you top a north-south trending ridge above a small rockslide. The views here do not compare to those at Mount Mitchell Viewpoint, but they are pleasant nonetheless, with a peek at a portion of Mt. Hood and nice looks to the east of rounded Mt. Wilson.

From the ridgeline the trail steeply descends a series of short rounded switchbacks to a crossing of remote gravel Road 5830 at 3.4 miles. From here the trail becomes sketchier as it descends gradually through a low tangle of huckleberry bushes. Watch carefully to avoid losing the trail and be sure to look back from time to time to locate landmarks for the return hike. After 0.4 mile you reach a shallow seasonal lake. *In late June and July the mosquitoes here (and for the rest of this hike) are so abundant that they make even a number like infinity seem like an absurd understatement.* Try to visit during a short window of opportunity in mid-June before the buzzing billions arrive, or simply wait until the bugs die down in August and September.

The trail disappears at this seasonal lake. In late summer and fall you can walk across the usually dry lake to the resumption of more distinct tread at the southeast

Mt. Hood from Mt. Mitchell Viewpoint

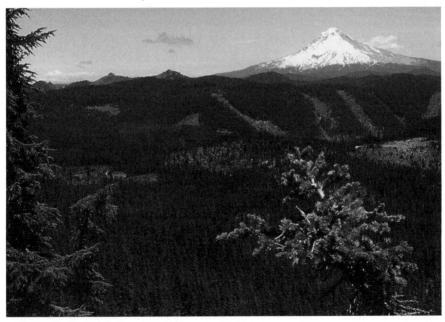

end. Earlier in the year, it is *slightly* easier, although still quite brushy, to bushwhack around the left side of the lake. Once relocated, the trail soon crosses an abandoned dirt road and then descends two switchbacks on faint tread, before entering the incredibly lush meadow at the north end of Cottonwood Meadows Lake. Willows surround this meadow, which in late June is choked with wildflowers, as well as bugs, unfortunately. Look for thousands of buttercups, false hellebores, marsh marigolds, groundsels, bluebells, and valerians, among others. Songbirds are also abundant, especially various brightly colored warblers and hummingbirds. There is a mediocre campsite near the head of this meadow.

The trail skirts the right side of the meadow and soon takes you to the open water of lovely Cottonwood Meadows Lake. At just 4 feet deep, the lake is too shallow for swimming, but it has a pretty setting surrounded by forested ridges and supports a population of brook trout to entice the angler. A very sketchy path continues beyond the lake to more meadows and through a clear-cut, but this section has little to recommend it. The lake is the logical turnaround point.

TRIP 19 Alder Flat Trail

Distance	1.8 miles, Out-and-back
Elevation Gain	250 feet
Hiking Time	1 hour
Optional Map	Green Trails *Fish Creek Mountain*
Usually Open	All year
Best Time	All year
Trail Use	Good for kids, dogs OK, wheelchair accessible, backpacking option, fishing
Agency	Clackamas River Ranger District, Mt. Hood National Forest
Difficulty	Easy
Note	Good in cloudy weather

HIGHLIGHTS This easy route gives hikers the opportunity to experience an increasingly rare ecosystem, the low-elevation, old-growth forest. Most of these forests were cut down decades ago, but here you can enjoy a small sample of what is still left. If this short path does not provide you with enough exercise, consider doing this trip in conjunction with the nearby Riverside Trail (Trip 20) for a full day of hiking.

DIRECTIONS Drive State Highway 224 southeast from Estacada for 25 miles to Milepost 49, just past the Timber Lake Work Center. The well-signed Alder Flat Trailhead parking lot is on your right.

The gentle Alder Flat Nature Trail descends through a peaceful, old-growth forest of Douglas fir and western hemlock, where small numbered posts mark places of interest. A thick mat of mosses crowds the forest floor along with Oregon grape, sword fern, and downed nurse logs. After just 0.2 mile, you pass above a medium-sized marsh created by beavers. From the lower end of the marsh, a worthwhile 0.1-mile side trail goes to the left. Along this route you will find evidence of beaver activity and several nest boxes for wood ducks.

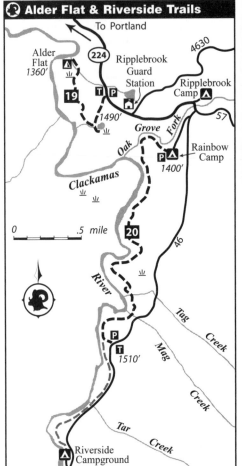

Alder Flat & Riverside Trails

To Portland

Alder Flat 1360'

224 Ripplebrook Guard Station

19

1490'

Grove *Fork*

Ripplebrook Camp

4630

57

Oak

Rainbow Camp

1400'

Clackamas

0   .5 mile

20

River

46

Tag

Creek

1510'

Mag *Creek*

Tar *Creek*

Riverside Campground

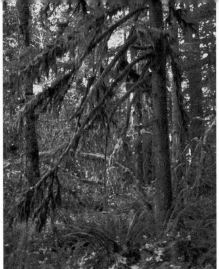

Forest along the Alder Flat Trail

After the marsh, the main trail curves right and goes slowly downhill through a glorious forest of big trees covered with draping mosses. Near the bottom of the hill, you will find a marshy area and a sluggish creek, as well as an ever-increasing number of western red cedar. The trail crosses a couple of wooden boardwalks before ending at Alder Flat, an attractive river-level bench with wooden picnic tables, and metal fire pits. Here, you can enjoy a fine lunch or dinner beside a lovely stream before returning to your car.

TRIP 20 Riverside Trail

Distance	4.8 miles, Out-and-back
Elevation Gain	400 feet
Hiking Time	2½ hours
Optional Map	Green Trails *Fish Creek Mountain*
Usually Open	All year
Best Time	Late September
Trail Use	Good for kids, dogs OK
Agency	Clackamas River Ranger District, Mt. Hood National Forest
Difficulty	Moderate
Note	Good in cloudy weather

see map on p.434

HIGHLIGHTS This short and pleasant outing is a winner any time of year, but it is probably most interesting in September when the salmon are spawning in the Clackamas River. In any season, however, you will enjoy stately old-growth forests, quiet trails, and some excellent high viewpoints above the water. The scenery is not as dramatic as on higher-elevation routes, but this is an excellent option for the quiet contemplation of nature.

DIRECTIONS Drive State Highway 224 southeast from Estacada for 25.5 miles to the Ripple-brook Guard Station. A little past the station, the road crosses a bridge, immediately after which you bear right at a fork. The new Riverside Trailhead is on the right about 1.6 miles from the bridge.

The path from the trailhead leads down 150 yards through a pretty forest to a junction with the main Riverside Trail. At this point, you can turn in either direction, but the route to the right is much more attractive and is the one described here.

The trail travels downhill through low-growing western red cedars and western hemlocks to the first of many viewpoints, this one above a bend in the Clackamas River. Still traveling downhill, you follow small Mag Creek to a bridged crossing of that stream and then begin the up-and-down pattern that will soon become this trail's trademark. The path ascends a ridge and then drops to a rocky beach beside the river, which is an ideal rest stop.

Next, you cross on a bridge over the often dry Tag Creek and then climb four short switchbacks to another viewpoint well above the river. From here the path wanders around in circuitous ups and downs through the hills above the river, before dropping to a superb rocky beach beside the water. You can eat lunch here or take a dip in the water, but you'd better make it a really quick dip, because the water is awfully cold!

Leaving this inviting beach, you cross a wooden boardwalk and climb to a final excellent viewpoint at the top of a cliff overlooking the river canyon. Stay well back from the drop-off, as the edges of this cliff are crumbly and unstable. This is a good turnaround point, but if you want to continue to Rainbow Camp, follow the path as it goes up and down through a forest of western red cedar and Douglas fir beside splashing Oak Grove Fork. It ends at a tiny parking area at the far end of the campground.

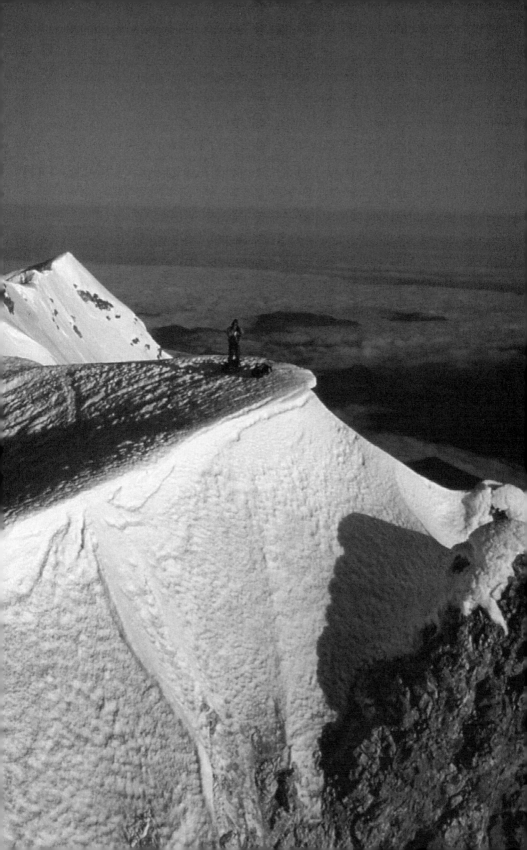

Appendix 1
Best Hikes by Theme

Birds & Wildlife

Chapter 3: Portland & the Willamette Valley
    Ridgefield Refuge: Oak to Wetlands Trail *(Trip 1)*
    Ridgefield Refuge: Kiwa Trail Loop *(Trip 3)*
    Oak Island Loop *(Trip 8)*
    Jackson Bottom Wetlands Loop *(Trip 11)*
    Audubon Sanctuary Loops *(Trip 20)*
    Sandy River Delta *(Trip 24)*
    Oxbow Regional Park: North Side *(Trip 25)*
    Mount Baldy & Baskett Slough Loop *(Trip 28)*
    Ankeny National Wildlife Refuge: Rail Trail Loop *(Trip 29)*

Mountains

Chapter 2: Southwest Washington
    Bluff Mountain Trail *(Trip 15)*

Chapter 6: Mount Hood Area
    McNeil Point via McGee Creek *(Trip 15)*
    Yocum Ridge *(Trip 20)*
    Timberline Lodge to Paradise Park *(Trip 36)*
    Mount Hood Climb *(Trip 38)*

Chapter 7: Clackamas River Area
    Cripple Creek & Serene Lake Loop *(Trip 17)*

Mountain Biking

Chapter 1: Coast Range
    Lester Creek Pinnacles *(Trip 8)*
    Central Gales Creek Trail *(Trip 15)*

Chapter 2: Southwest Washington
    Siouxon Creek Trail *(Trip 3)*
    Tarbell Trail to Hidden Falls *(Trip 7)*

Chapter 3: Portland & the Willamette Valley
    Henry Hagg Lake Loop *(Trip 10)*

Chapter 5: Eastern Columbia River Gorge
    Nestor Peak *(Trip 5)*
    Weldon Wagon Road *(Trip 7)*
    Hood River Mountain *(Trip 25)*

Waterfalls

Wildflowers

Appendix 2
Recommended Reading

Bookstore shelves are overflowing with books about the Pacific Northwest outdoors. It seems we Portlanders have an inexhaustible appetite for information about our beloved wilderness. Some books are better than others, of course, and owning them all would involve a lot of redundancy. Here are my recommendations for the best local books to have in your outdoor library.

Dayhiking Guides

With this book, you already own the most comprehensive guide to dayhikes close to Portland. You really don't need anything else—except for a new edition of it as changes occur in the future and the book is updated. There are, however, other good books with different purposes.

For coverage of hikes somewhat farther from Portland—up to two hours' driving time—your best choice is *100 Hikes in Northwest Oregon* by William L. Sullivan. It includes places like the east side of Mt. Hood, farther up the Clackamas River, and the Indian Heaven and Mt. St. Helens areas in Washington. If you are headed for the coast, Sullivan's *100 Hikes/Travel Guide Oregon Coast & Coast Range* is the best book covering this popular area.

If you want a different perspective on the wonderful trails of the Columbia River Gorge than what you find in this book, look for *Columbia Gorge Hikes: 42 Scenic Hikes* by Don and Roberta Lowe, the deans of Oregon guidebook authors. This old favorite was updated in 2000 with beautiful, all-color photographs, but it is has no maps and is in a large format that is awkward to carry on the trail. One useful and quaint book on the southern Mt. Hood area is *Hikes & Walks on Mt. Hood* by Sonia Buist and Emily Keller. Produced by LOLITS Press (an acronym for "Little Old Ladies in Tennis Shoes"), it covers unique hiking options on old and little-used roads, ski runs, and cross-country ski trails clustered around Government Camp and Timberline Lodge. It is a good choice if you are willing to expand your ideas about what qualifies as a "hiking" route.

Other Travel Guides

If you are interested in outdoor sports other than dayhiking, you might want to pick up some of the following outdoor guidebooks:

Long-distance backpackers looking for the best places to go for that 3-day to 2-week hiking vacation should pick up copies of *Backpacking Oregon* and *Backpacking Washington*, also by me and published by Wilderness Press.

Wildlife enthusiasts will get good value from two skinny volumes that designate areas for viewing wildlife in Oregon and Washington. Although far from a comprehensive list, the sites are usually reliable places to visit. *The Oregon Wildlife Viewing Guide* is written by James A. Yuskavitch, and the author of the *Washington Wildlife Viewing Guide* is Joe La Tourrette.

The bible on winter sports is Klindt Vielbig's *Cross-Country Ski Routes: Oregon,* which is consistently updated and valued by those who love this sport. The book covers southwest Washington as well as Oregon.

All the water in our area makes this a paradise for river runners. *Soggy Sneakers: A Guide to Oregon Rivers* by the Willamette Kayaking and Canoe Club and *Oregon River Tours* by John Garren are the two most useful books for this activity.

Those who prefer to power themselves along on two wheels will want *Bicycling the Backroads of Northwest Oregon* by Philip Jones and Jean Henderson.

Natural History

Two good, general-interest, natural history guides, which give an overview of the most common varieties of plants and animals are *The Audubon Society Nature Guide: Western Forests* and *A Field Guide to the Cascades & Olympics,* both by Stephen Whitney. The former has lovely color photography but does not include fish. With such wide coverage, it has room for a woefully inadequate number of mushrooms and wildflowers. The latter book is more specific to our region, but has only black and white drawings of many of the wildflowers and omits mushrooms and fungi entirely. Trees get adequate coverage in the general-interest guides, but if you are looking for more detail and comprehensive coverage, your best choice is probably *Northwest Trees* by Stephen Arno and Ramona Hammerly.

The best field guide for identifying birds is the *National Geographic Society's Field Guide to the Birds of North America.* Only the common species of reptiles, amphibians, and mammals are likely to be seen by most hikers, and these are adequately covered in the general-interest Whitney guides.

For the average hiker the best wildflower book for our area is an excellent new guide called *Wildflowers of the Pacific Northwest* by Mark Turner and Phyllis Gustafson. Unlike most wildflower books, which are filled with unpronounceable Latin names and have a layout only a professional botanist could understand, this one is organized by the color of the flower, making it much more useful for the amateur. The book also has excellent color photography. Although the maps are confusing and the index in poorly organized, the book is indispensable. Another good wildflower guide is Russ Jolley's *Wildflowers of the Columbia Gorge,* which also features color photos and includes useful recommendations on where to go for wildflower viewing in each season.

A fun guide you might consider is James Luther Davis's *Seasonal Guide to the Natural Year,* which you can use to plan trips around natural events such as animal migrations, fall color, and wildflower blooming.

Finally, an informative and endlessly fascinating book for history lovers is *Oregon Geographic Names* by Lewis A. McArthur. This classic is full of things like the meaning of the word *Wahtum* and how Starvation Creek got its name. It is more interesting to read than any other reference book you will probably ever own.

Appendix 3
Information Sources

Local Organizations

Friends of the Columbia Gorge
522 S.W. 5th Avenue, Suite 720
Portland, OR 97204
(503) 241-3762
www.gorgefriends.org

Friends of Powell Butte Nature Park
3908 S.E. 136th Avenue
Portland, OR 97236
www.friendsofpowellbutte.org

Friends of Tryon Creek State Park
11321 S.W. Terwilliger Boulevard
Portland, OR 97219
(503) 636-4398
www.tryonfriends.org

The Mazamas
527 S.E. 43rd Avenue
Portland, OR 97215
(503) 227-2345
www.mazamas.org

Oregon Chapter Sierra Club
2950 S.E. Stark Street, Suite 110
Portland, OR 97214
(503) 238-0442
www.oregon.sierraclub.org

Portland Audubon Society
5151 Cornell Road
Portland, OR 97210
(503) 292-6855
www.audubonportland.org

Ptarmigans Mountaineering Club
P.O. Box 1821
Vancouver, WA 98668
www.ptarmigans.org

Trails Club of Oregon
P.O. Box 1243
Portland, OR 97207
(503) 233-2740
www.trailsclub.org

Parks & Land Agencies

Ankeny National Wildlife Refuge
2301 Wintel Road
Jefferson, OR 97352
(503) 588-2701
www.fws.gov/willamettevalley/ankeny

Baskett Slough National Wildlife Refuge
10995 Highway 22
Dallas, OR 97338
(503) 623-2749
www.fws.gov/willamettevalley/baskett

Beacon Rock State Park
34841 State Route 14
Skamania, WA 98648
(509) 427-8265

**Bureau of Land Management:
Salem District**
1717 Fabry Road S.E.
Salem, OR 97306
(503) 375-5646
www.blm.gov/or/districts/salem

Clackamas County Parks Department
9101 S.E. Sunnybrook Boulevard
Clackamas, OR 97015
(503) 353-4414
www.co.clackamas.or.us/dtd/parks

Clark Parks & Recreation Department
P.O. Box 1995
Vancouver, WA 98668-1995
(360) 619-1111
www.ci.vancouver.wa.us/parks-recreation

Clatsop State Forest
92219 Highway 202
Astoria, OR 97103
(503) 325-5451
www.oregon.gov/ODF/FIELD/ASTORIA

Columbia River Gorge National Scenic Area
902 Wasco Avenue, Suite 200
Hood River, OR 97031
(541) 308-1700
www.fs.fed.us/r6/columbia

Gifford Pinchot National Forest
www.fs.fed.us/gpnf

Mount Adams Ranger District
2455 Highway 141
Trout Lake, WA 98650
(509) 395-3400

Jackson Bottom Wetlands Preserve
P.O. Box 3002
Hillsboro, OR 97123
(503) 681-6206
www.jacksonbottom.org

Mt. Hood Information Center
65000 E. Highway 26
Welches, OR 97067
(503) 622-4822
www.mthood.info/

Mt. Hood National Forest
www.fs.fed.us/r6/mthood

Clackamas River Ranger District
595 N.W. Industrial Way
Estacada, OR 97023
(503) 630-6861

Zigzag Ranger District
70220 E. Highway 26
Zigzag, OR 97049
(503) 622-3191

Mt. St. Helens National Volcanic Monument
42218 NE Yale Bridge Road
Amboy, WA 98601
(360) 499-7800
www.fs.fed.us/gpnf/mshnvm

The Nature Conservancy of Oregon
821 S.E. 14th Avenue
Portland, OR 97214
(503) 802-8100
www.nature.org/states/oregon

Nature of the Northwest Information Center
800 N. Oregon Street, Suite 177
Portland, OR 97232
(503) 872-2752
www.naturenw.org

Oregon State Parks
725 Summer Street N.E., Suite C
Salem, OR 97301-1002
(800) 551-6949
www.oregonstateparks.org

Milo McIver State Park
(503) 630-7150

Silver Falls State Park
(503) 873-4395

Stub Stewart State Park
(503) 324-0606

Tryon Creek State Natural Area
(503) 636-9886

Oxbow Regional Park
3010 S.E. Oxbow Parkway
Gresham, OR 97080
(503) 663-4708

Portland Parks & Recreation Bureau
1120 S.W. 5th Avenue, #1302
Portland, OR 97204
(503) 823-7529
www.portlandonline.com/parks

Ridgefield National Wildlife Refuge
P.O. Box 457
Ridgefield, WA 98642-0457
(360) 887-4106
www.fws.gov/ridgefieldrefuges

Santiam State Forest: Santiam Unit
22965 N. Fork Road S.E.
Lyons, OR 97358
(503) 859-2151
www.oregon.gov/ODF/FIELD/
NORTH_CASCADE

Sauvie Island Wildlife Area
18330 N.W. Sauvie Island Road
Portland, OR 97231
(503) 621-3488
www.dfw.state.or.us/wildlifearea/
sauvieisland.htm

Tillamook State Forest
www.oregon.gov/ODF/TSF

Forest Grove District Office
801 Gales Creek Road
Forest Grove, OR 97116
(503) 357-2191

Tillamook District Office
5005 3rd Street
Tillamook, OR 97141
(503) 842-2545

Tualatin Hills Park & Recreation District
15707 S.W. Walker Road
Beaverton, OR 97006-5941
(503) 645-6433
www.thprd.com

**Washington Department of
Natural Resources: Central Region
Yacolt State Forest**
P.O. Box 280
Castle Rock, WA 98611
(360) 577-2025
www.dnr.wa.gov/htdocs/lm/recreation/
yacoltburn

Appendixes

Map Sources

Nature of the Northwest
See listing in previous section.

Pittmon Map Co.
825 S.E. Hawthorne Blvd.
Portland, OR 97214
(503) 233-2207

REI (Recreational Equipment Inc.)
2235 N.W. Allie Avenue
Hillsboro, OR 97124
(503) 617-6072

REI (Recreational Equipment Inc.)
1405 N.W. Johnson Street
Portland, OR 97209
(503) 221-1938

REI (Recreational Equipment Inc.)
12160 SE 82nd Avenue
Portland, OR 97266
(503) 659-1156

REI (Recreational Equipment Inc.)
7410 S.W. Bridgeport Road
Tigard, OR 97224
(503) 624-8600

Appendix 4
Friends of Forest Park &
Friends of the Columbia Gorge

Several of the hikes in this book explore the beautiful trails through Forest Park. Like all urban preserves, this park needs committed and involved citizens to help maintain trails, keep out invasive nonnative plants, restore damaged habitats, and otherwise protect and preserve this irreplaceable treasure of the city of Portland. The Friends of Forest Park have done all of these things and more since 1946. I encourage hikers who enjoy the wild trails of this magnificent park to support and join this nonprofit organization and lend a hand in helping to protect, preserve, and enhance Forest Park.

Mailing Address:
Friends of Forest Park
P.O. Box 10934
Portland, OR 97296

Office Address:
Friends of Forest Park
2366 N.W. Thurman Street
Portland, OR 97208
Phone: (503) 223-5449
Fax: (503) 223-5637
info@friendsofforestpark.org
www.friendsofforestpark.org

More of the trails described in this book travel through the Columbia River Gorge than any other area. The magnificent landscapes of this nationally significant scenic treasure remain largely unspoiled and open to the public due, in part, to the tireless efforts of people dedicated to protecting this special place. Friends of the Columbia Gorge is a grassroots organization that works to protect and enhance the unique scenic, recreational, and biological features of this area, and it deserves your support.

Mailing Address:
Friends of the Columbia Gorge
522 S.W. 5th Ave., Ste. 720
Portland, OR 97204
(503) 241-3762
www.gorgefriends.org

Index

About the Author

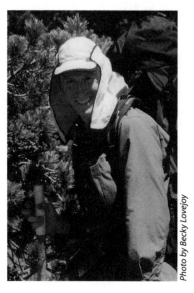

Photo by Becky Lovejoy

Douglas Lorain's family moved to the Pacific Northwest in 1969, and he has been obsessively hitting the trails of his home region ever since. With the good fortune to grow up in an outdoor-oriented family, he has vivid memories of countless camping, biking, birdwatching, and other trips in every corner of this spectacular area. Over the years he calculates that he has logged well over 30,000 trail miles in this corner of the continent, and despite a history that includes being bitten by a rattlesnake, shot at by a hunter, charged by a grizzly bear, and donating countless gallons of blood to "invertebrate vampires," he happily sees no end in sight.

Lorain is a photographer and recipient of the National Outdoor Book Award. His books cover only the best trips from the thousands of hikes and backpacking trips he has taken throughout Oregon, Washington, and Idaho. His photographs have been featured in numerous magazines, calendars, and books, and his other guidebook titles include *100 Classic Hikes in Oregon*, *Backpacking Idaho*, *Backpacking Oregon*, and *Backpacking Washington*.

Although he considers his real home to be on the trail, those few days he is forced to spend indoors, he lives in Portland, Oregon, with his wife, Becky Lovejoy.

More Pacific Northwest Books

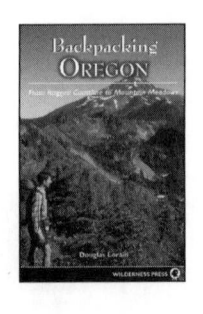

Backpacking Oregon
Douglas Lorain

The most intriguing backpacking trips along the Oregon Coast, through the Columbia Gorge, atop the High Cascades, Klamath, Siskiyou, Blue and Wallowa mountains, and into Hells Canyon. Adventures range from a weekend to over a week in length.

ISBN 978-0-89997-441-4

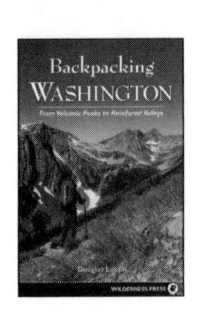

Backpacking Washington
Douglas Lorain

The premier backpacking opportunities across the Evergreen State. Co. 28 trips in Alpine Lakes, Blue Mountains, Glacier Peak Area, Mount Rain. Mount St. Helens, North Cascades, Northeastern Washington Mountains, Olympic Coast and Mountains, Pasayten Wilderness, Salmo-Priest Wilderness, and Southern Cascades.

ISBN 978-0-89997-423-1

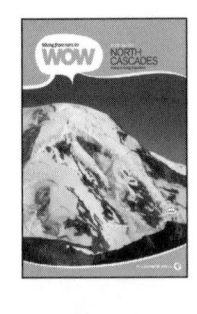

Hiking from Here to WOW: North Cascades
Kathy & Craig Copeland

In this full-color book, opinionated hikers Kathy and Craig Copeland describe 50 trails that epitomize the "*wonder of wilderness*." They visit cathedral forests, psychedelic meadows, spiky summits, colossal glaciers, and more on dayhikes and backpacking trips in Washington's Glacier Peak Wilderness and North Cascades National Park.

ISBN 978-0-89997-444-6

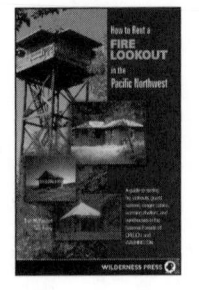

How to Rent a Fire Lookout in the Pacific Northwest
Tish McFadden & Tom Foley

The complete guide to 65 cabins or fire lookouts available for rent in Oregon and Washington fully describes each structure's heating, lighting, and cooking and sleeping facilities, as well as local attractions.

ISBN 0-89997-384-1

For ordering information, contact your local bookseller
or Wilderness Press, www.wildernesspress.com